Challenging Cases in Gynecologic Surgical Pathology

Ozlen Saglam

Challenging Cases in Gynecologic Surgical Pathology

Springer

Ozlen Saglam
Department of Pathology and Laboratory Medicine
Oregon Health & Science University
Portland, OR, USA

ISBN 978-3-031-51655-9 ISBN 978-3-031-51656-6 (eBook)
https://doi.org/10.1007/978-3-031-51656-6

This Springer imprint is published by the registered company Springer Nature Switzerland AG
The registered company address is: Gewerbestrasse 11, 6330 Cham, Switzerland

Paper in this product is recyclable.

To my mother, Sefika Seyda Gencer. A great teacher and a dear friend.
I am grateful for everything she did for me and my siblings.

Preface

The intent in preparation of this atlas is to illustrate unusual patterns of common gynecologic pathology cases and uncommon tumors of the gynecological tract with their relevant clinical work-up and differential diagnosis. The case presentations are from four anatomical sites: ovaries, endometrium, cervix, and vulva in order. After the case title, a typical clinical history is provided to facilitate clinicopathological correlation. The morphological features of the diagnostic entity with accompanying micrographs are under the "key diagnostic features" section. The ancillary studies include immunohistochemical and molecular tests commonly used in diagnostic work-up of a particular entity. In the differential diagnosis, a list of relevant benign and malignant entities with a summary of their morphological features and clinical work-ups is available. If one of the pathology cases illustrated in the atlas is in the list, the case number is referred to at the end. A summary sentence for the clinical significance of the diagnosis follows these sections. The case illustrations are by no means a complete review of gynecologic pathology. The emphasis is on developing a general approach to diagnose unusual patterns and rare tumors. The atlas is a practical review with relevant literature for further reading. I hope the reader finds the case presentations helpful and enjoyable for daily practice.

Portland, OR, USA　　Ozlen Saglam

Contents

Abbreviations

AA	Aggressive Angiomyxoma
AFP	Alpha-fetoprotein
AGCT	Adult granulosa cell tumor
APA	Atypical polypoid adenomyoma
APSN	Atypical placental site nodule
BCC	Basal cell carcinoma
BG	Bartholin glands
CA	Cellular angiofibroma
CCC	Clear cell carcinoma
CDLM	Cotyledonoid dissecting leiomyoma
CEA	Carcinoembryonic antigen
CF	Cellular fibroma
CHEC	Corded and hyalinized endometrioid carcinoma
CRS	Chemotherapy response score
DPL	Disseminated peritoneal leiomyomatosis
dVIN	Differentiated vulvar intraepithelial neoplasia
EHE	Epithelioid hemangioendothelioma
EIN	Endometrial intraepithelial neoplasia
ELMS	Epithelioid leiomyosarcoma
EMA	Epithelial membrane antigen
EMPD	Extramammary Paget disease
ER	Estrogen receptor
ERMS	Embryonal rhabdomyosarcoma
ESS	Endometrial stromal sarcoma
ETT	Epithelioid trophoblastic tumor
FAP	Familial adenomatous polyposis
FATWO	Female adnexal tumor of probable Wolffian origin
FEP	Fibroepithelial polyp
FH-leiomyoma	Fumarate hydratase deficient leiomyoma
GAS	Gastric-type adenocarcinoma
GTD	Gestational trophoblastic disease
HGSC	High-grade serous carcinoma
HIV	Human immunodeficiency virus
HMB45	Human melanoma black 45
HMWK	High molecular weight keratin
HP	Hidradenoma papilliferum (papillary hidradenoma)
hPL	Human placental lactogen
HPV	Human papillomavirus
IECA	Intraepithelial (non-invasive) carcinoma
IMT	Inflammatory myofibroblastic tumor
INSM1	Insulinoma associated protein 1
IVL	Intravenous leiomyomatosis

JGCT	Juvenile granulosa cell tumor
LCT	Leydig cell tumor
LEGH	Lobular endocervical glandular hyperplasia
LGESS	Low-grade endometrial stromal sarcoma
LGSC	Low-grade serous carcinoma
LMS	Leiomyosarcoma
LP	Lichen planus
LS	Lichen sclerosus
LSC	Lichen simplex chronicus
MA	Mullerian adenosarcoma
MBT	Mucinous borderline tumor
MC	Molluscum contagiosum
MELF	Microcytic elongated and fragmented
MH	Mesonephric hyperplasia
MLMS	Myxoid leiomyosarcoma
MMGCT	Malignant mixed germ cell tumor
MMR	Mismatch repair
MST	Ovarian microcytic stromal tumor
(NH) of Bartholin Glands: (BG)	Nodular hyperplasia
NEC	Neuroendocrine carcinoma
NEEC	Mixed neuroendocrine and endometrioid carcinoma
PAM	Polypoid adenomyoma
pCEA	Polyclonal carcinoembryonic antigen
PEComa	Perivascular epithelioid cell neoplasm
PHH3	Phosphohistone H3
PJS	Peutz-Jeghers syndrome
PNL2	Melanoma associated antigen
PR	Progesterone receptor
PSN	Placental site nodule
PTH	Papillary tubal hyperplasia
RCC	Renal cell carcinoma
SB	Sarcoma botryoids
SBT	Borderline serous tumor
SCC	Squamous cell carcinoma
SCCOHT	Small cell carcinoma of the ovary, hypercalcemic type
SCNEC	Small cell neuroendocrine carcinoma of the cervix
SCT	Steroid cell tumor
SET	Solid endometrioid-like and transitional
SF1	Steroidogenic factor 1
SFT	Solitary fibrous tumor
SIL	Squamous intraepithelial lesion
SLCT	Sertoli-Leydig cell tumor
SMA	Smooth muscle actin
SMILE	Stratified mucin-producing intraepithelial lesion
SPT	Solid pseudopapillary tumor
SS	Synovial sarcoma
STIC	Serous tubal intraepithelial carcinoma
TCGA	The cancer genome atlas
TTF1	Thyroid transcription factor 1
UTROSCT	Uterine tumor resembling ovarian sex cord stromal tumor
VKA	Vulvar keratoacanthoma
WHO	World Health Organization
WNET	Well-differentiated neuroendocrine tumor
YST	Yolk sac tumor

Part I

The Ovarian and Fallopian Tube Pathology Cases

1 Epithelial Ovarian Lesions

1.1 Endometrioid Carcinoma with Spindle Cells (ECSC)

1.1.1 A 47-Year-Old Woman with a Pelvic Mass

1.1.1.1 Key Diagnostic Features

- Low-grade adenocarcinoma with prominent spindle cell component (Fig. 1.1) (up to 90% of the lesion) [1].
- The nuclear features of spindle cells are similar to those of epithelial/glandular cells (low-grade) without any or rare mitotic activity.
- The spindle cells merge with the glandular component throughout the lesion (Fig. 1.2). They are not spatially distinct from each other.
- Spindle cells usually grow in a diffuse pattern. Focally, there might be nuclear palisading, necrosis (Fig. 1.3), or keratinization within the spindle cell areas.
- Histological grading depends on the grade of the adenocarcinoma component (FIGO grading) by expert consensus [1]. There is no established grading system.

1.1.1.2 Ancillary Studies

- Keratin is focal or diffuse positive in spindle cell component [1].
- P16 is patchy positive.
- P53: normal/wild-type staining in both components.
- ER/PR: positive in glandular component.

1.1.1.3 Differential Diagnosis

- Sex cord-stromal tumors with spindle cell component or heterologous elements (adult granulosa cell tumor and Sertoli-Leydig cell tumor)
  - The presence of focal typical endometrioid-type carcinoma, squamous differentiation within the spindle cells, adenofibroma component or endometriosis in the background, and intraluminal mucin within the glandular epithelium are the morphological features that support the endometrioid carcinoma diagnosis.

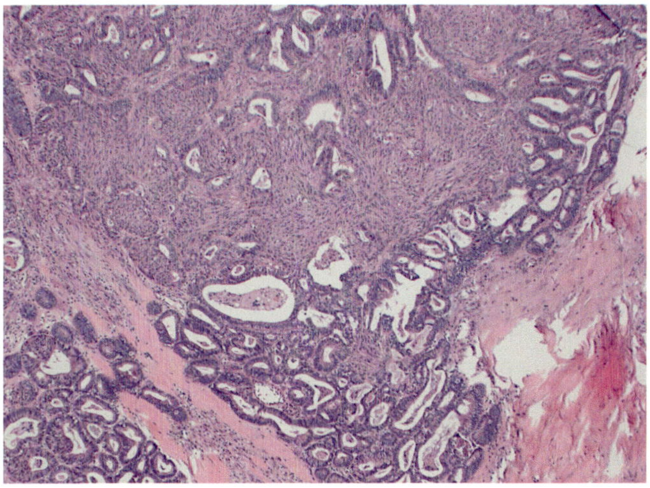

Fig. 1.1 Endometrioid carcinoma with spindle cells. The spindle cell component and adenocarcinoma are spatially continuous with each other (40×)

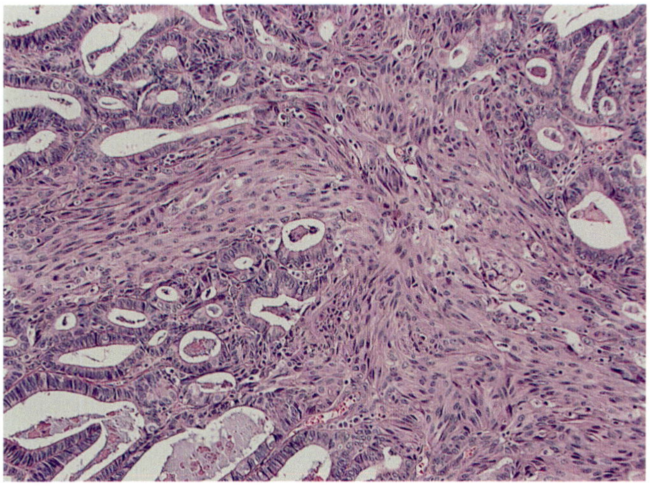

Fig. 1.2 The spindle cells have bland nuclei. There is no mitotic activity. They merge with the glandular component (100×)

O. Saglam, *Challenging Cases in Gynecologic Surgical Pathology*, https://doi.org/10.1007/978-3-031-51656-6_1

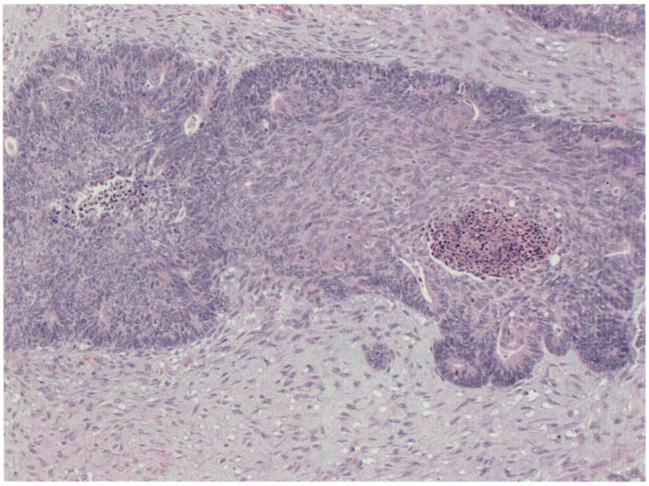

Fig. 1.3 There is focal necrosis within the spindle cell component. The peripheral nuclei are palisading (perpendicular to the surrounding stroma) (100×)

- EMA is positive in ECSC and negative in sex cord tumors. Inhibin and calretinin are positive in sex cord tumors.

- Female adnexal tumor of probable Wolffian origin [2]
  - AKA Wolffian tumor of the ovary.
  - The location of FATWO is in the broad ligament or ovarian hilum.
  - Well-circumscribed lesions with variable patterns, usually in combination.
  - Lobulation, hallow tubules, retiform (sieve-like) appearance, cystic areas, and diffuse sheaths of spindle cells are the frequent histological patterns.
  - Pankeratin is positive; EMA, CK7, GATA3, PAX8, CD10, SF-1, calretinin, inhibin, ER, PR, and WT1 are variably expressed in FATWO [3].
- Low-grade endometrial stromal sarcoma (LGESS) with glandular differentiation
  - The glandular component is focal. The neoplastic cells resemble stromal cells of normal proliferative type endometrium. The vascular pattern is delicate, like spiral arterioles of the endometrium, with tumor cells arranged in concentric whorls around them. Thick bands of collagen and hyalinization are components of the neoplasm [4].
  - CD10 is positive in LGESS.
- Carcinosarcoma
  - Epithelial and mesenchymal components are high-grade tumors (rare cases might present with low-grade carcinoma).
  - Two components are usually spatially distinct.
  - P53 is a mutant type in both components [5].

1.1.1.4 Clinical Significance

- Endometrioid adenocarcinomas with spindle cells are low-grade tumors (FIGO grade 1 or 2).

1.2 Endometrioid Carcinoma with Sertoliform Pattern

1.2.1 A 55-Year-Old Woman with Torsion of Left Ovarian Mass

1.2.1.1 Key Diagnostic Features

- Usually, a mixture of typical endometrioid-type adenocarcinoma and areas resembling Sertoli cells in solid-tubular structures (Fig. 1.4). There might be small cavities resembling Call-Exner bodies [6] that can mimic Adult Granulosa Cell Tumor [7].
- Cytological atypia is mild to moderate.
- Well-differentiated conventional endometrioid adenocarcinoma usually merges with the sertoliform component in some foci (Fig. 1.5).
- The presence of mucinous, squamous, or secretory-type changes in the glandular component is supportive of endometrioid adenocarcinoma diagnosis.
- The histological grade depends on the conventional endometrioid carcinoma component [8].

1.2.1.2 Ancillary Studies

- Inhibin and calretinin are negative in areas resembling sex cord elements [9, 10].

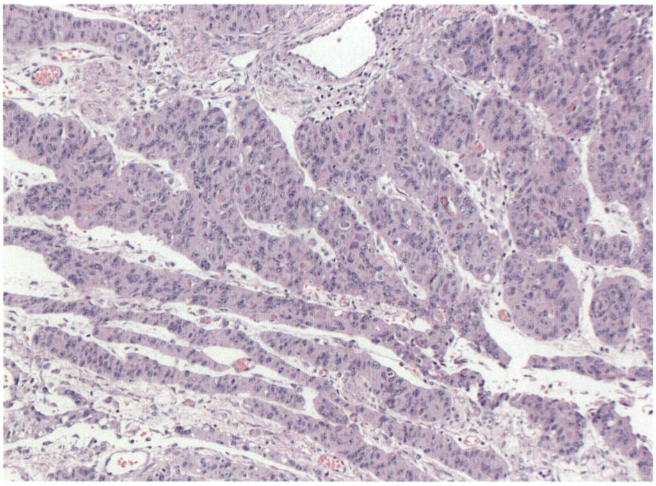

Fig. 1.4 Slender cords and trabeculae are anastomosing within a fibrotic stroma (100×)

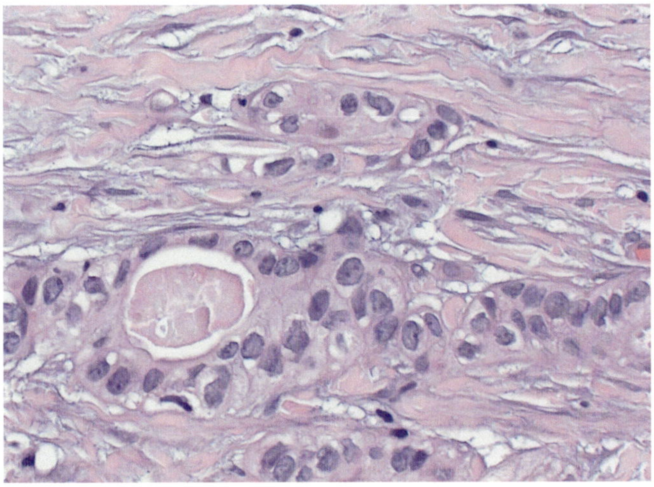

Fig. 1.5 The glandular component is merging the sertoliform areas. Cytological atypia is mild to moderate and similar in both elements (100×)

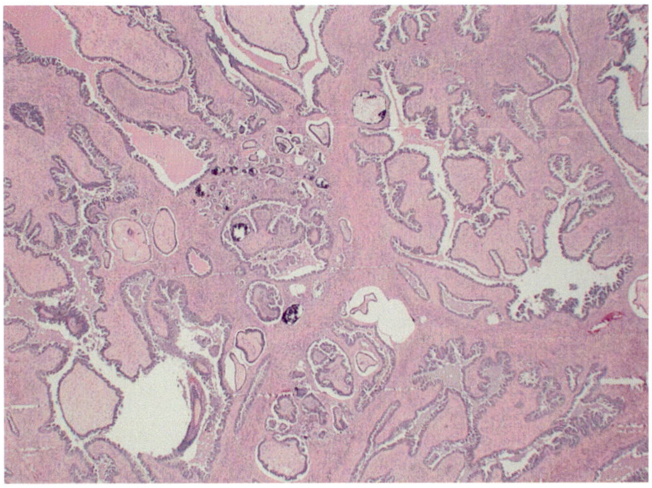

Fig. 1.6 LGSC at the center of the image with a background of SBT (20×)

1.2.1.3 Differential Diagnosis

- Sertoli cell tumor
  - The sex cord-like elements in endometrioid adenocarcinoma are usually embedded in a hyalinized stroma.
  - The presence of mucin or squamous differentiation, associated endometriosis, and an adenofibroma component support the adenocarcinoma diagnosis.
  - EMA is negative, and sex cord markers (inhibin, calretinin, and SF1) are positive in Sertoli cell tumors.
- Collision tumors with components of epithelial and sex cord tumors [11]
  - Extremely rare.
  - The components are discrete, and each has diagnostic morphologic and immunophenotypic features.
- Well-differentiated neuroendocrine tumor
  - Similar trabecular and acinar architectural patterns.
  - Coarse nuclear chromatin (salt and pepper appearance).
  - Synaptophysin, chromogranin, INSM1: positive [10].
  - See Part I, Sect. 4.1.

1.2.1.4 Clinical Significance

- In small series, survival is favorable and depends on the grade of adjacent conventional endometrioid carcinoma component [12].

1.3 Low-Grade Serous Carcinoma (LGSC) in the Background of Serous Borderline Tumor (SBT)

1.3.1 A 34-Year-Old Woman with a Pelvic Mass

1.3.1.1 Key Diagnostic Features

- Areas of stromal invasion (5 mm or more) in the background of a borderline tumor (Fig. 1.6), mild to moderate nuclear atypia (<3-fold variation in nuclear size), and mitotic rate <12 per 10 high-power fields [13].

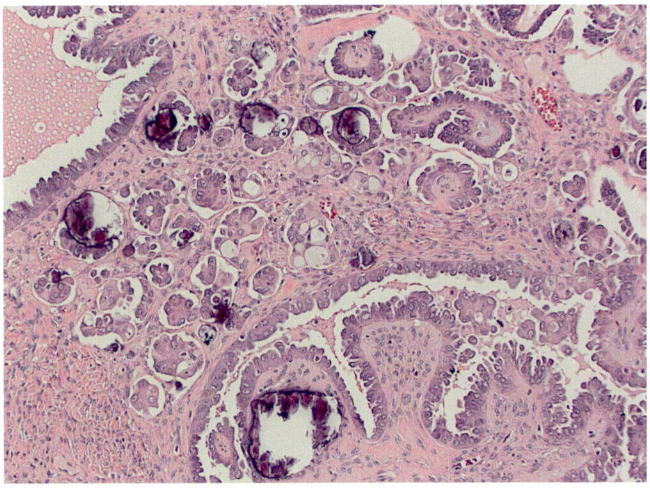

Fig. 1.7 Micropapillary pattern of invasion in LGSC is characterized by small, uniform papillae with cores containing little or no stroma surrounded by empty spaces (200×)

- Stromal invasion patterns include micropapillary (Fig. 1.7), compact cell nests, inverted macropapillae (Fig. 1.8), glandular (Figs. 1.9 and 1.10), cribriform (Fig. 1.11), cystic, solid sheets with slit-like spaces, and single cells [14–16].
- LGSC is associated with SBT in 84% of cases [14]. Epithelial and glandular proliferation in SBT may focally merge with LGSC.

1.3.1.2 Ancillary Studies

- Positive immunostains: PAX8, WT-1, ER, p16 (patchy) [17].
- P53: normal/wild type.

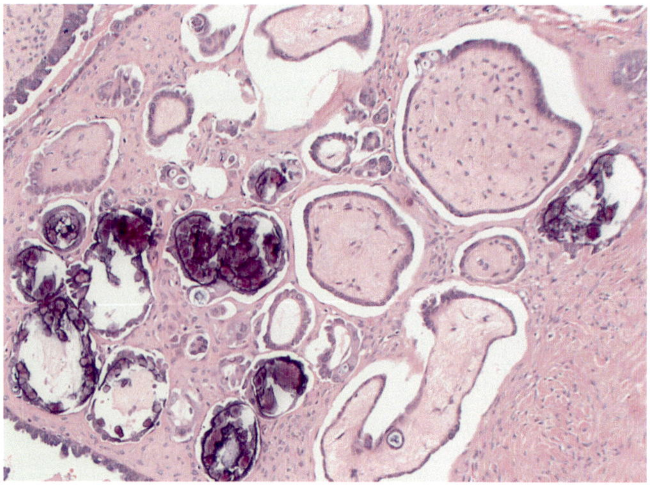

Fig. 1.8 Inverted macropapillary pattern of invasion in LGSC. This area contains large and small papillae, single cells, and psammomatous calcifications (200×)

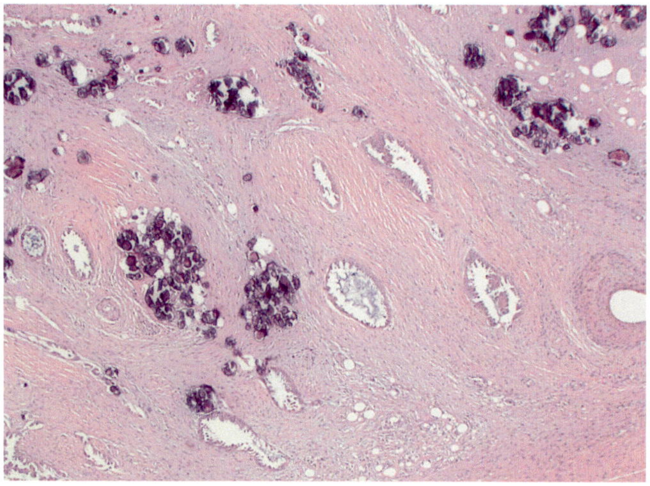

Fig. 1.9 The glandular pattern of invasion in LGSC. Well-formed and cystically dilated glands within a desmoplastic stroma are associated with abundant calcifications. Angulated glands with tapered ends are in the field (40×)

1.3.1.3 Differential Diagnosis

- SBT
  - Intracystic or exophytic lesions with ovarian surface involvement.
  - Papillae are architecturally complex, with hierarchical branching and variable amounts of stromal cores.
  - The lining epithelium has low-grade nuclear features. Eosinophilic cells, either budding from papillae or in free-floating clusters, can be present.
  - No stromal reaction.
- SBT with microinvasion

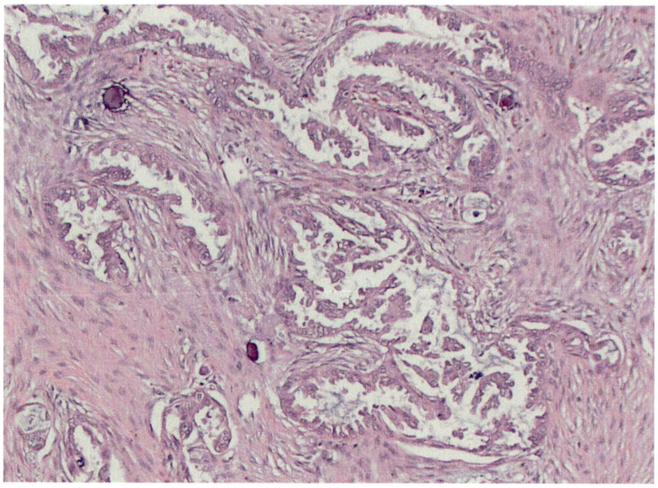

Fig. 1.10 Infiltrative glandular epithelium with disorganized papillae. The papillae do not follow a hierarchical order from primary to secondary to tertiary papillae (200×)

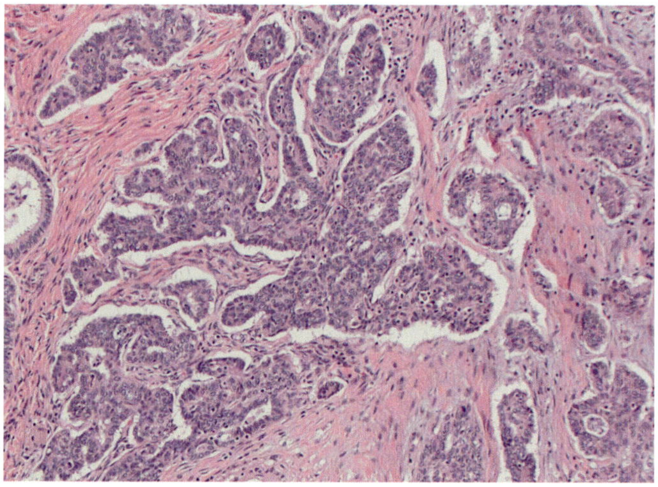

Fig. 1.11 Cribriform architectural pattern of LGSC (200×)

  - Small cluster of cells or single cells with dense eosinophilic cytoplasm without desmoplastic reaction within the ovarian stroma
  - <5 mm in the largest dimension in a single focus by definition
- Microinvasive LGSC
  - Similar patterns of LGSC with maximum tumor dimension measuring less than 5 mm [18].

1.3.1.4 Clinical Significance

- LGSC has an indolent clinical course. Women younger than 35 years with LGSC and those with persistent disease at completion of primary therapy have the worst outcomes [19].

1.4 Lymph Node Involvement by Serous Borderline Tumor

1.4.1 A 42-Year-Old Woman Underwent a Staging Procedure for Ovarian SBT

1.4.1.1 Key Diagnostic Features

- This finding is more common in subcapsular spaces of lymph nodes than in parenchyma.
- Papillary clusters or glandular structures (Fig. 1.12) and single cells (Fig. 1.13) resemble non-invasive epithelial implants. There is frequently background endosalpingiosis (Fig. 1.14) and no reactive changes in the lymph node parenchyma.

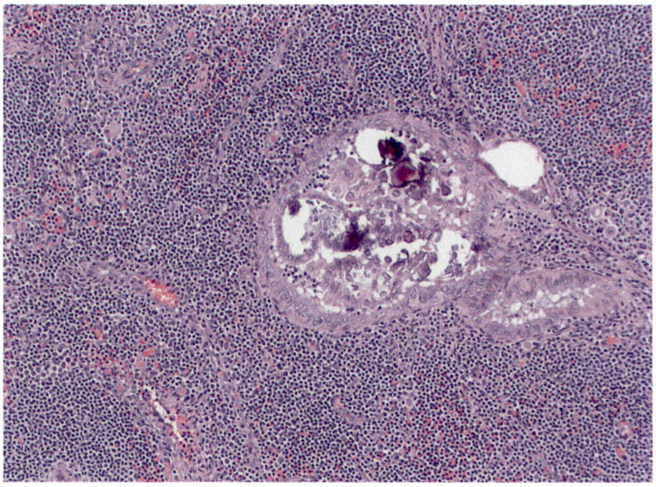

Fig. 1.12 Intraglandular pattern of a lymph node involvement by SBT. The gland contains papillae with tufting (200×)

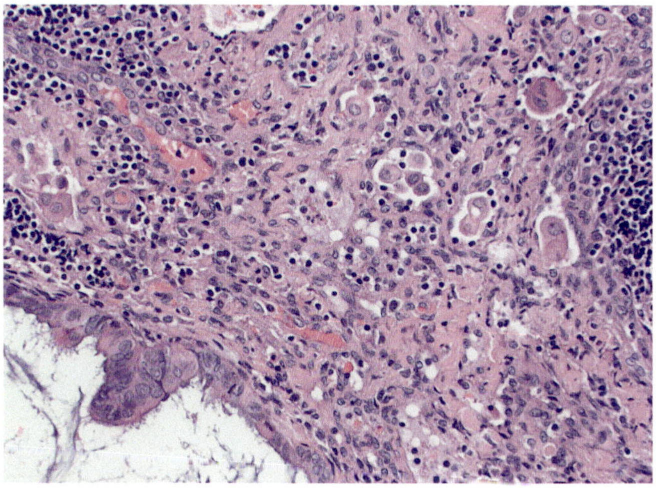

Fig. 1.13 Lymph node parenchyma contains aggregates of single cells with ample eosinophilic cytoplasm (200×)

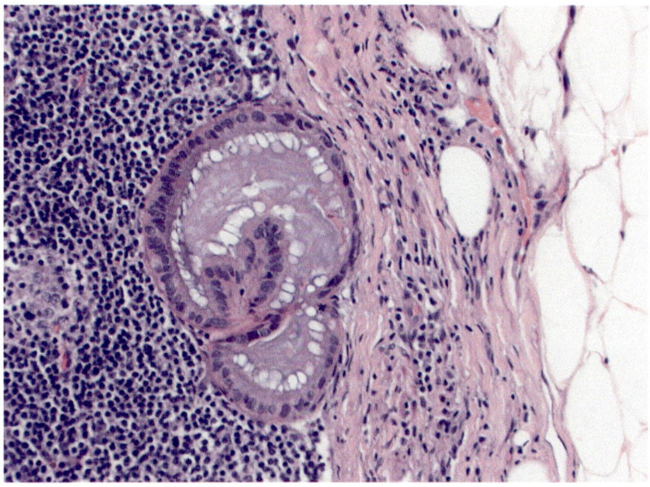

Fig. 1.14 Endosalpingiosis is frequently present in the background of SBT involving lymph nodes (200×)

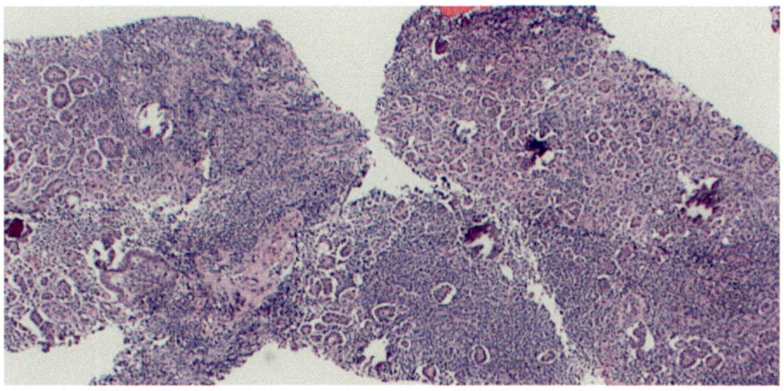

Fig. 1.15 Destructive micropapillary architectural pattern of nodal LGSC in a core biopsy specimen (100×)

- When the morphological features are similar to those of LGSC, it is considered an N1 disease (Figs. 1.15 and 1.16).
- The lymph node involvement in SBT is the most common in pelvic lymph nodes (58%), followed by mesenteric/omental (29%), para-aortic (26%), and supradiaphragmatic lymph nodes (6%) [20].

1.4.1.2 Ancillary Studies

N/A.

1.4.1.3 Differential Diagnosis

- Nodal low-grade serous carcinoma associated with ovarian SBT (N1 disease) [21]
  - An exuberant proliferation of serous epithelial cells exceeding 50% of an intermediate power field (×10) and exhibiting destructive invasion of nodal parenchyma (Figs. 1.15 and 1.16).
  - Architectural features of nodal LGSC include micropapillae, cell clusters, papillae, and solid nests.

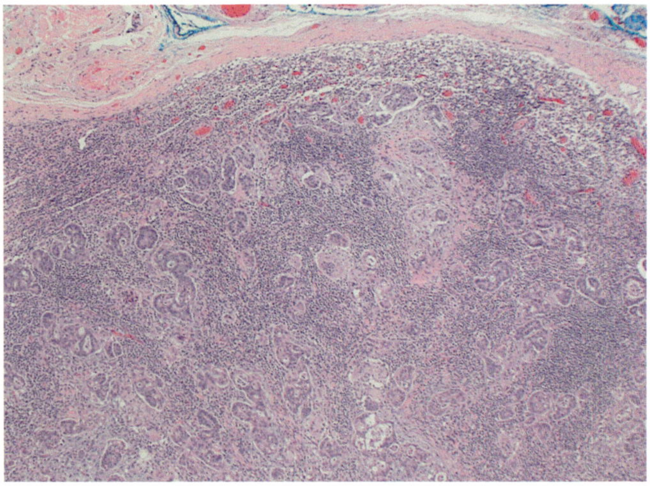

Fig. 1.16 Metastatic LGSC from an ovarian primary disease. The cellularity of serous-type epithelium is high with foci of surrounding fibrotic reaction (40×)

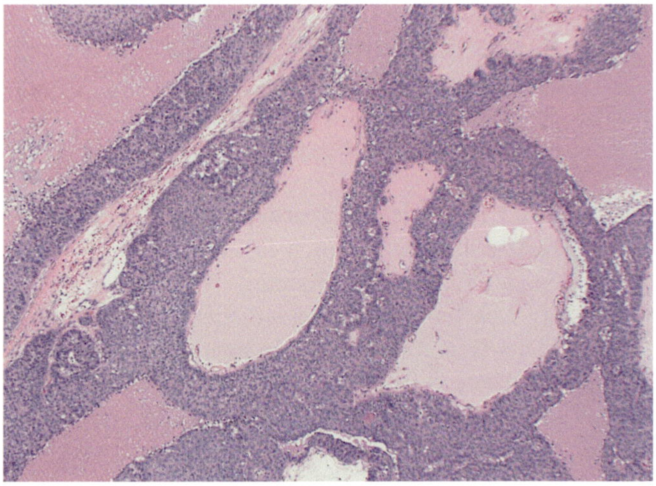

Fig. 1.17 Transitional cell-like growth pattern (40×)

- Nodal endosalpingiosis
  - Simple glandular formations in lymph nodes lined by a single layer of tubal-type epithelium (Fig. 1.14).
  - Simple papillary structures lined by a single layer of tubal-type epithelium with focal piling up are permitted in the definition of nodal endosalpingiosis.

1.4.1.4 Clinical Significance

- The prognosis of patients with borderline tumors of the ovary and nodal involvement is excellent [22].

1.5 High-Grade Serous Carcinoma (HGSC) with Solid Endometrioid-Like and Transitional (SET) Pattern

1.5.1 A 49-Year-Old Woman with a Known History of *BRCA1* Mutation

1.5.1.1 Key Diagnostic Features

- HGSC associated with homologous recombination deficiencies frequently demonstrates a combination of morphological features described as Solid Endometrioid-like and Transitional (SET) pattern [23, 24] (Figs. 1.17, 1.18, and 1.19).
- A higher mitotic index, high numbers of tumor-infiltrating inflammatory cells, and the presence of necrosis are also associated with *BRCA1*-inactivated tumors.
- *The BRCA1* mutation rate is 45% in non-classic HGSC (SET or ambiguous patterns) and 8% in classic HGSC. A comparable association does not exist with *BRCA2* mutations [24].

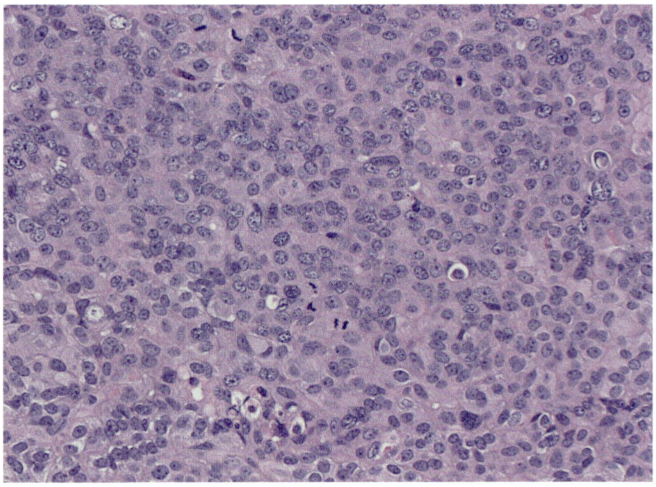

Fig. 1.18 Solid areas with high mitotic index (200×)

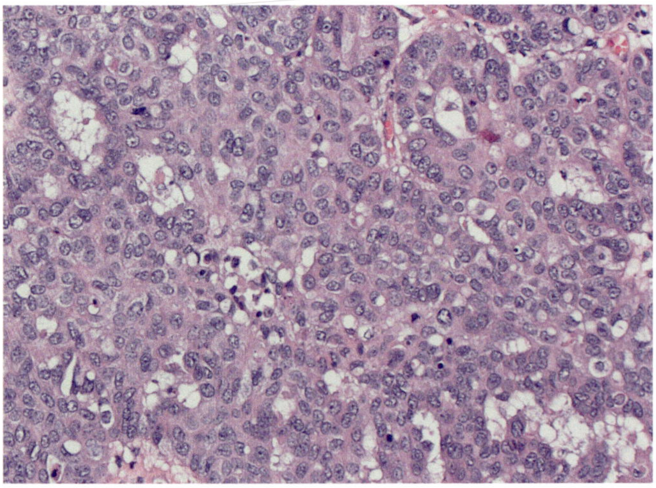

Fig. 1.19 Areas of pseudoglandular/endometrioid-like pattern without any true acini formation (200×)

1.5.1.2 Ancillary Studies

- There is no difference in expression of p53, ER, and PR by immunohistochemistry among the microscopic tumor patterns of HGSC (SET predominant or not) [25].

1.5.1.3 Differential Diagnosis

- High-grade endometrioid adenocarcinoma
  - A true gland/acini formation with polarization of nuclei around spaces supports endometrioid adenocarcinoma diagnosis, but the finding might be focal.
- Metastatic high-grade urothelial cell carcinoma
  - High-grade nuclear features, including nuclear pleomorphism, hyperchromasia, high nuclear/cytoplasmic ratio, and frequent mitotic figures
  - Positive immunostains: GATA3, CK7, CK20, p63, and p40
- Undifferentiated carcinoma
  - Dyscohesive sheets of cells without any glandular differentiation.
  - Broad zones of necrosis, cells with plasmacytoid morphology, abrupt keratinization, multinucleation, and focal spindling can be present.
  - See Part II, Sect. 6.12 (endometrial undifferentiated carcinoma).

1.5.1.4 Clinical Significance

- Mutations involving homologous recombination pathways have a significant influence on platinum sensitivity and survival [26, 27].

1.6 High-Grade Serous Carcinoma with Treatment Effect

1.6.1 A 69-Year-Old Woman with HGSC Treated with Platinum-Based Chemotherapy

1.6.1.1 Key Diagnostic Features

- The morphologic features of treated HGSC include enlarged nuclei, reduced nuclear-cytoplasmic ratio, bizarre nuclear outlines, nuclear chromatin clumping, and loss of details of chromatin (Figs. 1.20 and 1.21). Cytoplasmic alterations are intense eosinophilia, vacuolation, or foamy cell change. The stromal changes are fibrosis, inflammation, collections of foamy histiocytes, cholesterol cleft formation, hemosiderin deposition, fat necrosis, and dystrophic calcification [28] (Figs. 1.22 and 1.23).
- Chemotherapy Response Score (CRS) is a three-tiered scoring system based on an assessment of a section of omentum that shows the least response to chemotherapy [29, 30].

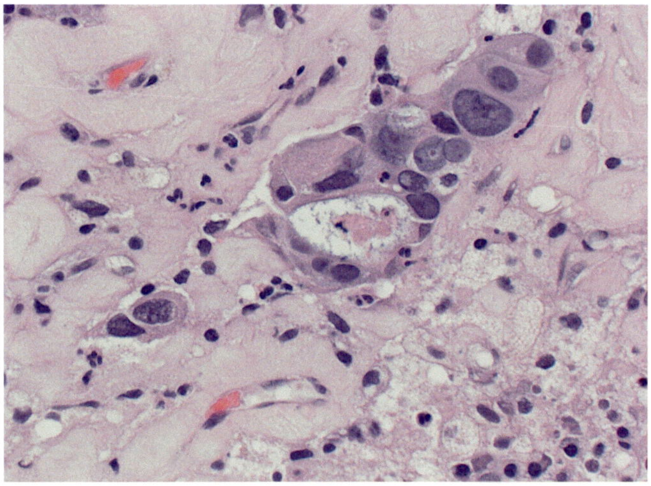

Fig. 1.20 The cytological features after neoadjuvant therapy are reduced N/C ratios, macronuclei, binucleation, eosinophilic, and foamy cytoplasm (200×)

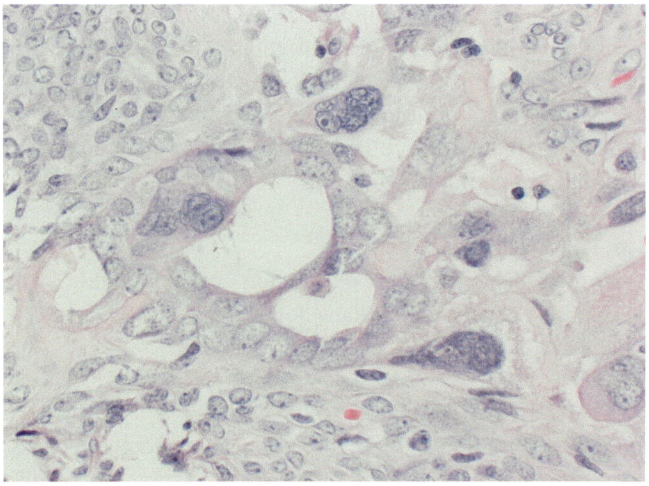

Fig. 1.21 Multinucleation of the tumor cells with loss of nuclear details and smudgy chromatin (200×)

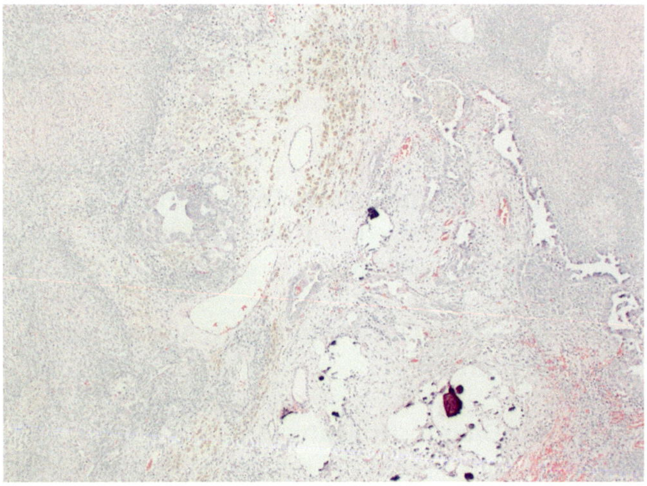

Fig. 1.22 Stromal changes after neoadjuvant therapy include areas of fibrosis, calcifications, and hemosiderin depositions (40×)

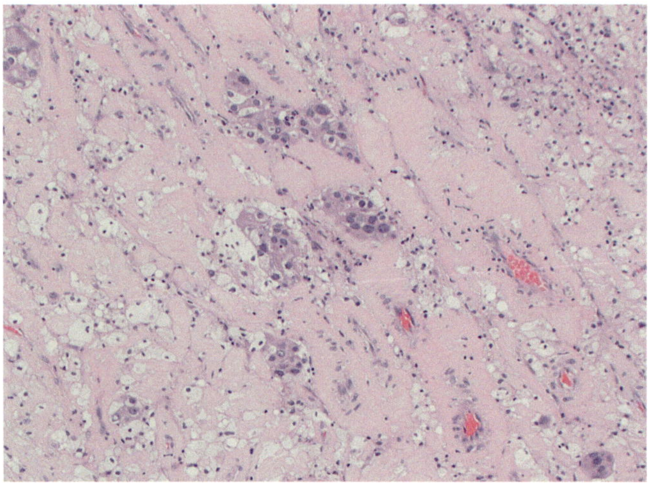

Fig. 1.23 Scant neoplastic cells within histiocytic infiltrates (100×)

- CRS 1: No or minimal tumor response (viable tumor with no or minimal regression).
- CRS 2: Appreciable tumor response amidst viable tumor, both readily identifiable and regularly distributed.
- CRS 3: Complete or near-complete response with no residual tumor or minimal irregularly scattered tumor foci seen as individual cells, cell groups, or nodules up to 2 mm in maximum size.

1.6.1.2 Ancillary Studies

- Immunohistochemical expression of p53 and WT1 remains largely concordant before and after chemotherapy [31].

1.6.1.3 Differential Diagnosis

- Accurate tumor typing and grading are difficult after neoadjuvant chemotherapy. However, biomarker expression is not affected by treatment. If the pretreatment biopsy is not available, positive staining with PAX8, WT-1, and p53 is supportive of HGSC diagnosis.

1.6.1.4 Clinical Significance

- Only CRS3 is significantly associated with improved progression-free survival and overall survival [30].

1.7 High-Grade Serous Carcinoma with Microcytic Pattern (Mucinous Differentiation)

1.7.1 A 71-Year-Old Woman with Abdominal Distention

1.7.1.1 Key Diagnostic Features

- Predominantly microcystic pattern and mucinous material within the lumen of microcysts [32] (Fig. 1.24).

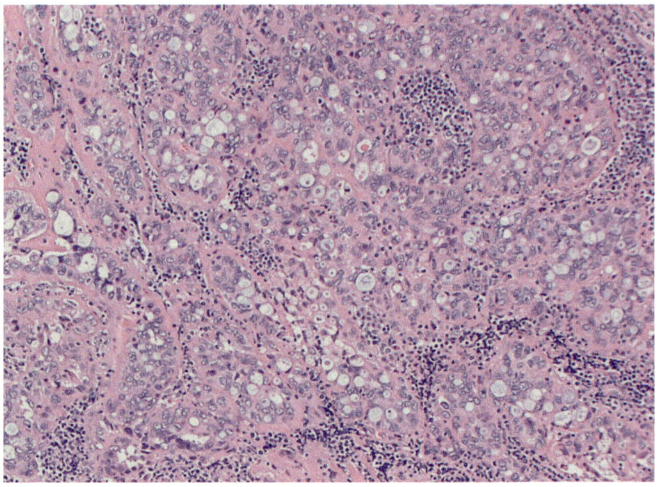

Fig. 1.24 High-grade ovarian serous carcinoma in microcytic pattern (100×)

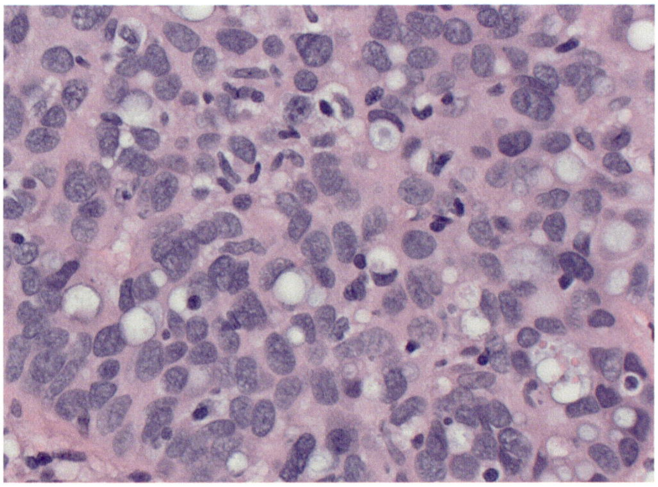

Fig. 1.25 Signet ring-type cells (200×)

- Rare signet ring cells: +/− (Fig. 1.25).
- Nuclear pleomorphism (size variability) >3-folds as conventional HGSC (Fig. 1.26).
- Usual patterns of serous carcinoma can be focal. The microcystic pattern is associated with the SET pattern of HGSC in recent studies [33].

1.7.1.2 Ancillary Studies

- PAS highlights intracytoplasmic mucin.
- CK7: positive, CK20, and neuroendocrine markers: negative [32].
- P53: mutation pattern staining.

1.7.1.3 Differential Diagnosis

- Endometrioid carcinoma with microglandular pattern (see Fig. 1.27)
  - Resembles endocervical microglandular hyperplasia.

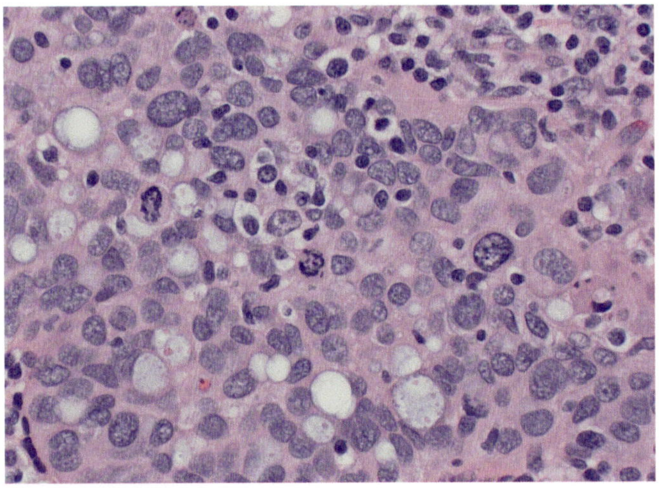

Fig. 1.26 The nuclear size variation is more than threefolds (200×)

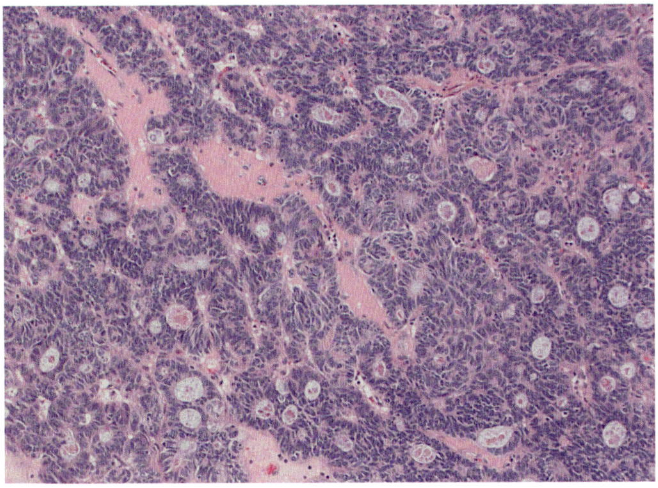

Fig. 1.27 Low-grade endometrioid carcinoma in microglandular pattern. Nuclei are columnar, and cytological atypia is minimal (100×)

  - Nuclei are columnar, and cytological atypia is minimal.
- Metastatic mucinous carcinoma
  - Typically exhibits single or small groups of signet ring cells infiltrating ovarian stroma. Only rarely microcystic pattern is part of the lesion.
  - Clinical and imaging correlation contributes to diagnosis.
  - Positive results with PAX8, p53, and CK7 by immunohistochemistry support primary ovarian tumor.
- Mucinous carcinoid
  - There might be a background teratoma.
  - Usually metastatic, rare case reports for primary mucinous carcinoid of the ovaries [34].
  - The morphological features vary with the degree of differentiation.
  - In well-differentiated tumors, variable-sized glands lined by goblet cells infiltrate the ovarian stroma. Cells might have red cytoplasmic granules. A solid growth pattern, signet ring-type cells, and high mitotic activity are the morphological features of carcinoma arising in mucinous carcinoids.
  - Immunoreactivity for neuroendocrine markers (synaptophysin, chromogranin, and CD56).

1.7.1.4 Clinical Significance

- Relatively rare pattern of HGSC without known clinical significance

1.8 Mucinous Borderline Tumor with Intraepithelial (Non-invasive) Carcinoma (MBT with IECA)

1.8.1 A 42-Year-Old Woman with a Pelvic Mass Lesion

1.8.1.1 Key Diagnostic Features

- Architectural patterns include cribriform intraglandular proliferations, intraglandular bridges, or finger-like projections of solid cellular masses without connective tissue support [35] (Figs. 1.28 and 1.29).
- The nuclear features are diagnostic. Nuclei are enlarged, vesicular and display prominent nucleoli. There is a loss of polarization around the basement membrane and stratification of nuclei [36]. Mitotic figures are frequent (Fig. 1.30).

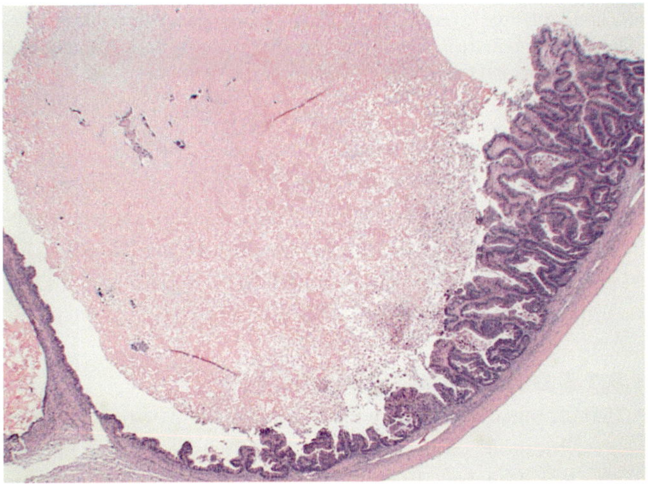

Fig. 1.28 Ovarian mucinous borderline tumor with focal finger-like projections and back-to-back glandular crowding. There is ovarian stroma between cystically dilated glands (20×)

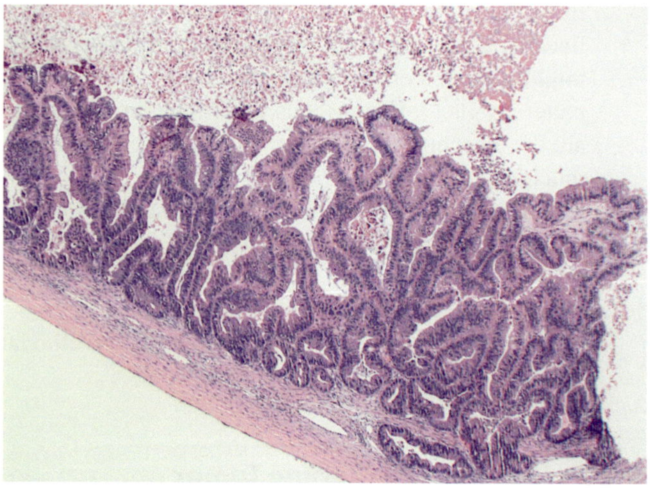

Fig. 1.29 The area of glandular crowding in higher power view (100×)

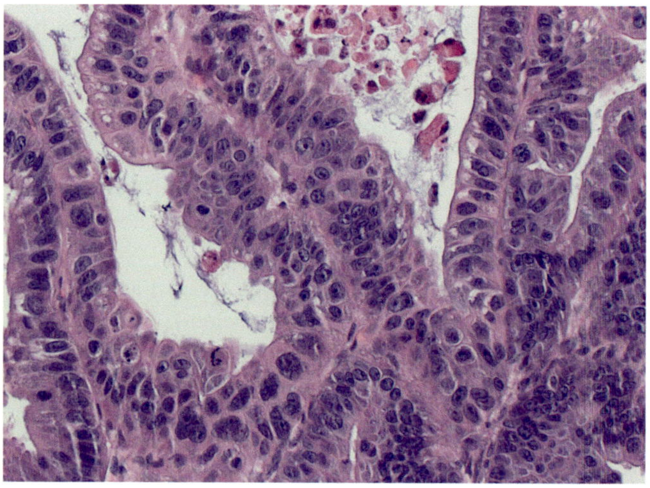

Fig. 1.30 The glands are lined by cells with large round nuclei, which pile up in multiple layers. There is a loss of polarization around the basement membrane and a lack of intracytoplasmic mucin in the IECA. Nucleoli are prominent, and the mitotic figures are frequent (200×)

1.8.1.2 Ancillary Studies

- There is an overlap in the immunophenotype of mucinous ovarian lesions and metastatic gastrointestinal tract neoplasms. The ovarian mucinous tumors are usually diffusely positive for CK7, and CK20, CEA, and CDX2 might be focal or diffuse positive [37].

1.8.1.3 Differential Diagnosis

- Mucinous carcinoma with an expansile growth pattern
  - Mucinous carcinoma with an expansile growth pattern is architecturally complex and often has a labyrinthine arrangement of glands, cysts, or papillae lined by malignant epithelium with minimal or no intervening normal ovarian stroma (Fig. 1.31).
  - The area of multiple closely approximated glands separated by only thin strands of ovarian stroma should measure at least 5 mm.

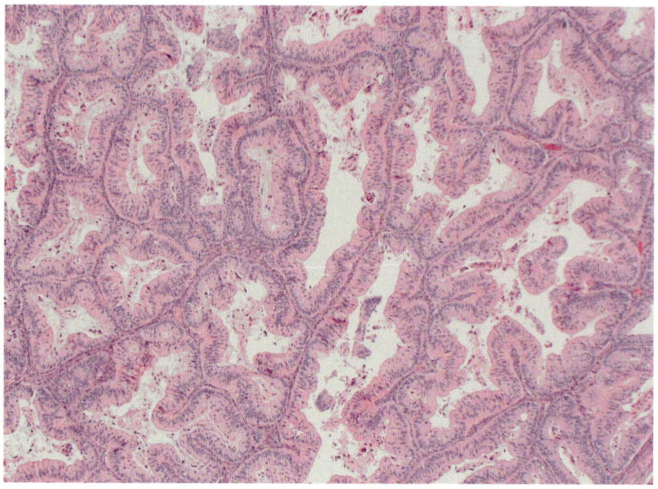

Fig. 1.31 Mucinous carcinoma by expansion/confluent growth pattern. Cystically dilated glands are back to back and occupy an area measuring at least 5 mm. There is minimal or absent stroma between complex glands (40×)

- Metastatic adenocarcinomas from the gastrointestinal tract
  - Metastatic lesions have areas composed of highly differentiated glands with an orderly growth pattern that may closely mimic IECA, borderline tumor, and even cystadenoma [38, 39]. The morphological features that are consistent with metastatic carcinoma are the following:
    - Bilateral tumors
    - Microscopic foci of ovarian surface involvement by carcinoma cells
    - Nodular growth pattern
    - An infiltrative pattern of stromal invasion and single-cell invasion
    - Ovarian hilar involvement and vascular invasion

1.8.1.4 Clinical Significance

- The presence of IECA in an MBT should prompt additional sampling as the IECA may be an indicator of invasive carcinoma in other foci of the specimen. The presence and the percentage (≥10%) of IECA in the background of MBT are associated with tumor recurrences [40]. The latter finding might be related to inadequate tissue sampling.

1.9 Serous Borderline Tumor (SBT) with Extraovarian Disease (Implants)

1.9.1 Biopsies Obtained at the Staging Procedure for Serous Borderline Tumor

1.9.1.1 Key Diagnostic Features

- Epithelial non-invasive implants: Similar to morphological features of SBT, the serous epithelium forms hierarchically branching papillae. They might present on the surface of the peritoneum or, more commonly, in smoothly contoured sub-mesothelial invaginations (Fig. 1.32) and between omental fat lobules [41]. The invaginations are lined by a single layer of flattened to cuboidal cells that resemble mesothelial or tubal epithelial cells (Fig. 1.33).
- Desmoplastic non-invasive implants: There is a sharp demarcation between desmoplastic implants and peritoneal surfaces and underlying soft tissue (Fig. 1.34). At high-power examination, distorted glands (Fig. 1.35), groups of cells, or single eosinophilic cells (Fig. 1.36) are present within a fibrous or granulation tissue. Desmoplastic implants on the ovarian surface are called auto-implants.
- Invasive epithelial implants (extraovarian low-grade serous carcinoma (LGSC)): Destructive invasion of the underlying tissue is the key morphological feature. Patterns are similar to those of LGSC of the ovaries: (1) Inverted macropapillary (Fig. 1.37) (2) Micropapillary (3) Cribriform (4) Glandular patterns. The empty spaces (retraction artifact) around the epithelium and stromal fibroblastic reaction (Fig. 1.38) are associated with invasive epithelial implants.

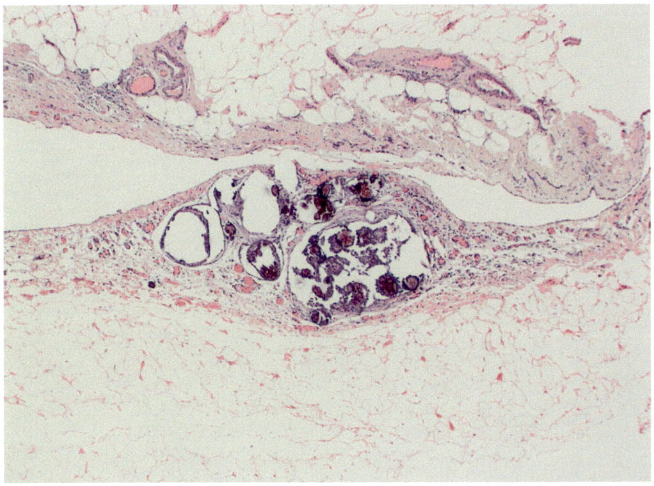

Fig. 1.32 Non-invasive epithelial implant with calcifications underneath the omental surface as smooth-contoured invaginations (40×)

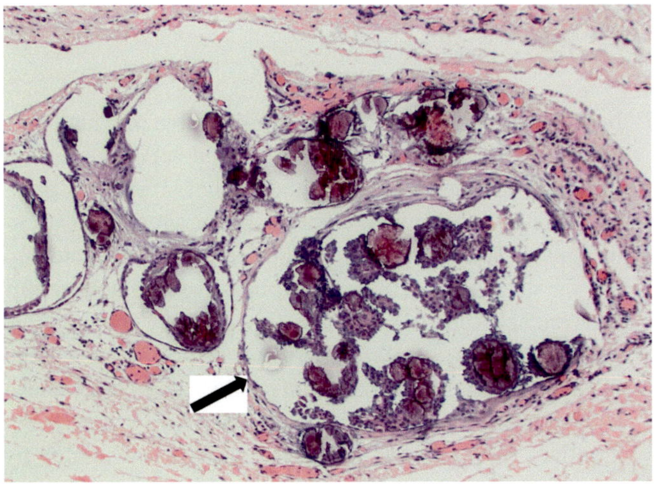

Fig. 1.33 The neoplastic cells in papillary architecture are confined within a mesothelium-lined space (arrow). There is no stromal reaction (200×)

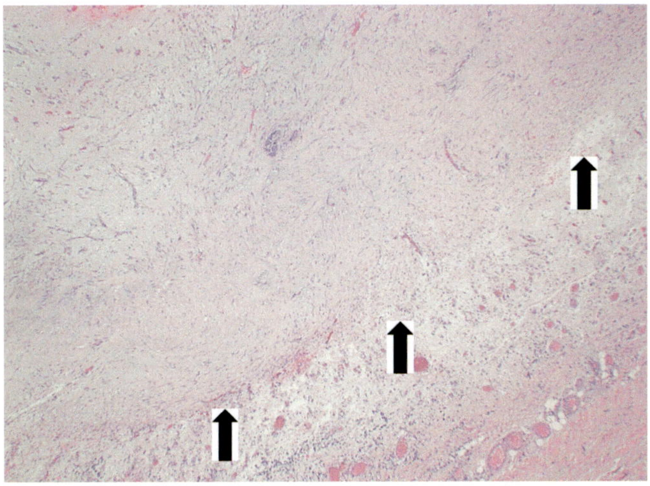

Fig. 1.34 There is a sharp demarcation between desmoplastic implants and underlying soft tissue (arrows) (40×)

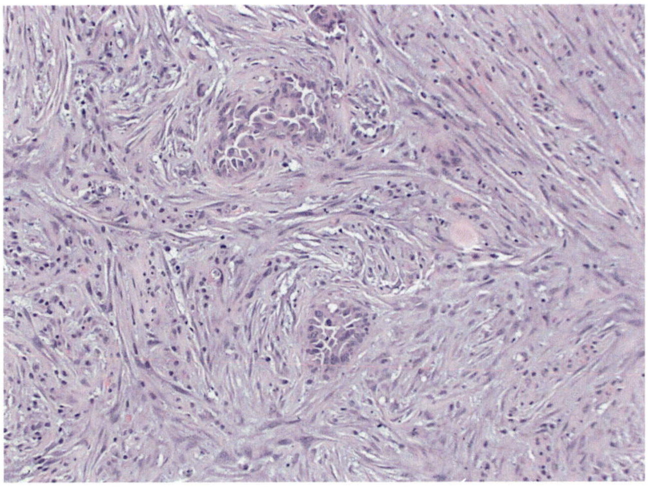

Fig. 1.35 Glands within a desmoplastic implant are compressed and distorted by the surrounding dense fibrous stroma (200×)

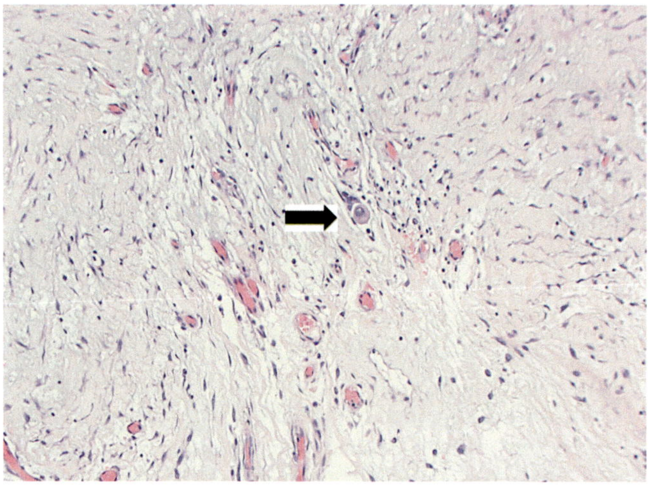

Fig. 1.36 There might be a single (arrow) or group of cells with dense eosinophilic cytoplasm within a desmoplastic implant (200×)

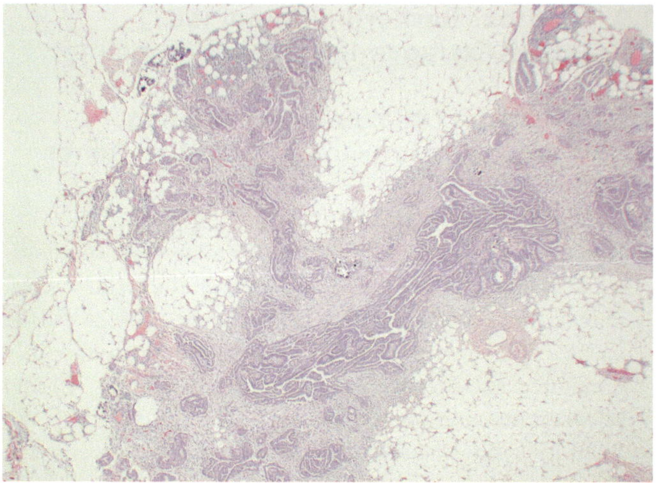

Fig. 1.38 Invasive epithelial implant (LGSC): The neoplastic epithelium is surrounded by fibroblastic reaction in an omental section. The neoplastic glands engulf/surround the omental fat (40×)

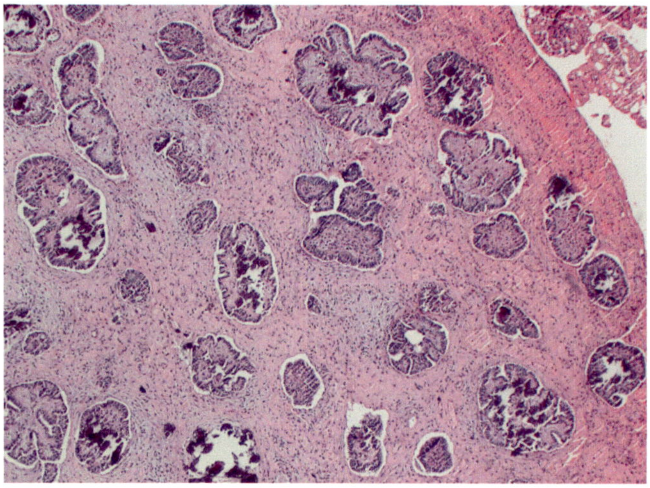

Fig. 1.37 Invasive epithelial implants (LGSC): Inverted macropapillary pattern. The empty spaces surround the papillary neoplastic epithelium (40×)

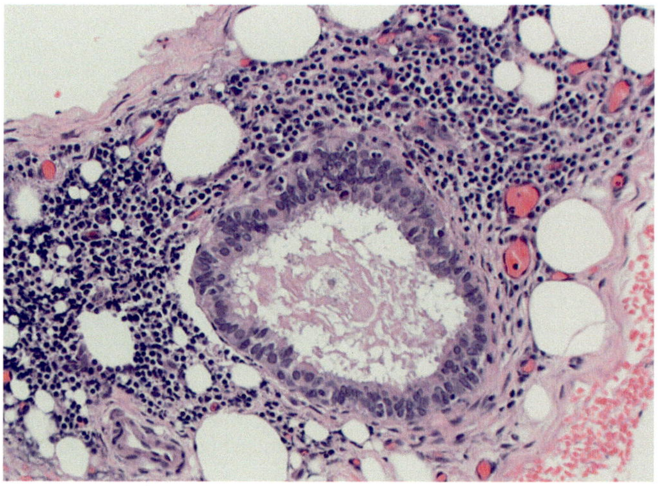

Fig. 1.39 A focus of background endosalpingiosis (200×)

1.9.1.2 Ancillary Studies

- The majority of peritoneal implants, non-invasive or invasive, harbor identical *KRAS* or *BRAF* mutations that are also present in the associated SBT [42].
- Endosalpingiosis might represent a precursor lesion of some peritoneal implants [43] (Fig. 1.39).

1.9.1.3 Differential Diagnosis

- Invasive and non-invasive implants are commonly found together [44].
- In small biopsies, underlying tissue is absent in about 25% of implants [45]. The absence of underlying tissue generally indicates the implant is easily stripped away and thus non-invasive [46].
- In the omentum, desmoplastic non-invasive implants may produce fibrous adhesions between fat lobules, causing difficulty in determining whether actual invasion is present. Non-invasive implants follow the omental fibrovascular septae. They are not expansile and do not infiltrate into the surrounding fat. In contrast, invasive implants engulf and replace omental adipose tissue [44]. The invasive implants have a greater proportion of proliferating neoplastic epithelial cells that often produce complex glandular, micropapillary, and cribriform patterns.
- Papillary tufts or nests of epithelial cells surrounded by clefts in non-invasive implants should be distinguished from solid nests of micropapillary invasive implants. The papillary tufts in non-invasive implants have scalloped

borders, are usually composed of cells with columnar or eosinophilic cytoplasm, and appear compressed by the stroma. Similar nests are often present without clefts that merge with the surrounding stroma, and the nests often vary in size and shape. In contrast, solid nests of invasive implants/LGSC usually have smoother contours, are composed of cuboidal cells with a higher nuclear to cytoplasmic ratio, appear uncompressed, and are more uniform [47].

1.9.1.4 Clinical Significance

- Invasive implants are equivalent to LGSC [48]. Identification of invasive implants/LGSC is the most important adverse prognostic factor for patients with SBT.

1.10 Borderline Brenner Tumor with Mucinous Metaplasia

1.10.1 Large Cystic Ovarian Neoplasm by Imaging Studies

1.10.1.1 Key Diagnostic Features

- Large cystic lesions with alternating papillary architecture (Fig. 1.40).
- The lining epithelium resembles papillary urothelial neoplasm.
- Mucinous or squamous metaplasia and background benign Brenner tumor might be present.
- Neoplastic cells usually have slightly enlarged nuclei with nuclear grooves. Overlapping of nuclei and loss of polarization to the basement membrane are other cytological features (Figs. 1.41 and 1.42).

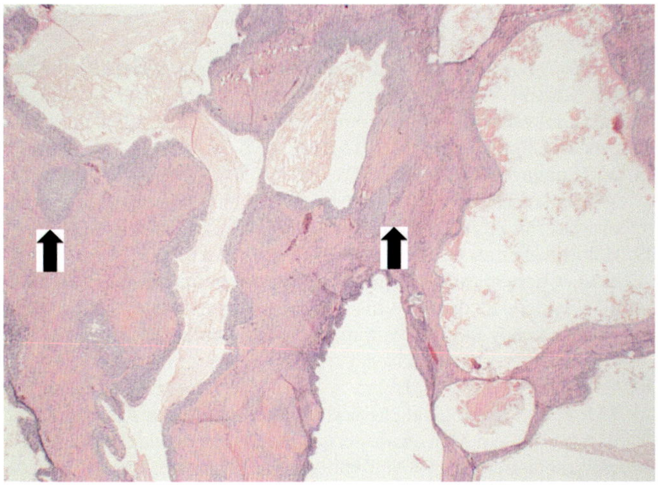

Fig. 1.40 A large cystic neoplasm. In the background, there are groups of nodular transitional type epithelium (Brenner tumor) (arrows) (40×)

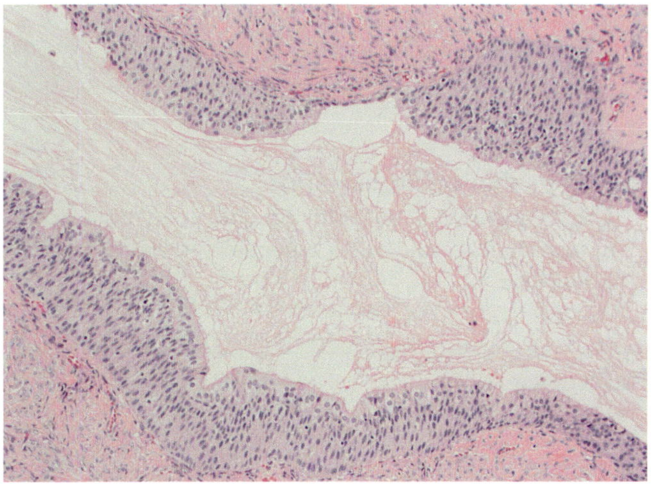

Fig. 1.41 The lining epithelium resembles papillary urothelial neoplasm. At the luminal site, the mucinous-type epithelium overlies at the top of the stratified epithelium (100×)

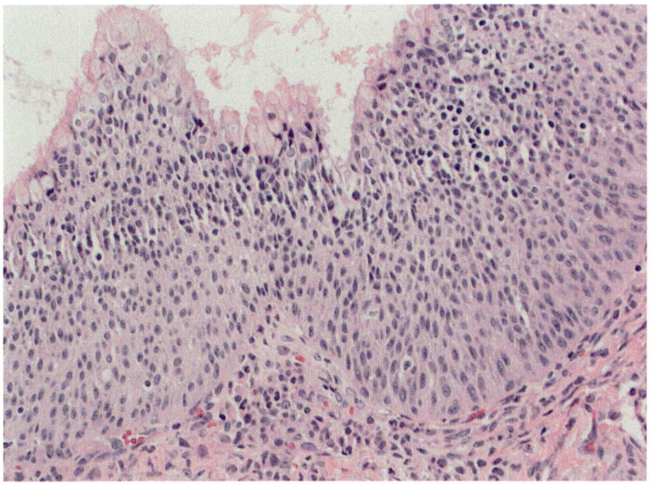

Fig. 1.42 The neoplastic cells are enlarged with hyperchromatic nuclei; some have nuclear grooves. The metaplastic mucinous epithelium is on the luminal side of the multi-layered stratified epithelium (200×)

1.10.1.2 Ancillary Studies

- Positive immunostains: p63, GATA3 [49, 50]
- P53: normal staining pattern [51]
- Loss of p16 expression due to *CDKN2A* mutation [52]

1.10.1.3 Differential Diagnosis

- Metastatic urothelial carcinoma
  - Bilateral and multinodular growth pattern
  - Lack of background benign Brenner tumor
- High-grade serous carcinoma with solid endometrioid-like and transitional (SET) pattern

– Nuclei are highly atypical (size variation >3 times).
– Pseudoglandular areas.
– Mutation pattern p53 expression.
– See Part I, Sect. 1.5.

1.10.1.4 Clinical Significance

- The prognosis is good, with rare late recurrences [53]. It is important to rule out a potential invasive carcinoma component.

References

1. Tornos C, Silva EG, Ordonez NG, Gershenson DM, Young RH, Scully RE. Endometrioid carcinoma of the ovary with a prominent spindle-cell component, a source of diagnostic confusion. A report of 14 cases. Am J Surg Pathol. 1995;19(12):1343–53.
2. Young RH, Scully RE. Ovarian tumors of probable wolffian origin. A report of 11 cases. Am J Surg Pathol. 1983;7(2):125–35.
3. Bennett JA, Ritterhouse LL, Furtado LV, Lastra RR, Pesci A, Newell JM, et al. Female adnexal tumors of probable Wolffian origin: morphological, immunohistochemical, and molecular analysis of 15 cases. Mod Pathol. 2020;33(4):734–47.
4. McCluggage WG, Ganesan R, Herrington CS. Endometrial stromal sarcomas with extensive endometrioid glandular differentiation: report of a series with emphasis on the potential for misdiagnosis and discussion of the differential diagnosis. Histopathology. 2009;54(3):365–73.
5. Fadare O, Parkash V. Pathology of endometrioid and clear cell carcinoma of the ovary. Surg Pathol Clin. 2019;12(2):529–64.
6. Young RH, Prat J, Scully RE. Ovarian endometrioid carcinomas resembling sex cord-stromal tumors. A clinicopathological analysis of 13 cases. Am J Surg Pathol. 1982;6(6):513–22.
7. Fujibayashi M, Aiba M, Iizuka E, Igarashi A, Muraoka M, Takagi K. Granulosa cell tumor-like variant of endometrioid carcinoma of the ovary exhibiting nuclear clearing with biotin activity: a subtype showing close macroscopic, cytologic, and histologic similarity to adult granulosa cell tumor. Arch Pathol Lab Med. 2005;129(10):1288–94.
8. Talia KL, McCluggage WG. The diverse morphology and immunophenotype of ovarian endometrioid carcinomas. Pathology. 2023;55(3):269–86.
9. Misir A, Sur M. Sertoliform endometrioid carcinoma of the ovary: a potential diagnostic pitfall. Arch Pathol Lab Med. 2007;131(6):979–81.
10. Zhao C, Bratthauer GL, Barner R, Vang R. Comparative analysis of alternative and traditional immunohistochemical markers for the distinction of ovarian sertoli cell tumor from endometrioid tumors and carcinoid tumor: a study of 160 cases. Am J Surg Pathol. 2007;31(2):255–66.
11. Schoolmeester JK, Keeney GL. Collision tumor of the ovary: adult granulosa cell tumor and endometrioid carcinoma. Int J Gynecol Pathol. 2012;31(6):538–40.
12. Ordi J, Schammel DP, Rasekh L, Tavassoli FA. Sertoliform endometrioid carcinomas of the ovary: a clinicopathologic and immunohistochemical study of 13 cases. Mod Pathol. 1999;12(10):933–40.
13. Malpica A, Deavers MT, Lu K, Bodurka DC, Atkinson EN, Gershenson DM, et al. Grading ovarian serous carcinoma using a two-tier system. Am J Surg Pathol. 2004;28(4):496–504.
14. Ahn G, Folkins AK, McKenney JK, Longacre TA. Low-grade serous carcinoma of the ovary: clinicopathologic analysis of 52 invasive cases and identification of a possible noninvasive intermediate lesion. Am J Surg Pathol. 2016;40(9):1165–76.
15. Silva EG, Deavers MT, Malpica A. Patterns of low-grade serous carcinoma with emphasis on the nonepithelial-lined spaces pattern of invasion and the disorganized orphan papillae. Int J Gynecol Pathol. 2010;29(6):507–12.
16. Yemelyanova A, Mao TL, Nakayama N, Shih Ie M, Kurman RJ. Low-grade serous carcinoma of the ovary displaying a macropapillary pattern of invasion. Am J Surg Pathol. 2008;32(12):1800–6.
17. Köbel M, Luo L, Grevers X, Lee S, Brooks-Wilson A, Gilks CB, et al. Ovarian carcinoma histotype: strengths and limitations of integrating morphology with immunohistochemical predictions. Int J Gynecol Pathol. 2019;38(4):353–62.
18. Seidman JD, Savage J, Krishnan J, Vang R, Kurman RJ. Intratumoral heterogeneity accounts for apparent progression of noninvasive serous tumors to invasive low-grade serous carcinoma: a study of 30 low-grade serous tumors of the ovary in 18 patients with peritoneal carcinomatosis. Int J Gynecol Pathol. 2020;39(1):43–54.
19. Gershenson DM, Bodurka DC, Lu KH, Nathan LC, Milojevic L, Wong KK, et al. Impact of age and primary disease site on outcome in women with low-grade serous carcinoma of the ovary or peritoneum: results of a large single-institution registry of a rare tumor. J Clin Oncol. 2015;33(24):2675–82.
20. McKenney JK, Balzer BL, Longacre TA. Lymph node involvement in ovarian serous tumors of low malignant potential (borderline tumors): pathology, prognosis, and proposed classification. Am J Surg Pathol. 2006;30(5):614–24.
21. Djordjevic B, Malpica A. Ovarian serous tumors of low malignant potential with nodal low-grade serous carcinoma. Am J Surg Pathol. 2012;36(7):955–63.
22. Seidman JD, Kurman RJ. Ovarian serous borderline tumors: a critical review of the literature with emphasis on prognostic indicators. Hum Pathol. 2000;31(5):539–57.
23. Soslow RA, Han G, Park KJ, Garg K, Olvera N, Spriggs DR, et al. Morphologic patterns associated with BRCA1 and BRCA2 genotype in ovarian carcinoma. Mod Pathol. 2012;25(4):625–36.
24. Ritterhouse LL, Nowak JA, Strickland KC, Garcia EP, Jia Y, Lindeman NI, et al. Morphologic correlates of molecular alterations in extrauterine Müllerian carcinomas. Mod Pathol. 2016;29(8):893–903.
25. Uner H, Demir M, Goksuluk D, Kars A, Uner M, Usubutun A. Evidence for diverse prognosis in high-grade serous ovarian carcinoma: solid, pseudoendometrioid, and transitional-like; so-called "set morphology" and progesterone receptor status. Turk Patoloji Derg. 2022;38(3):240–50.
26. Pennington KP, Walsh T, Lee M, Pennil C, Novetsky AP, Agnew KJ, et al. BRCA1, TP53, and CHEK2 germline mutations in uterine serous carcinoma. Cancer. 2013;119(2):332–8.
27. Candido-dos-Reis FJ, Song H, Goode EL, Cunningham JM, Fridley BL, Larson MC, et al. Germline mutation in BRCA1 or BRCA2 and ten-year survival for women diagnosed with epithelial ovarian cancer. Clin Cancer Res. 2015;21(3):652–7.
28. McCluggage WG, Lyness RW, Atkinson RJ, Dobbs SP, Harley I, McClelland HR, et al. Morphological effects of chemotherapy on ovarian carcinoma. J Clin Pathol. 2002;55(1):27–31.
29. Böhm S, Faruqi A, Said I, Lockley M, Brockbank E, Jeyarajah A, et al. Chemotherapy response score: development and validation of a system to quantify histopathologic response to neoadjuvant chemotherapy in tubo-ovarian high-grade serous carcinoma. J Clin Oncol. 2015;33(22):2457–63.
30. Cohen PA, Powell A, Böhm S, Gilks CB, Stewart CJR, Meniawy TM, et al. Pathological chemotherapy response score is prognostic in tubo-ovarian high-grade serous carcinoma: a systematic review and meta-analysis of individual patient data. Gynecol Oncol. 2019;154(2):441–8.
31. Casey L, Köbel M, Ganesan R, Tam S, Prasad R, Böhm S, et al. A comparison of p53 and WT1 immunohistochemical expression pat-

terns in tubo-ovarian high-grade serous carcinoma before and after neoadjuvant chemotherapy. Histopathology. 2017;71(5):736–42.
32. Che M, Tornos C, Deavers MT, Malpica A, Gershenson DM, Silva EG. Ovarian mixed-epithelial carcinomas with a microcystic pattern and signet-ring cells. Int J Gynecol Pathol. 2001;20(4):323–8.
33. Hatano Y, Tamada M, Asano N, Hayasaki Y, Tomita H, Morishige KI, et al. High-grade serous ovarian carcinoma with mucinous differentiation: report of a rare and unique case suggesting transition from the "SET" feature of high-grade serous carcinoma to the "STEM" feature. Diagn Pathol. 2019;14(1):4.
34. Hsu WW, Mao TL, Chen CH. Primary ovarian mucinous carcinoid tumor: a case report and review of literature. Taiwan J Obstet Gynecol. 2019;58(4):570–3.
35. Riopel MA, Ronnett BM, Kurman RJ. Evaluation of diagnostic criteria and behavior of ovarian intestinal-type mucinous tumors: atypical proliferative (borderline) tumors and intraepithelial, microinvasive, invasive, and metastatic carcinomas. Am J Surg Pathol. 1999;23(6):617–35.
36. Hart WR. Mucinous tumors of the ovary: a review. Int J Gynecol Pathol. 2005;24(1):4–25.
37. Vang R, Gown AM, Wu LS, Barry TS, Wheeler DT, Yemelyanova A, et al. Immunohistochemical expression of CDX2 in primary ovarian mucinous tumors and metastatic mucinous carcinomas involving the ovary: comparison with CK20 and correlation with coordinate expression of CK7. Mod Pathol. 2006;19(11):1421–8.
38. Lash RH, Hart WR. Intestinal adenocarcinomas metastatic to the ovaries. A clinicopathologic evaluation of 22 cases. Am J Surg Pathol. 1987;11(2):114–21.
39. Young RH, Hart WR. Metastases from carcinomas of the pancreas simulating primary mucinous tumors of the ovary. A report of seven cases. Am J Surg Pathol. 1989;13(9):748–56.
40. Khunamornpong S, Settakorn J, Sukpan K, Suprasert P, Siriaunkgul S. Mucinous tumor of low malignant potential ("borderline" or "atypical proliferative" tumor) of the ovary: a study of 171 cases with the assessment of intraepithelial carcinoma and microinvasion. Int J Gynecol Pathol. 2011;30(3):218–30.
41. Bell DA, Weinstock MA, Scully RE. Peritoneal implants of ovarian serous borderline tumors. Histologic features and prognosis. Cancer. 1988;62(10):2212–22.
42. Ardighieri L, Zeppernick F, Hannibal CG, Vang R, Cope L, Junge J, et al. Mutational analysis of BRAF and KRAS in ovarian serous borderline (atypical proliferative) tumours and associated peritoneal implants. J Pathol. 2014;232(1):16–22.
43. Moore WF, Bentley RC, Berchuck A, Robboy SJ. Some mullerian inclusion cysts in lymph nodes may sometimes be metastases from serous borderline tumors of the ovary. Am J Surg Pathol. 2000;24(5):710–8.
44. Hart WR. Borderline epithelial tumors of the ovary. Mod Pathol. 2005;18(Suppl 2):S33–50.
45. Bell KA, Smith Sehdev AE, Kurman RJ. Refined diagnostic criteria for implants associated with ovarian atypical proliferative serous tumors (borderline) and micropapillary serous carcinomas. Am J Surg Pathol. 2001;25(4):419–32.
46. Eichhorn JH, Bell DA, Young RH, Scully RE. Ovarian serous borderline tumors with micropapillary and cribriform patterns: a study of 40 cases and comparison with 44 cases without these patterns. Am J Surg Pathol. 1999;23(4):397–409.
47. Bell DA. Low-grade serous tumors of ovary. Int J Gynecol Pathol. 2014;33(4):348–56.
48. Board WCoTE. Female genital tumours. Lyon: International Agency for Research on Cancer; 2020.
49. Liao XY, Xue WC, Shen DH, Ngan HY, Siu MK, Cheung AN. p63 expression in ovarian tumours: a marker for Brenner tumours but not transitional cell carcinomas. Histopathology. 2007;51(4):477–83.
50. Esheba GE, Longacre TA, Atkins KA, Higgins JP. Expression of the urothelial differentiation markers GATA3 and placental S100 (S100P) in female genital tract transitional cell proliferations. Am J Surg Pathol. 2009;33(3):347–53.
51. Cuatrecasas M, Catasus L, Palacios J, Prat J. Transitional cell tumors of the ovary: a comparative clinicopathologic, immunohistochemical, and molecular genetic analysis of Brenner tumors and transitional cell carcinomas. Am J Surg Pathol. 2009;33(4):556–67.
52. Kuhn E, Ayhan A, Shih Ie M, Seidman JD, Kurman RJ. The pathogenesis of atypical proliferative Brenner tumor: an immunohistochemical and molecular genetic analysis. Mod Pathol. 2014;27(2):231–7.
53. Hallgrìmsson J, Scully RE. Borderline and malignant Brenner tumours of the ovary. A report of 15 cases. Acta Pathol Microbiol Scand Suppl. 1972;233:56–66.

2 Fallopian Tube Lesions

2.1 Papillary Tubal Hyperplasia (PTH)

2.1.1 A 46-Year-Old Woman with SBT of the Left Ovary

2.1.1.1 Key Diagnostic Features

- A proliferative lesion of the fallopian tubes (Fig. 2.1).
- Small rounded clusters of tubal epithelial cells and small papillae either floating in the lumen or protruding from the tubal mucosa with or without associated psammoma bodies [1] (Figs. 2.2 and 2.3). The fallopian tube epithelium might have foci of tufting (Fig. 2.4).
- PTH might be associated with salpingitis.

2.1.1.2 Ancillary Studies

N/A.

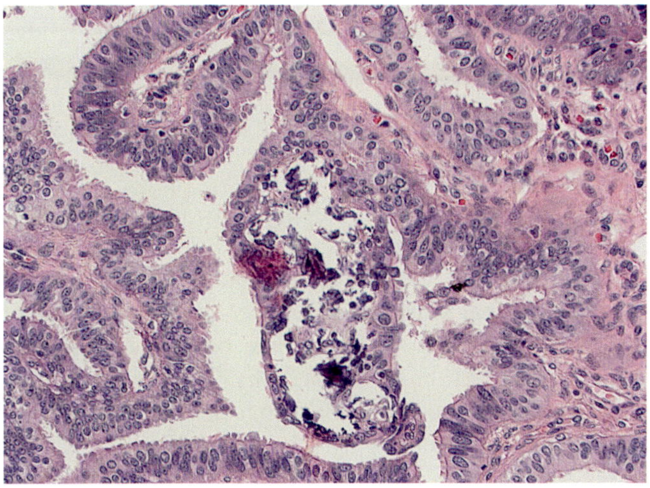

Fig. 2.2 The ciliated fallopian tube epithelium surrounds calcifications (200×)

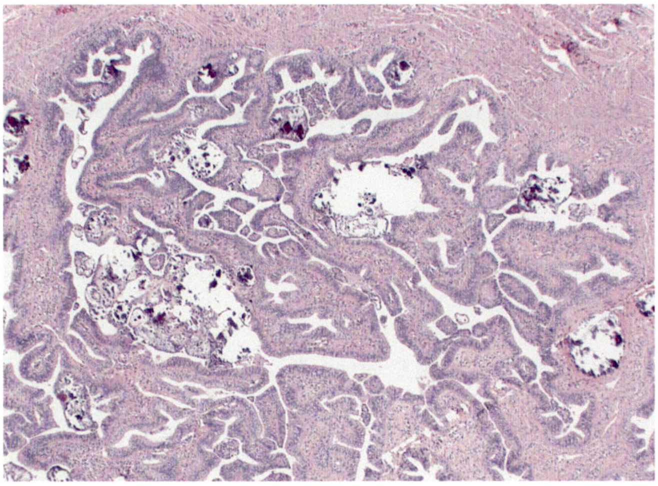

Fig. 2.1 The fallopian tube lumen has multiple loose papillary fragments and associated psammomatous calcifications. The complex fragments represent neoplastic tissue from ovarian SBT. Smaller ones are PTH lined by fallopian tube epithelium (40×)

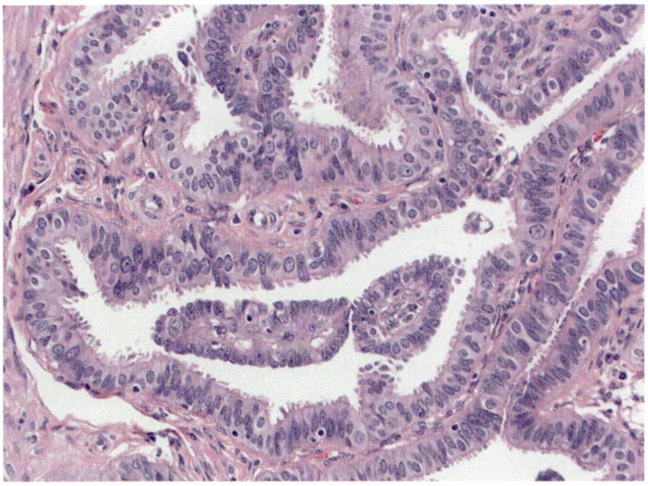

Fig. 2.3 Detached papillary fragments (PTH) within the lumen of the fallopian tube (200×)

O. Saglam, *Challenging Cases in Gynecologic Surgical Pathology*, https://doi.org/10.1007/978-3-031-51656-6_2

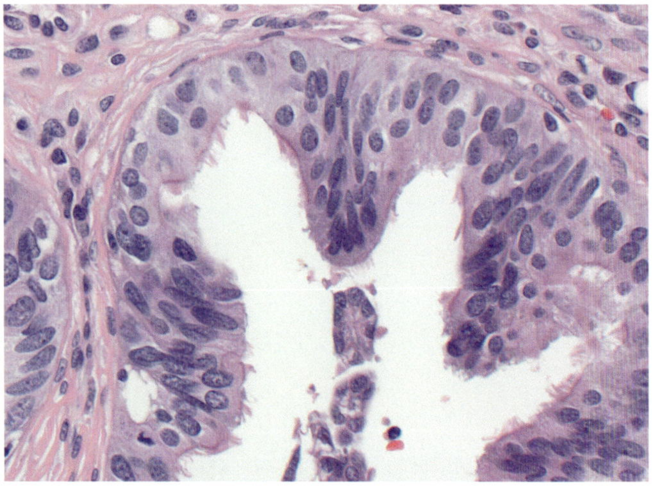

Fig. 2.4 Tufting of the epithelium (200×)

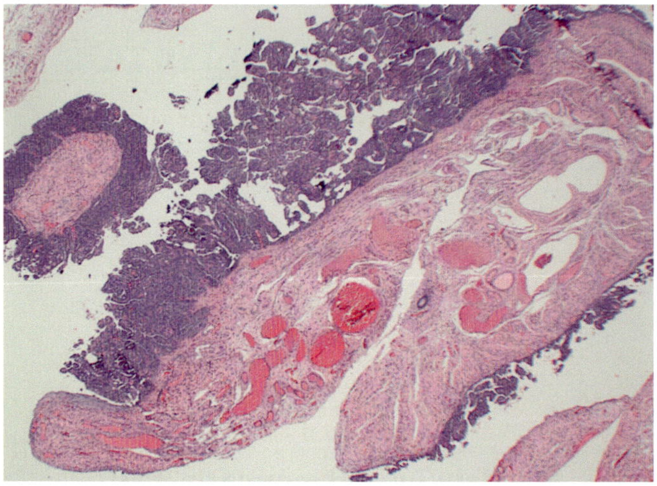

Fig. 2.5 The fimbriated end of the fallopian tube is involved by HGSC (40×)

2.1.1.3 Differential Diagnosis

- In the presence of SBT, they might be misinterpreted as noninvasive implants.

2.1.1.4 Clinical Significance

- The association of PTH with the borderline tumors of ovaries varies from 68 to 5% in the literature [2, 3]. PTH is proposed as a precursor lesion of SBT, noninvasive implants, and endosalpingiosis [1]. PTH with a gonadoblastoma is described in a patient with Ovotesticular Disorder of Sexual Development [4].

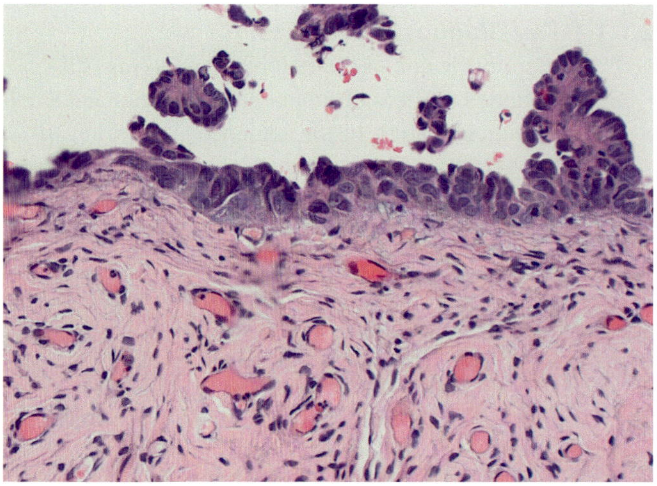

Fig. 2.6 The background STIC with morphological features of nuclear stratification, loss of polarity and cilia, marked nuclear enlargement, and prominent nucleoli (200×)

2.2 High-Grade Serous Carcinoma in the Background of Serous Tubal Intraepithelial Carcinoma (STIC)

2.2.1 A 56-Year-Old Woman with *BRCA* 1 Mutation

2.2.1.1 Key Diagnostic Features

- The morphological features are identical to those of ovarian high-grade serous carcinoma.
- There might be a dominant or mixture of papillary, solid, or endometrial-like architectural patterns (Fig. 2.5).
- STIC usually localizes at the tuboperitoneal junction [5] and supports the primary fallopian tube carcinoma diagnosis.
- STIC is characterized by a proliferation of nonciliated epithelium showing nuclear stratification, loss of polarity, marked nuclear pleomorphism, prominent nucleoli, and mitotic figures (Fig. 2.6).

2.2.1.2 Ancillary Studies

- Diffuse p53 expression (>75%) and high Ki67 labeling index [6].

2.2.1.3 Differential Diagnosis

- Non-gynecological and nontubal gynecological cancers can colonize in the fallopian tube mucosa and mimic STIC [7].
- In a study ten out of 100 metastatic non-gynecological cancers, including primary colon and breast adenocarcinomas, involved only the fimbriated end of the fallopian tube, and 29% of metastatic disease is localized in the tubal mucosa [8].

- Cervical and endometrial carcinomas can colonize the tubal mucosa and mimic a primary tubal carcinoma [7, 9].
- P53 and p16 expressions might overlap with STIC and metastatic carcinoma. PAX-8, WT-1, CK7, specific markers for a potential primary site, and HPV molecular studies for cervical cancer might be useful.

2.2.1.4 Clinical Significance

- HGSC of the fallopian tubes is staged and treated similarly to ovarian and peritoneal serous carcinomas.

2.3 Mucinous Metaplasia of Bilateral Fallopian Tubes in Peutz-Jeghers Syndrome (PJS)

2.3.1 A Patient with PJS Selected to Have Hysterectomy and Bilateral Salpingo-Oophorectomy

2.3.1.1 Key Diagnostic Features

- A field change/transition in the epithelium of the Mullerian type (fallopian tube epithelium) to the bland mucinous epithelium (Fig. 2.7) [10]. The lack of atypia and mitotic figures is supportive of a metaplastic process (Fig. 2.8). Clinical and imaging correlation is required, and a mass lesion is not associated with mucinous metaplasia.
- Gastric-type mucinous adenocarcinoma of the endocervix, ovarian sex cord tumor with annular tubules, oxyphilic Sertoli cell tumor [11], synchronous or metachronous mucinous neoplasia of the ovaries, fallopian tube, endometrium, and peritoneum may occur in the gynecological tract of patients with PJS (germline mutation of *STK11*) [12, 13].

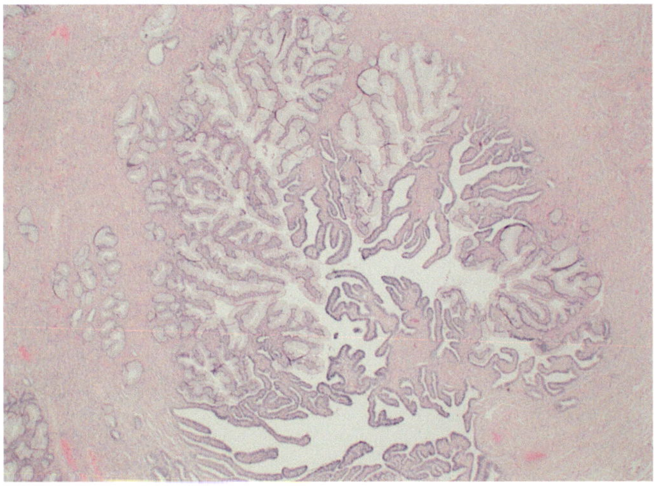

Fig. 2.7 Alternating bland pyloric-type mucinous epithelium and Mullerian-type/fallopian tube epithelium (40×)

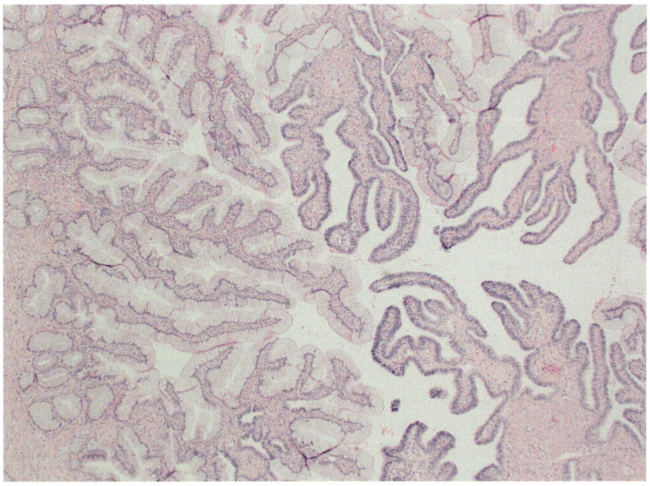

Fig. 2.8 A field change/transition from ciliated epithelium to mucinous epithelium, which has abundant pink cytoplasm and basally located bland nuclei. There is no cytological atypia or mitotic activity (100×)

- It might be challenging to exclude metastasis or direct extension of mucinous tumors from mucinous metaplasia.

2.3.1.2 Ancillary Studies

- HPV studies might be useful to rule out usual-type endocervical adenocarcinoma.
- P53 might be positive (mutation pattern) in gastric-type endocervical adenocarcinoma.
- Metastatic mucinous carcinomas from the gastrointestinal tract and pancreas usually have overlapping immunostaining profiles with the mucinous lesions of the gynecological tract.

2.3.1.3 Differential Diagnosis

- Metastatic carcinoma or direct extension of mucinous type endocervical adenocarcinoma
  - Features support metastatic disease or direct extension from mucinous-type endocervical adenocarcinoma: (1) short interval between cervical and ovarian tumors. (2) Similar histologic findings in cervical and ovarian tumors. (3) Deep invasion of cervical tumor. (4) Presence of lymphovascular invasion [10]. Features argue against metastatic carcinoma: (1) Absence of tumor emboli in lymphovascular spaces. (2) The early stage of invasive components. (3) The existence of intervening mucinous metaplasia in additional foci. (4) Uneventful clinical course [13].

2.3.1.4 Clinical Significance

- No treatment is required for benign mucinous metaplasia of fallopian tubes or ovaries. The finding should trigger a genetic consultation for PJS.

References

1. Kurman RJ, Vang R, Junge J, Hannibal CG, Kjaer SK, Shih Ie M. Papillary tubal hyperplasia: the putative precursor of ovarian atypical proliferative (borderline) serous tumors, noninvasive implants, and endosalpingiosis. Am J Surg Pathol. 2011;35(11):1605–14.
2. Robey SS, Silva EG. Epithelial hyperplasia of the fallopian tube. Its association with serous borderline tumors of the ovary. Int J Gynecol Pathol. 1989;8(3):214–20.
3. Horn LC, Angermann K, Hentschel B, Einenkel J, Höhn AK. Frequency of papillary tubal hyperplasia (PTH), salpingoliths and transition from adenoma to borderline ovarian tumors (BOT): a systematic analysis of 74 BOT with different histologic types. Pathol Res Pract. 2017;213(4):305–9.
4. Şimşek E, Binay Ç, Demiral M, Tokar B, Kabukçuoğlu S, Üstün M. Gonadoblastoma and papillary tubal hyperplasia in ovotesticular disorder of sexual development. J Clin Res Pediatr Endocrinol. 2016;8(3):351–5.
5. Seidman JD. Serous tubal intraepithelial carcinoma localizes to the tubal-peritoneal junction: a pivotal clue to the site of origin of extrauterine high-grade serous carcinoma (ovarian cancer). Int J Gynecol Pathol. 2015;34(2):112–20.
6. Sugimoto S, Uchiyama T, Kawahara N, Ohbayashi C, Kobayashi H. Immunohistochemical expression status of p53, CD44v9, and Ki-67 in a series of fallopian tube lesions of high-grade serous carcinoma. Int J Gynecol Pathol. 2021;40(5):419–26.
7. Singh R, Cho KR. Serous tubal intraepithelial carcinoma or not? Metastases to fallopian tube mucosa can masquerade as in situ lesions. Arch Pathol Lab Med. 2017;141(10):1313–5.
8. Rabban JT, Vohra P, Zaloudek CJ. Nongynecologic metastases to fallopian tube mucosa: a potential mimic of tubal high-grade serous carcinoma and benign tubal mucinous metaplasia or nonmucinous hyperplasia. Am J Surg Pathol. 2015;39(1):35–51.
9. Reyes C, Murali R, Park KJ. Secondary involvement of the adnexa and uterine corpus by carcinomas of the uterine cervix: a detailed morphologic description. Int J Gynecol Pathol. 2015;34(6):551–63.
10. Young RH, Scully RE. Mucinous ovarian tumors associated with mucinous adenocarcinomas of the cervix. A clinicopathological analysis of 16 cases. Int J Gynecol Pathol. 1988;7(2):99–111.
11. Ferry JA, Young RH, Engel G, Scully RE. Oxyphilic Sertoli cell tumor of the ovary: a report of three cases, two in patients with the Peutz-Jeghers syndrome. Int J Gynecol Pathol. 1994;13(3):259–66.
12. Anjarwalla S, Rollason TP, Rooney N, Hirschowitz L. Atypical mucinous metaplasia and intraepithelial neoplasia of the female genital tract—a case report and review of the literature. Int J Gynecol Cancer. 2007;17(5):1147–50.
13. Mikami Y, Kiyokawa T, Sasajima Y, Teramoto N, Wakasa T, Wakasa K, et al. Reappraisal of synchronous and multifocal mucinous lesions of the female genital tract: a close association with gastric metaplasia. Histopathology. 2009;54(2):184–91.

3 Sex Cord-Stromal Tumors of the Ovaries and Benign Mimickers

3.1 Cellular Fibroma (CF)

3.1.1 A 62-Year-Old Woman with a Large, Solid, and Cystic Pelvic Mass

3.1.1.1 Key Diagnostic Features

- Intensely but not uniformly hypercellular tumors (patchy hypercellular). Densely cellular areas merge with edematous hypocellular areas [1] (Figs. 3.1 and 3.2).
- Mitotic counts might be 4 or more per 10 high-power fields (AKA mitotically active cellular fibroma) [2] (Fig. 3.3).
- Fascicular arrangement of cytologically bland spindle cells might have scattered histiocytes and luteinized cells with abundant clear to eosinophilic cytoplasm between fascicules.
- The border between ovarian stroma and CF is usually irregular (Fig. 3.4). There might be adhesions to peritoneal surfaces or extraovarian tumor.

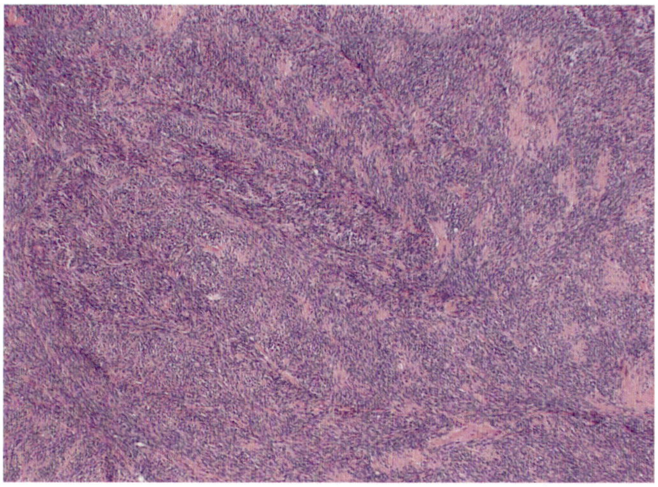

Fig. 3.1 Hypercellular areas separated by collagen fibers are composed of spindle cells in a fascicular pattern (40×)

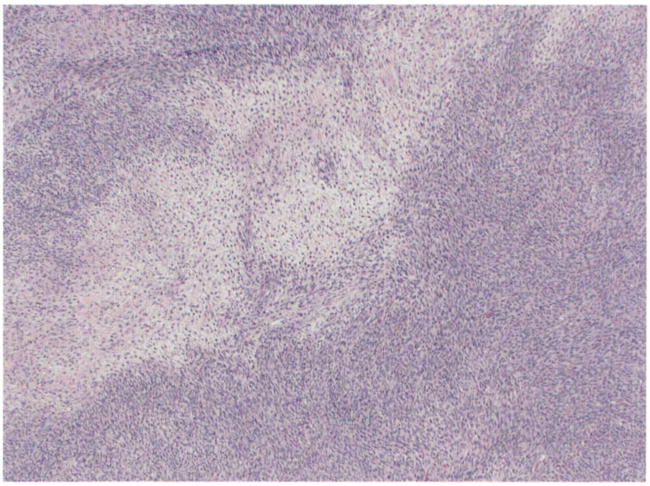

Fig. 3.2 Densely cellular areas are merging with hypocellular foci (40×)

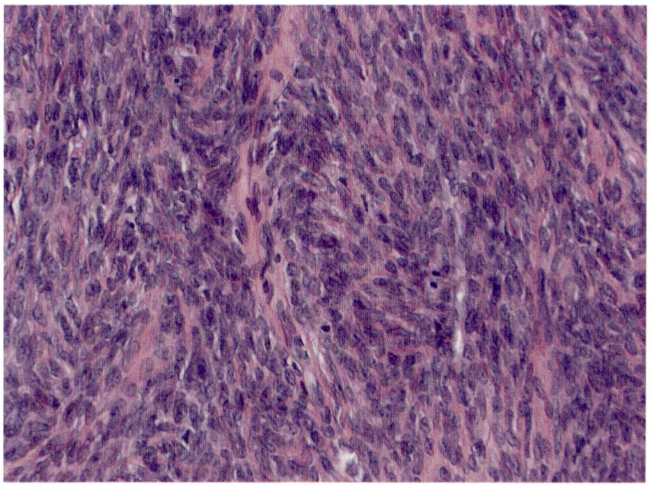

Fig. 3.3 The mitotic figures are 4 or more per 10 high-power fields in mitotically active CF (200×)

O. Saglam, *Challenging Cases in Gynecologic Surgical Pathology*, https://doi.org/10.1007/978-3-031-51656-6_3

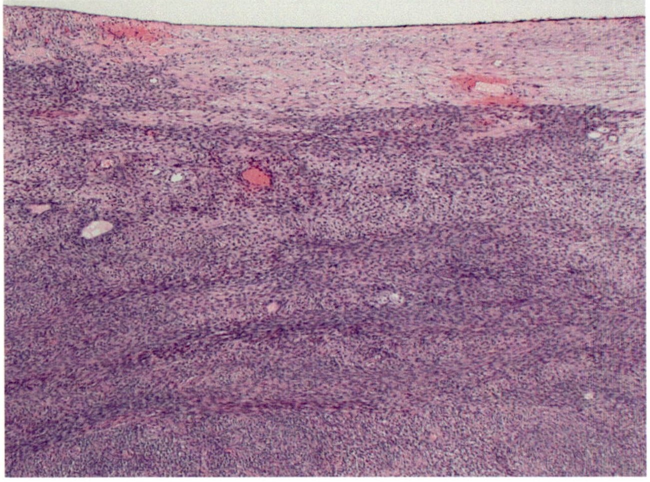

Fig. 3.4 The border of the lesion with the ovarian stroma is irregular (100×)

3.1.1.2 Ancillary Studies

- Inhibin and calretinin can be focal positive in ovarian fibromas [3].
- Reticulin wraps individual fibroblasts.

3.1.1.3 Differential Diagnosis

- Fibrosarcoma
  - Extremely rare in the ovaries
  - Uniformly cellular
  - Moderate to severe cytological atypia
  - High mitotic activity
- Adult granulosa cell tumors with fibromatous background (diffuse pattern)
  - Identification of granulosa cells (>10% of the lesion) supports the diagnosis.
  - See Part I, Sect. 3.5.
- Ovarian endometrial stromal sarcoma (ESS)
  - Associated with endometriosis in some cases.
  - The presence of typical neoplastic endometrial stromal cells and the characteristic network of numerous small arterioles support the ESS diagnosis [4].
  - CD10 is positive in low-grade ESS.
- Ovarian fibromatosis
  - Sparsely cellular with abundant intercellular collagen.
  - Follicular derivatives are surrounded by collagenous tissue. Their architecture is not disrupted by the surrounding proliferation [5].

3.1.1.4 Clinical Significance

- CF should be considered as a tumor with low malignant potential. Tumor size, presence or absence of capsular rupture, and pelvic adhesions dictate the prognosis [1].

3.2 Cystic Adult Granulosa Cell Tumor (AGCT)

3.2.1 A 52-Year-Old Woman with a Large Cystic Pelvic Mass

3.2.1.1 Key Diagnostic Features

- Cystic lesions with variable wall thickness (Fig. 3.5). The cyst wall might be focally denuded.
- Markedly thickened granulosa layer of the cyst wall (more than ten cell layers) usually has heterogeneous growth patterns, predominantly trabecular, corded (Fig. 3.6), or microfollicular (Fig. 3.7) patterns [6].

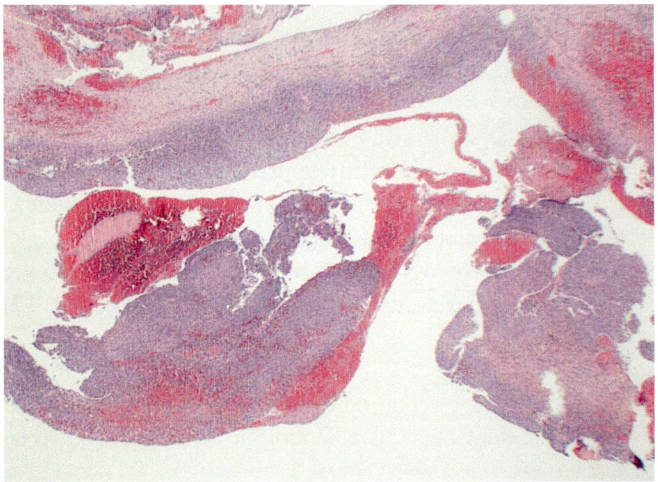

Fig. 3.5 Cystic ovarian lesion (40×)

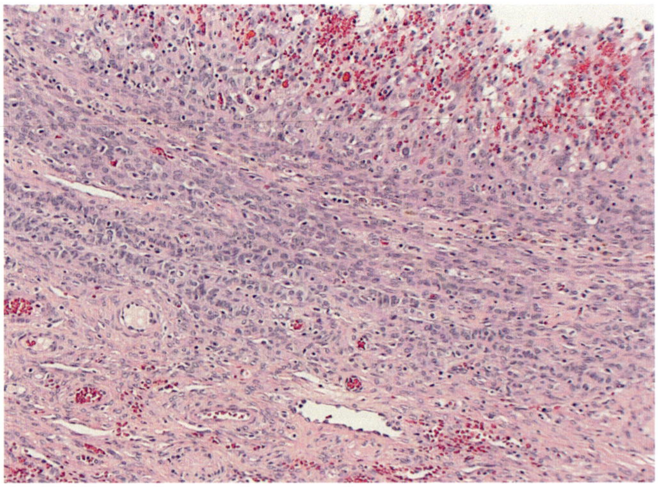

Fig. 3.6 The wall of the cyst exhibits granulosa cells growing in cords and trabeculae (200×)

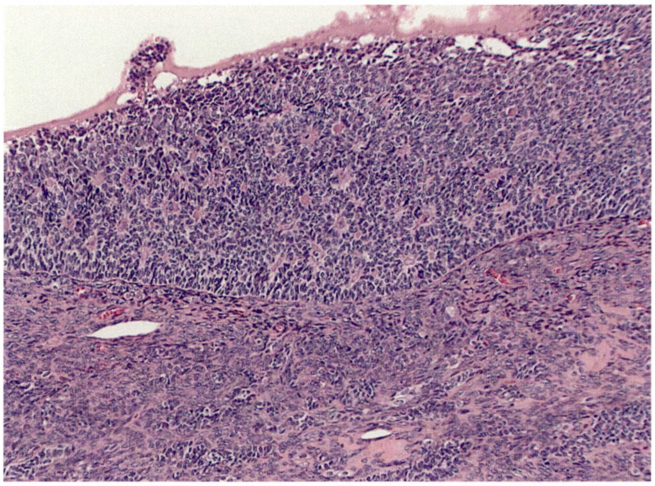

Fig. 3.7 This focus has Call-Exner bodies in the cyst wall (200×)

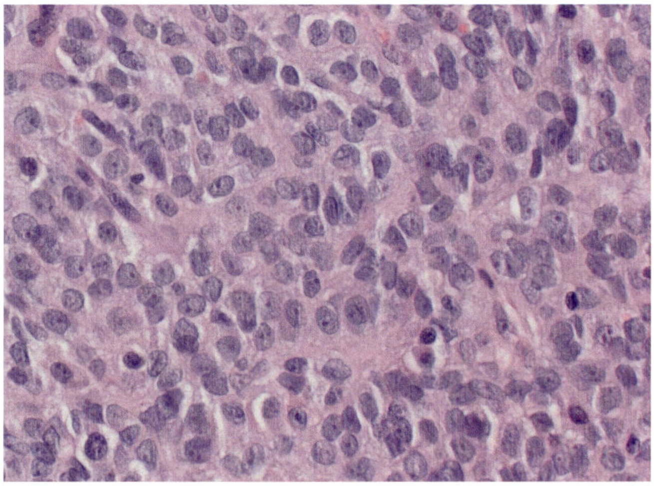

Fig. 3.8 The cyst wall is thick and made of more than ten layers of granulosa cells. The granulosa cells have pale nuclei and nuclear grooves (400×)

- Intracystic papillae, nodularity in the cyst wall, or invagination into the cyst wall might be present [7].
- Cytological features are typical of AGCT with pale nuclei and nuclear grooves (Fig. 3.8). The nuclear grooves may become inconspicuous in luteinized AGCT, and additional sampling may be necessary for the identification of nonluteinized granulosa cells.

3.2.1.2 Ancillary Studies

- Sex cord markers (inhibin calretinin, FOXL2, WT1 and CD56) are expressed in cystic AGCT.
- *FOXL2* sequencing may show a false-negative result in cystic AGCT because of the limited number of neoplastic cells in the sample.

3.2.1.3 Differential Diagnosis

- Large follicular cysts
  - The smaller size (<8 cm), thinner cell layers in the cyst wall, absence of architectural variability of AGCT, lack of typical cytological features (pale nuclei and nuclear grooves), lack of intracystic papillary projections, lack of Call-Exner bodies, and absence of *FOXL2* mutation are features that support the diagnosis [8].
- Unilocular juvenile granulosa cell tumor (JGCT)
  - Papillary structures protruding into the cyst lumen or confluent nodules in the cyst wall can also be present in JGCT.
  - Typical large follicles with basophilic secretions are usually present within the cystic JGCT.
  - Cytological features are the key to a correct diagnosis. The neoplastic cells have moderate to abundant cytoplasm and some with vacuolization. The nuclei are round and hyperchromatic without grooves in JGCT. The mitotic figures are abundant.

3.2.1.4 Clinical Significance

- Androgenic manifestations are associated with 25–52% of cystic AGCT [7, 9].

3.3 Sertoli Leydig Cell Tumor (SLCT) with Heterologous Elements

3.3.1 A 30-Year-Old Woman with Hirsutism

3.3.1.1 Key Diagnostic Features

- SLCT with moderate to poorly differentiated histological features (depending on the degree of tubular differentiation) (Figs. 3.9 and 3.10) might contain heterologous elements.
- They are frequently cystic in gross examination [10].
- Among the large case series with SLCT, the presence of heterologous elements varies from 5 to 22% [11, 12].
- Heterologous elements can be in the form of gastrointestinal-type epithelium (most common) (Figs. 3.11 and 3.12), carcinoid, skeletal muscle, cartilage (cellular and fetal type), and neuroblastoma [12, 13].
- The mucinous epithelium might be in the spectrum of benign to low-grade adenocarcinoma. Insular or mucinous-goblet cell carcinoids, usually of microscopic size, occasionally arise from the mucinous epithelium [1].

3.3.1.2 Ancillary Studies

- Inhibin, calretinin, cytokeratin, SF1, WT1, FOXL2: positive [14]
- *DICER1* mutant SLCT is more likely to have heterologous elements [15].

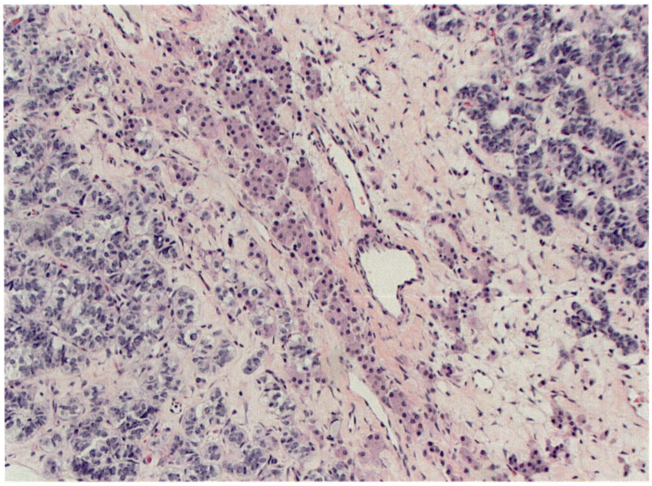

Fig. 3.9 SLCT, intermediate grade. The neoplastic cells with eosinophilic cytoplasm around the blood vessels are Leydig cells. The Sertoli cells form trabeculae and cords (100×)

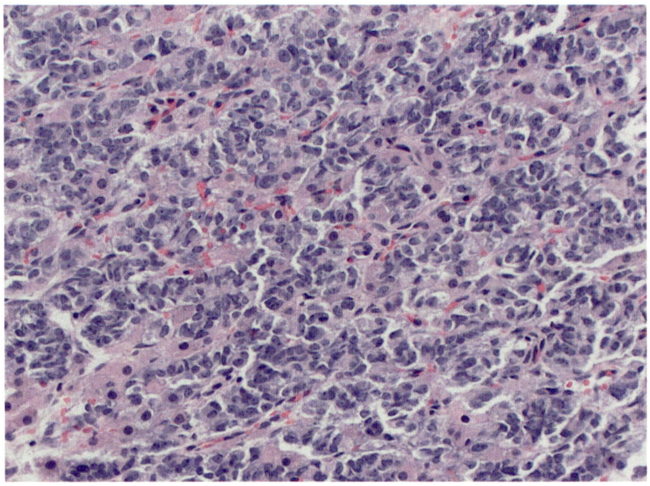

Fig. 3.10 In this field, Sertoli and Leydig cells are in close proximity (200×)

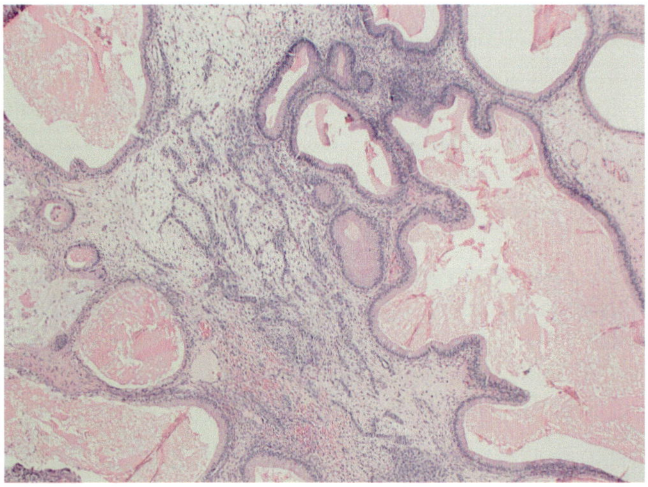

Fig. 3.11 Enteric type epithelium and Sertoli cells (40×)

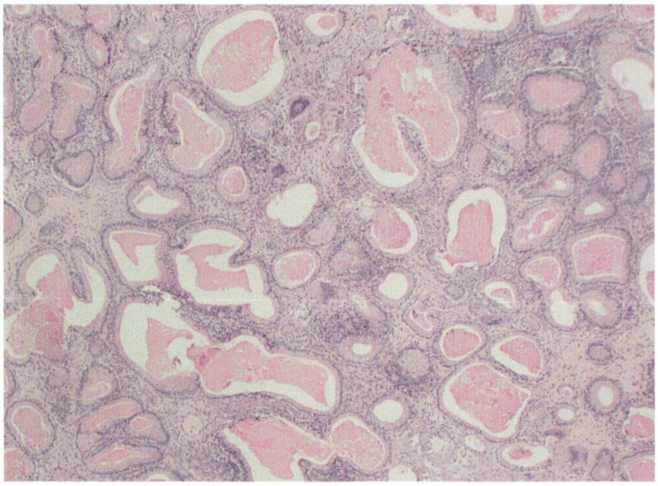

Fig. 3.12 Low-grade mucinous adenocarcinoma is the heterologous elements in an intermediate-grade SLCT (40×)

3.3.1.3 Differential Diagnosis

- Carcinosarcoma (CS) of the ovaries
  - SLCT typically occurs in young women (<30 years of age). CS is a disease of postmenopausal women. The epithelial and mesenchymal components of CS are almost always high-grade neoplasms.
- Mucinous cysts
  - A large heterologous mucinous component may mimic a mucinous cystadenoma. Sertoli and Leydig might not be sampled or overlooked.

3.3.1.4 Clinical Significance

- Heterologous elements are often associated with intermediate to poorly differentiated SLCT, and they are one of the poor prognostic features [12, 16].

3.4 Juvenile Granulosa Cell Tumor (JGCT)

3.4.1 A 17-Year-Old Girl with Abdominal Pain and Distension

3.4.1.1 Key Diagnostic Features

- The architectural patterns in JGCT are variable, including follicular (Fig. 3.13), nodular (Fig. 3.14), diffuse, reticular, and pseudopapillary (rare) patterns.
- Follicles contain basophilic or eosinophilic secretions (Fig. 3.15).
- The neoplastic cells have round, vesicular, hyperchromatic nuclei and abundant eosinophilic or pale cytoplasm (Fig. 3.16).
- The mitotic activity might be brisk with atypical forms [17].

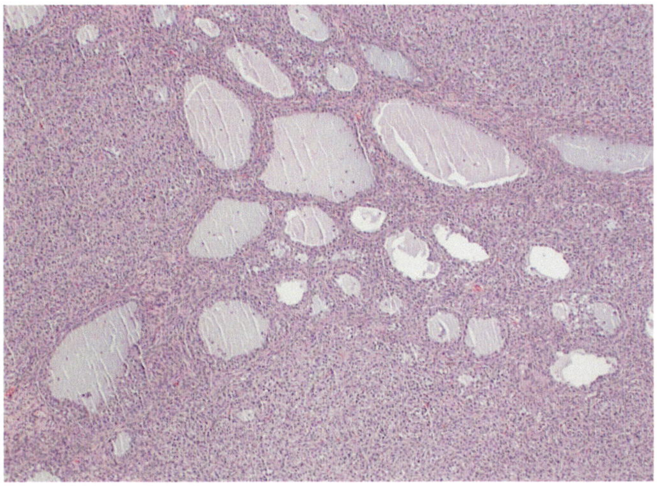

Fig. 3.13 Follicle formation in varying sizes is a typical pattern of JGCT. Mixed follicular and solid growth patterns in this field (40×)

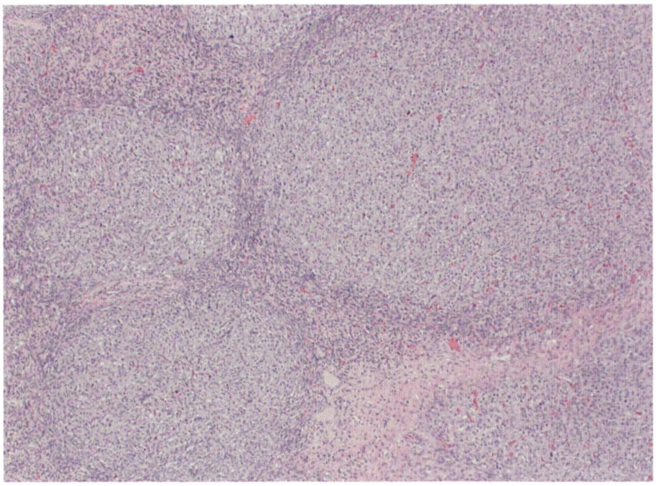

Fig. 3.14 Nodular pattern of JGCT (40×)

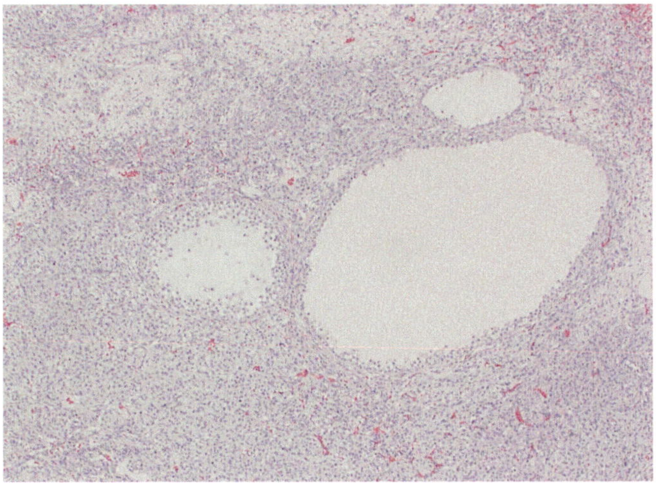

Fig. 3.15 Cystically dilated follicles contain basophilic secretions (100×)

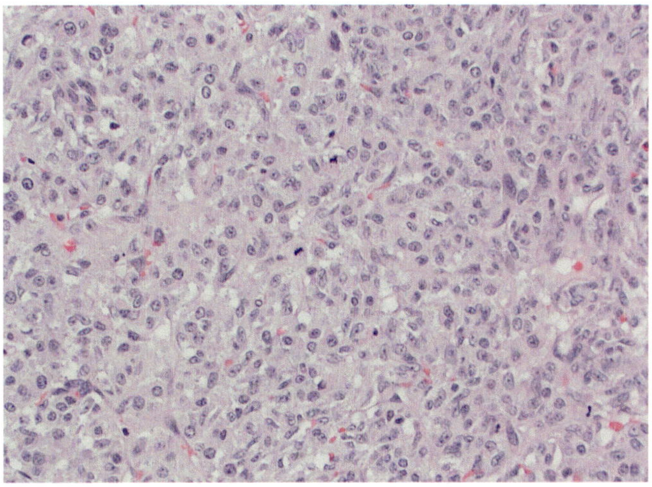

Fig. 3.16 The neoplastic cells contain abundant eosinophilic cytoplasm. Nuclei are vesicular with rare nuclear grooves. The mitotic activity is high (200×)

3.4.1.2 Ancillary Studies

- Inhibin, calretinin, FOXL2 [18]: Positive by immunohistochemistry. However, *FOXL2* somatic mutation is absent in JGCT [19].

3.4.1.3 Differential Diagnosis

- Yolk Sac Tumor (reticular pattern)
  - YST might be associated with other germ cell elements, such as mature or immature teratoma. The reticular pattern resembles a honeycombed structure of communicating spaces lined by primitive epithelial cells. The presence of Schiller–Duval bodies, syncytiotrophoblastic cells, positivite germ cell markers (SALL4, glypican 3), AFP, and negativite inhibin and calretinin support the diagnosis.
- Small cell carcinoma, hypercalcemic type (SCCHT) (follicular pattern)
  - SCCHT might have cells with abundant eosinophilic cytoplasm (large cell variant). The neoplastic cells in JGCT have uniformly eosinophilic, pale, or clear cytoplasm. JGCT has a theca cell component and is positive for sex cord markers (inhibin and calretinin).
  - See Part I, Sect. 5.1.
- Dysgerminoma (follicular pattern)
  - In poorly preserved specimens, artifactual spaces resemble follicles of JGCT [20]. Nests of large, uniform polygonal cells with clear or eosinophilic cytoplasm are separated by fibrous septae containing lymphocytic infiltrates in dysgerminoma.
  - Positive markers for dysgerminoma: OCT3/4, SALL4, CD117, and D2-40.

3.4.1.4 Clinical Significance

- Recurrences are early (in the first 3 years) and more common in cases with tumor rupture, positive peritoneal cytology, and extraovarian spread [17]. Ollier disease (enchondromatosis) and Maffucci syndrome (enchondromatosis and vascular lesions) are associated with JGCT [21].

3.5 Adult Granulosa Cell Tumor (AGCT) with Prominent Fibromatous Component (Diffuse Pattern)

3.5.1 A 70-Year-Old Woman with a 3-Month History of Abdominal Pain

3.5.1.1 Key Diagnostic Features

- AGCT with an extensive stromal component resembling cellular fibroma at low-power examination (Fig. 3.17).
- The granulosa cell groups in insular or follicular patterns are within the intersecting fascicles of spindle cells [22] (Fig. 3.18). These foci might be apparent after extensive sampling in some cases.
- The granulosa cells have pale vesicular nuclei, with or without grooves (Fig. 3.19).

3.5.1.2 Ancillary Studies

- Reticulin invests groups of granulosa cells (Fig. 3.20) and single fibroblasts.
- Inhibin (more specific) and calretinin are positive in granulosa cells [23].

3.5.1.3 Differential Diagnosis

- AGCT with sarcomatous transformation

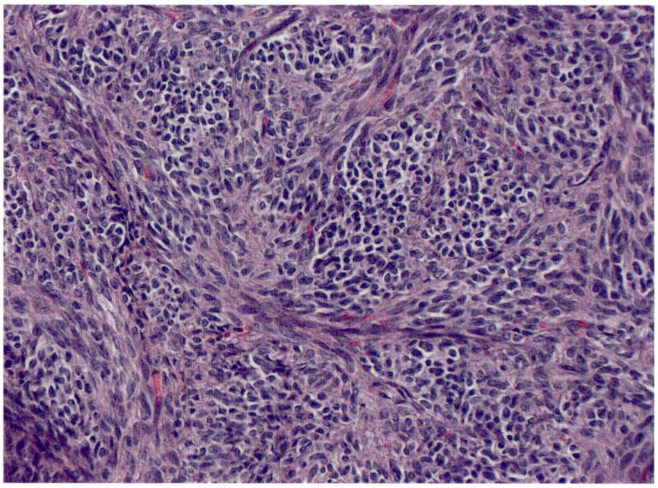

Fig. 3.18 Groups of granulosa cells in a nested pattern within the fibrous stroma (200×)

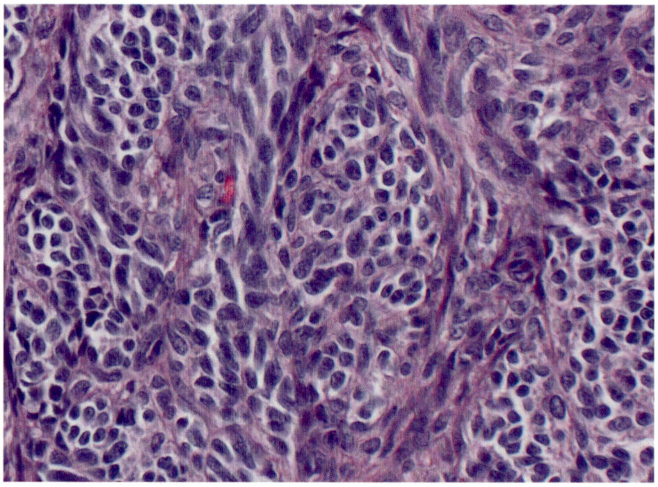

Fig. 3.19 The granulosa cells have typical pale nuclei and nuclear grooves (400×)

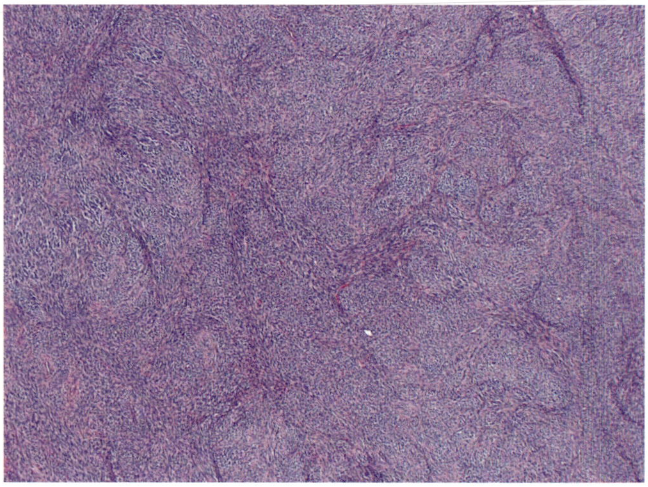

Fig. 3.17 AGCT with prominent fibromatous stroma (40×)

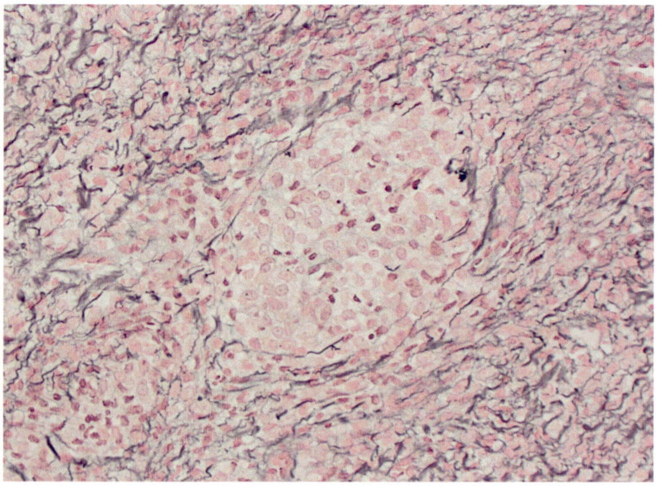

Fig. 3.20 Reticulin stain wraps around a group of granulosa cells (center) and individual fibroblasts (periphery) (200×)

- Focal areas of markedly pleomorphic cells (spindle and epithelioid), increased mitotic activity with atypical forms, sometimes resembling carcinoma, are present in a background of otherwise typical AGCT [24].

- Cellular fibroma
  - Fascicular arrangements of spindle cells with no or mild cytological atypia.
  - Mitotic rate up to 4 per 10 high-power fields.
  - See Part I, Sect. 3.1.

3.5.1.4 Clinical Significance

- Early stage (stage I) AGCT has an excellent prognosis. The recurrence rate is higher in long-term follow-up, with a rate of 20–30% for all stages [25, 26].

3.6 Luteinized Adult Granulosa Cell Tumor

3.6.1 A 50-Year-Old Woman with Postmenopausal Bleeding

3.6.1.1 Key Diagnostic Features

- Diffuse growth of granulosa cells with abundant eosinophilic or clear cytoplasm [27]
- The dominant pattern is large nodules separated by thin fibrous septa (Fig. 3.21). Ords or ribbons of cells are other architectural patterns (Fig. 3.22).
- Cytological features include central round, pale nuclei with prominent nucleoli and occasional grooves (Fig. 3.23).
- Varying amounts of unluteinized component display characteristic nuclear features (scant cytoplasm, pale nuclei, and prominent nuclear grooves).

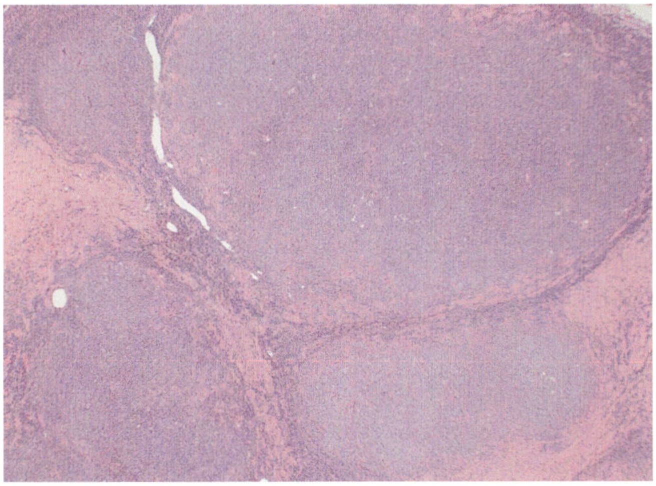

Fig. 3.21 Collagenous septa separate the large nodules (20×)

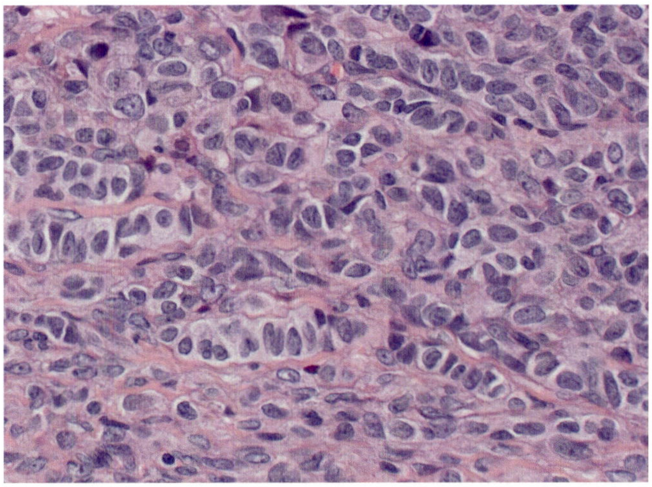

Fig. 3.22 The neoplastic cells form cords and trabeculae (100×)

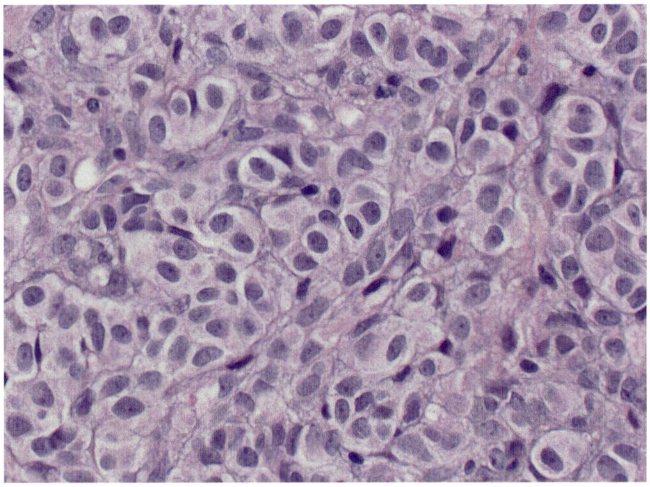

Fig. 3.23 The neoplastic cells have abundant clear to pinkish cytoplasm. Nucleoli are prominent. Nuclear grooves are scant (200×)

3.6.1.2 Ancillary Studies

- Positive immunostains: Sex cord markers (Inhibin, calretinin, and WT-1)
- Negative immunostains: Melan A and EMA

3.6.1.3 Differential Diagnosis

- Juvenile granulosa cell tumor
  - Mixed solid and follicular growth pattern.
  - Nuclei are hyperchromatic.
  - High mitotic rate.
  - See Part I, Sect. 3.4.
- Fibroma with luteinized cells
  - Focal finding (luteinized cells make less than 10% of the lesion).
  - The neoplastic cells lack pale nuclei.
  - Reticulin wraps single cells (fibroblasts).

- Steroid cell tumors
  - Lack of characteristic architectural patterns of AGCT.
  - Scattered cells with spongy (vacuolated) cytoplasm.
  - Positive for Melan A.
  - See Part I, Sect. 3.9.
- Metastatic malignant melanoma
  - Correlation with clinical history is supportive of the diagnosis.
  - Malignant melanomas can express inhibin [28] in addition to melanocytic markers (S-100, Melan A, HMB-45).

3.6.1.4 Clinical Significance

- Luteinized AGCT can present as a functioning tumor like other morphological patterns of AGCT. There might be associated endometrial hyperplasia or well-differentiated endometrial adenocarcinoma [29].

3.7 Stromal Hyperplasia and Hyperthecosis (SHHT)

3.7.1 A 49-Year-Old Woman with Bilateral Ovarian Enlargement by Imaging Studies

3.7.1.1 Key Diagnostic Features

- Bilateral diffuse proliferation of monotonous stromal spindle cells of the ovaries (stromal hyperplasia) and scattered luteinized cells either as single cells or in groups (hyperthecosis) (Fig. 3.24).
- Luteinized cell groups do not form gross mass lesions (<1 cm) (Figs. 3.25 and 3.26).
- The stromal proliferation incorporates normal ovarian structures.

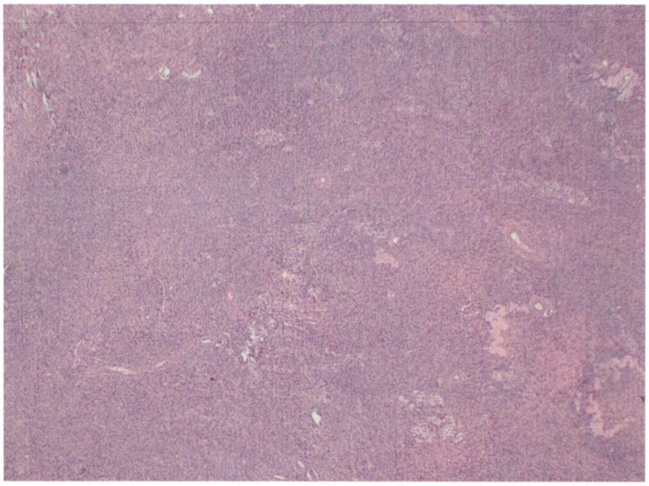

Fig. 3.24 Diffuse proliferation of bland stromal cells (20×)

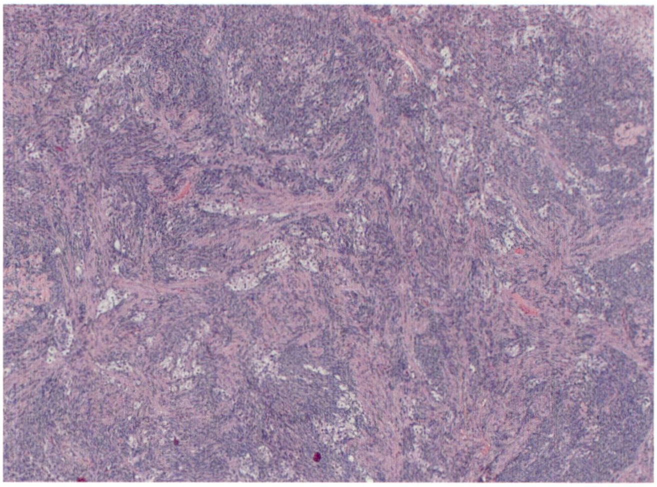

Fig. 3.25 Hypercellular areas are intercepted by groups of luteinized cells (40×)

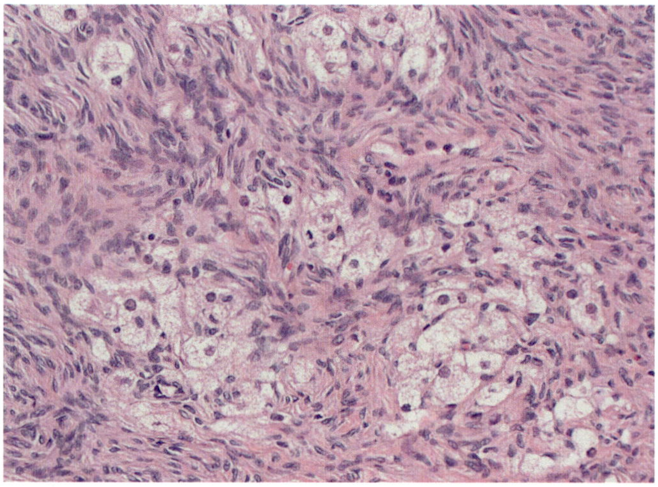

Fig. 3.26 Luteinized stromal cells with foamy cytoplasm and small round nuclei (200×)

- The luteinized cells can be functional and associated with endocrine manifestations, endometrial hyperplasia, and endometrial carcinoma [30–32].

3.7.1.2 Ancillary Studies

- Luteinized stromal cells express inhibin and calretinin.

3.7.1.3 Differential Diagnosis

- Fibroma
  - Usually, unilateral lesions with a distinct mass formation.
  - Intersecting fascicules of bland spindle cells.
  - Hyalinization and calcifications are associated with fibroma.
  - Rare tumors might have minor sex cord elements (<10% of the lesion) or melanin pigment.

3.7.1.4 Clinical Significance

- SHHT is a non-neoplastic cause of ovarian hyperandrogenism with unknown etiology. Polycystic ovarian disease and SHHT can be a component of Hyperandrogenism, Insulin Resistance, and Acanthosis Nigricans syndrome (HAIR-AN syndrome) [33].

3.8 Leydig Cell Tumor (LCT)

3.8.1 A 54-Year-Old Woman Underwent a Hysterectomy for Pelvic Prolapse. Samples from an Incidental Ovarian Mass (1.6 cm) Lesion

3.8.1.1 Key Diagnostic Features

- Predominantly located in the ovarian hilum.
- Well-circumscribed nodule composed of large cells with abundant eosinophilic cytoplasm (Fig. 3.27).
- Lipochrome pigment is a common finding (Fig. 3.28).
- Rod-shaped eosinophilic Reinke crystals are diagnostic of LCT (Fig. 3.29).
- Clustering of nuclei forms "nuclear free" zones (Fig. 3.30).
- Fibrinoid changes in the vessels are frequently present.
- Bilateral involvement of the ovaries and association with cystadenomas are reported [34, 35].

3.8.1.2 Ancillary Studies

- Inhibin, calretinin, and Melan A are positive in LCT [36–38].

3.8.1.3 Differential Diagnosis

- Hilar cell hyperplasia
  - Microscopic lesions (<5 mm)

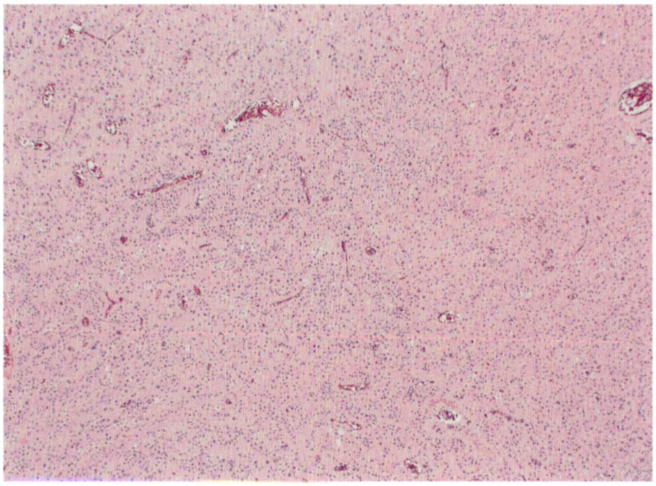

Fig. 3.27 Diffuse proliferation of eosinophilic cells within the ovarian hilum (40×)

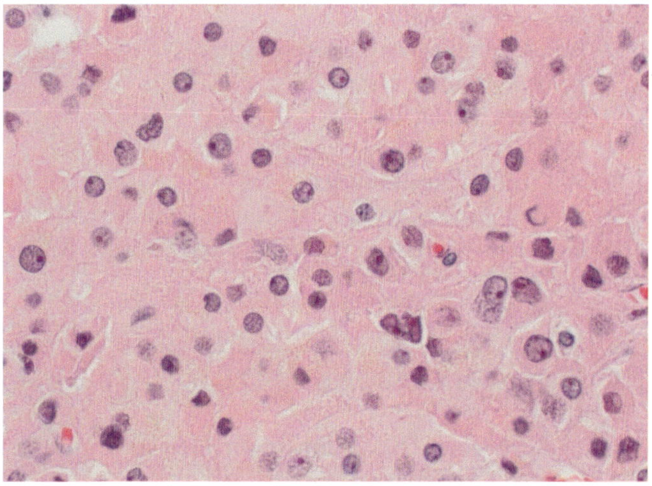

Fig. 3.28 The neoplastic cells have yellow lipochrome pigment (200×)

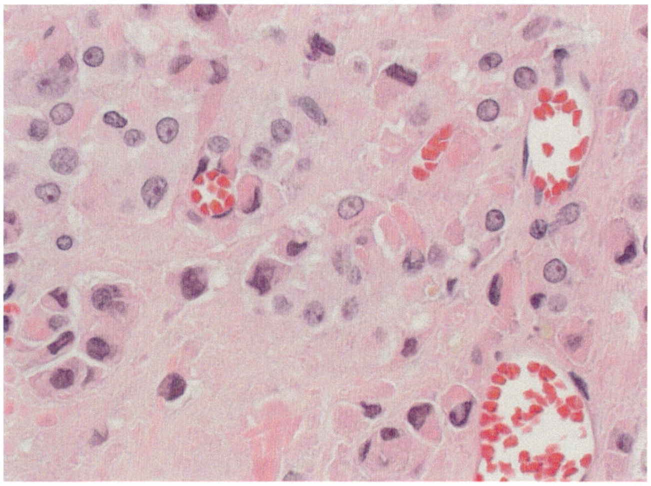

Fig. 3.29 Multiple eosinophilic rod-shaped Reinke crystals are in this field (200×)

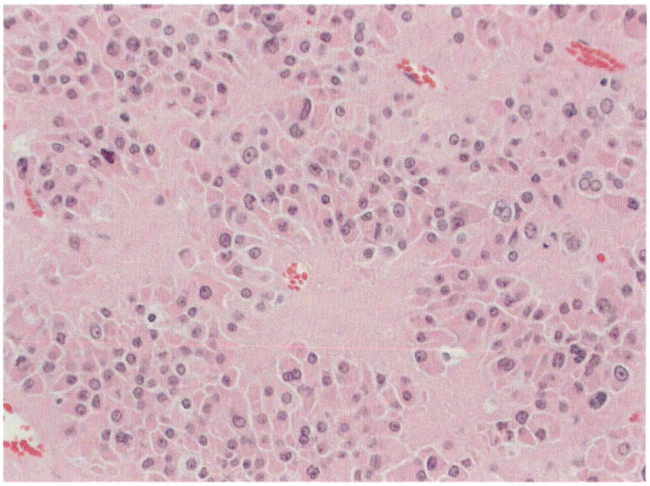

Fig. 3.30 Nuclei cluster together and leave nuclear-free zones (200×)

- Steroid cell tumors
  - Located in the ovarian parenchyma.
  - Lack of Reinke crystals.
  - See Part I, Sect. 3.9.

3.8.1.4 Clinical Significance

- The initial manifestation is androgenic in more than 60% of the cases. The clinical course is almost always benign [39].

3.9 Steroid Cell Tumor (SCT)

3.9.1 A 50-Year-Old Woman with Hirsutism and Clitoromegaly

3.9.1.1 Key Diagnostic Features

- The architectural patterns include diffuse/expansile, nested (Fig. 3.31), pseudoglandular (Fig. 3.32), and trabecular (Fig. 3.33) structures.
- The neoplastic cells are polygonal with well-defined borders and an abundant eosinophilic or clear (vacuolated) cytoplasm (Fig. 3.34). Nuclei are round and centrally located with prominent nucleoli. Similar to other endocrine tumors, scattered atypical cells are often present. Significant cytological atypia and necrosis are rare findings.
- The stroma might be scant or fibromatous. In rare case reports, they present as mixed tumors, i.e., fibroma and steroid cell tumors [40].

3.9.1.2 Ancillary Studies

- Positive staining by inhibin, calretinin Melan A, HMB45, and AR [36, 41]. FOXL2 expression is rare (1 out of 11 SCT) [18].

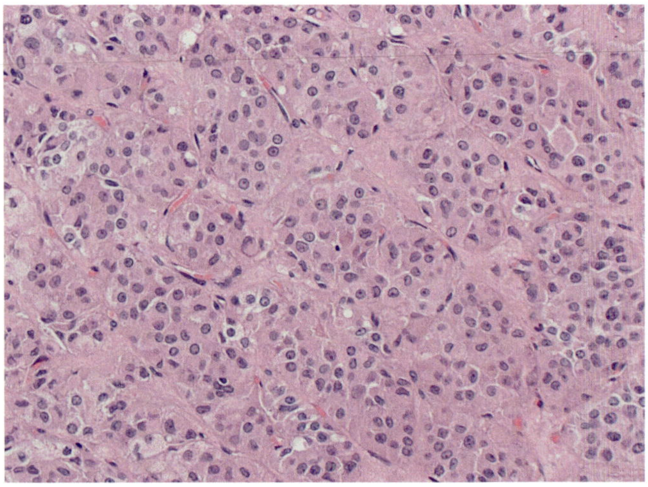

Fig. 3.31 SCT with nested pattern. The cells have abundant eosinophilic cytoplasm and centrally located nuclei with prominent nucleoli (100×)

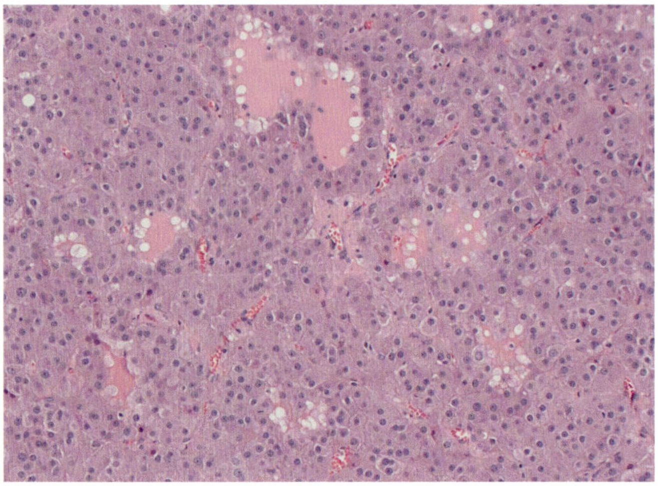

Fig. 3.32 Areas with pseudoglandular architecture (100×)

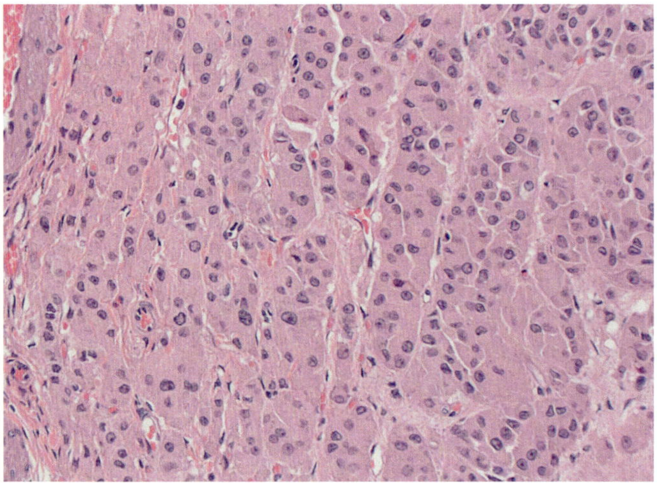

Fig. 3.33 Trabecular pattern (100×)

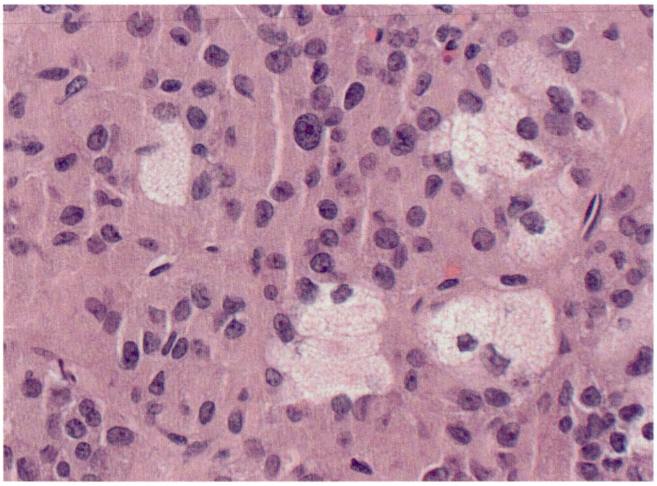

Fig. 3.34 Scattered cells with foamy cytoplasm and variable nuclear atypia (200×)

3.9.1.3 Differential Diagnosis

- Leydig cell tumor (LCT)
  - The presence of Reinke crystals in the cytoplasm is diagnostic for LCT.
  - See Part I, Sect. 3.8.
- Fibroma with luteinized cells
  - Predominantly spindle cell proliferation arranged in a fascicular pattern with a minor component of luteinized cells (<10% of the lesion) [20].
  - Nests of pale and luteinized cells in a background of fibromatous stroma might be associated with androgenic clinical symptoms [42].
- Pregnancy luteoma
  - Multiple lesions in half of the cases and bilateral in one-third [43].
  - Well-circumscribed nodules, which might contain follicle-like spaces.
  - Cells contain little or no lipids. The cytoplasm is abundant, and nuclei are central with prominent nucleoli.
  - After delivery, luteoma degenerates and leaves scar tissue within the ovarian parenchyma.
- Clear cell carcinoma (CCC), oncocytic type
  - A CCC is rarely composed of cells with predominantly eosinophilic cytoplasm. Typical architectural and cytological features are present with adequate sampling in almost all cases
- Metastatic Renal Cell Carcinoma (RCC)
  - Neoplastic cells lack endocrine atypia. Clinical correlation is useful for appropriate work-up of histological RCC subtypes.
  - AMACR, vimentin, CD10, and RCC (variable): positive in oncocytic RCC.

3.9.1.4 Clinical Significance

- SCT is a functional tumor and can produce androgens, ACTH, and rarely estrogens. The clinical behavior is uncertain, and some morphological features, including tumor size (>7 cm), presence of necrosis and hemorrhage, high mitotic activity (2 or more per 10 high-power field), and significant cytological atypia, are associated with malignant behavior [43].

3.10 Microcytic Stromal Tumor (MST)

3.10.1 A 59-Year-Old Woman with a 10 cm Right Ovarian Mass

3.10.1.1 Key Diagnostic Features

- In a typical tumor, there is a lobular arrangement of solid cellular foci, hyalinized fibrous stroma, and microcysts (Fig. 3.35) [44].
- Microcysts are characterized by small round to oval cystic areas and may coalesce to form larger spaces (Fig. 3.36).
- Cytological features are variable from monotonous (Fig. 3.37) to focal, highly atypical cells with multiple nuclei (Fig. 3.38). Intracytoplasmic vacuoles are frequently present and may result in a signet-ring cell morphology.
- Unusual morphological features are nested, tubular, and corded arrangements and spindle cell elements [45].

3.10.1.2 Ancillary Studies

- Positive immunostains: CD10, FOXL2, WT-1, SF-1, beta-catenin (nuclear and cytoplasmic), Cyclin D1 [46]
- Negative immunostains: EMA, inhibin, calretinin, ER, and PR

3.10.1.3 Differential Diagnosis

- Sex cord-stromal tumors with eosinophilic cytoplasm (steroid cell tumor, sclerosing stromal tumor, juvenile granulosa cell tumor, and luteinized adult granulosa cell tumor)

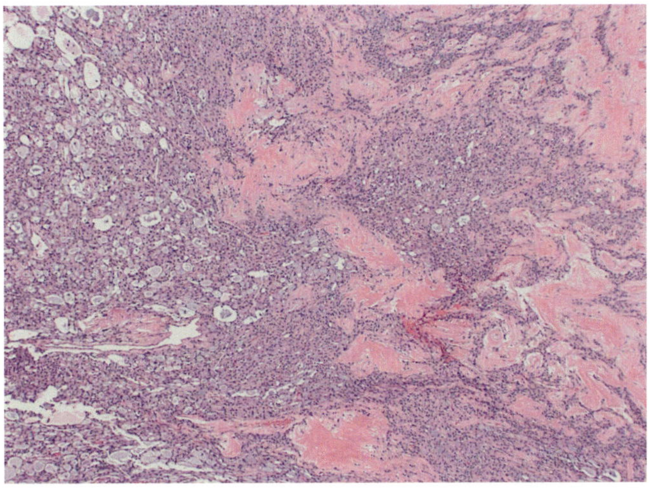

Fig. 3.35 The lesion has three components: (1) Hyalinized stroma. (2) Solid cellular areas. (3) Microcysts (40×)

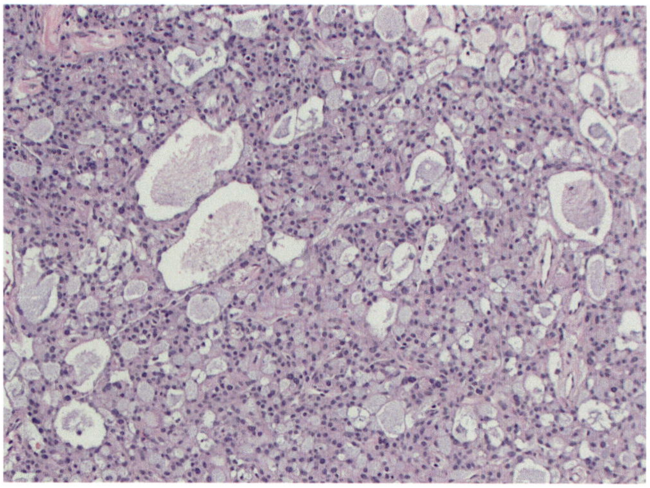

Fig. 3.36 Epithelioid cells forming small cystic spaces in variable sizes (100×)

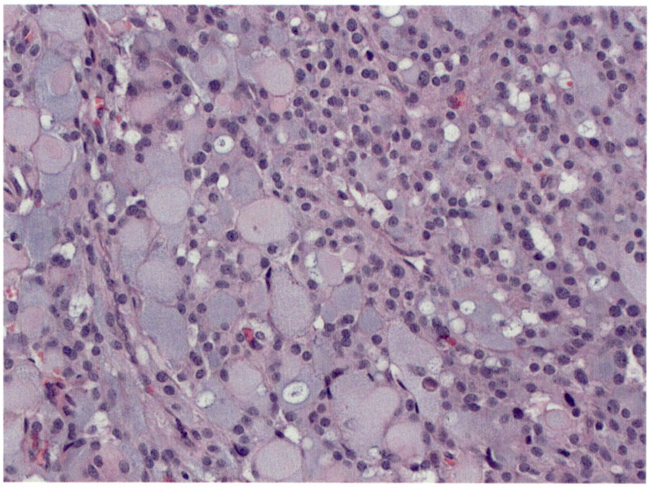

Fig. 3.37 The neoplastic cells are monotonous. Cystic areas merged with solid cellular component (100×)

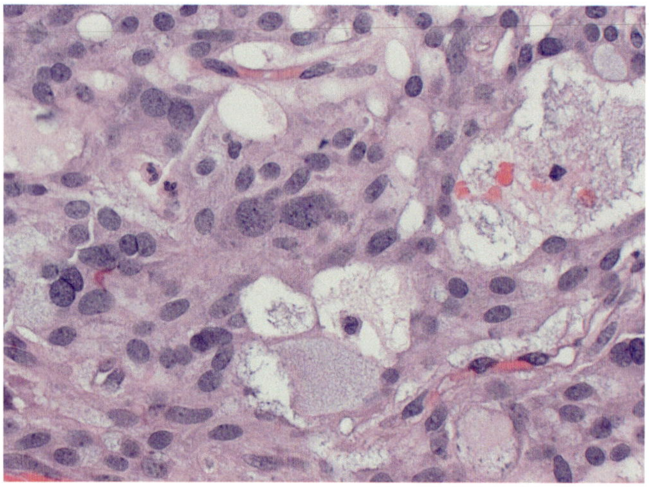

Fig. 3.38 In some foci, cytological atypia and binucleation of neoplastic cells might be present (200×)

  - Foci of typical cytological features are confirmatory of diagnosis
  - All sex cord-stromal tumors express at least focally inhibin and calretinin
- Yolk sac tumor (reticular pattern)
  - The reticular pattern is a meshwork of anastomosing spaces forming cysts in variable sizes.
  - Multiple morphological patterns are usually present with adequate sampling in YST.
  - Schiller-Duval bodies (large central vessels lined by tumor cells forming papillary structures) might be present.
  - Positive staining with germ markers (SALL4 and glypican-3) and AFP.
- Solid pseudopapillary tumor of the ovary (SPT)
  - Resembles pancreatic counterpart.
  - Distinctive pseudopapillary architecture due to dyscohesion of neoplastic cells.
  - SPT of the ovary also harbors *CTNNB1* mutations and expresses nuclear beta-catenin by immunohistochemistry [47].
  - Positive for CD10, Alpha-1 antitrypsin, PR, and WT1 (variable) immunostains [48].

3.10.1.4 Clinical Significance

- MST may be an extracolonic manifestation of familial adenomatous polyposis (FAP) syndrome, especially in bilateral ovarian involvements [49–51]. Endometrioid tubal intraepithelial neoplasia is associated with MST of the ovary [51]. *CTNNB1* (β-catenin) and *APC* genemutations are identified in most MST samples [52–54]. The latter finding indicates that the Wnt/β-catenin pathway plays a crucial role in the tumorigenesis of MST. *CTNNB1* and *APC* gene mutations are mutually exclusive [50]

3.11 Gynandroblastoma

3.11.1 A 22-Year-Old Nulliparous Woman with a History of Menstrual Irregularities

3.11.1.1 Key Diagnostic Features

- Rare sex cord-stromal tumor with elements of female and male differentiation.
- The diagnosis of gynandroblastoma should be reserved only for samples that contain a substantial amount of easily recognizable ovarian and testicular elements [55] (Fig. 3.39).
- The most common combination is Sertoli-Leydig cell tumor (SLCT) (Fig. 3.40) and juvenile granulosa cell tumor (JGSC) [1].

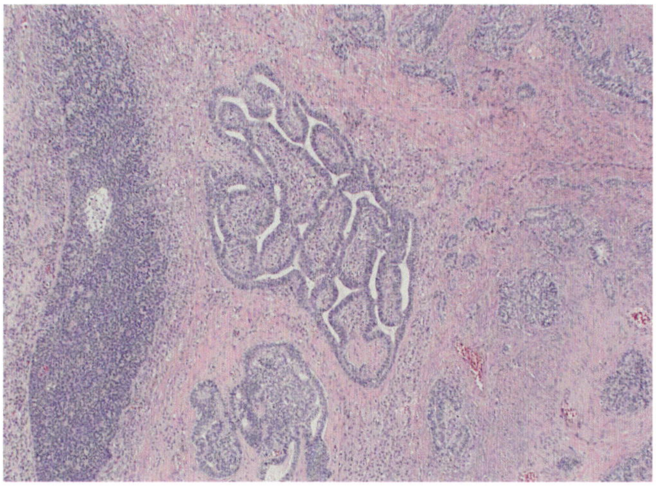

Fig. 3.39 Sex cord-stromal tumor with SLCT (right) and AGCT (left) components. The first component is predominant in this field (40×)

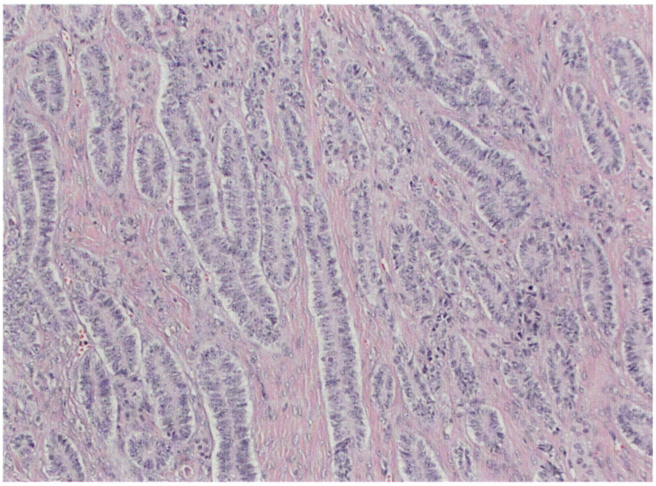

Fig. 3.40 The tubules of intermediate-grade SLCT (100×)

3.11.1.2 Ancillary Studies

- Sex cord markers such as inhibin, calretinin, and FOXL2 are positive in both components, and EMA is negative [56, 57].
- Gynandroblastoma containing components of SLCT and JGCT but not gynandroblastoma containing AGCT (Figs. 3.41 and 3.42) harbors *DICER1* hot-spot mutation [57].

3.11.1.3 Differential Diagnosis

- Depends on the morphologic components of the tumor.
- See Part I, Sects. 3.2, 3.3, 3.4, 3.5, and 3.6 (sex cord-stromal tumors).

3.11.1.4 Clinical Significance

- Ovarian gynandroblastomas have the potential to metastasize, and they are tumors of low malignant potential [56].

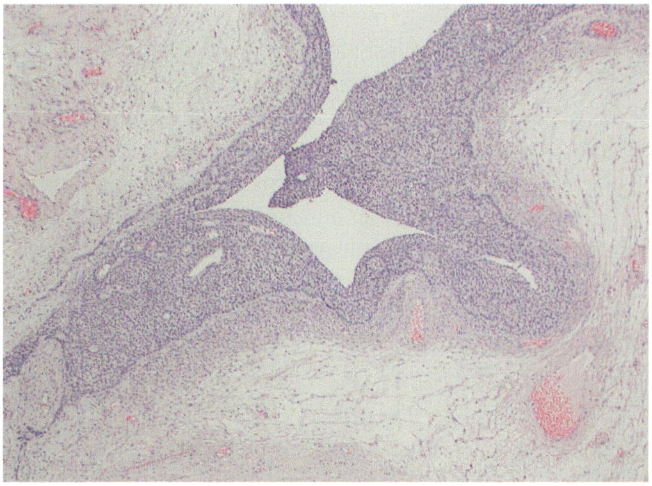

Fig. 3.41 AGCT with macrocystic pattern (100×)

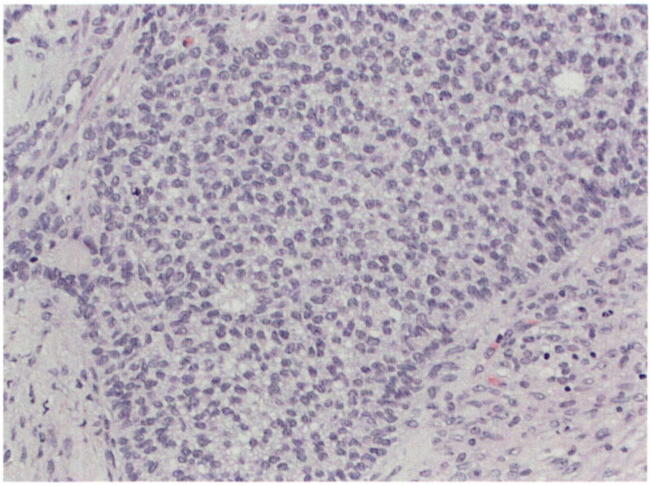

Fig. 3.42 Granulosa cells are forming acini-like structures (Call-Exner bodies). Nuclei are pale, and some have grooves (200×)

3.12 Sertoli-Leydig Cell Tumor with Retiform Pattern

3.12.1 A 5-Year-Old Girl with a Mother, Who is a Carrier of *DICER 1* Mutation

3.12.1.1 Key Diagnostic Features

- A network of elongated branching tubules resembling rete testis (Fig. 3.43).
- The lumens of tubules are usually narrow (slit-like spaces) or might be focally dilated with eosinophilic secretion mimicking thyroid follicles.
- Tubules are lined by cuboidal epithelium with scant cytoplasm (Fig. 3.44). The mitotic activity is low. The tumor cells might have hobnail-like nuclei in some areas.

- Either short, blunt, or branching papillae are present within the lumen (Figs. 3.45, 3.46, and 3.47).
- Gonadal stroma (immature mesenchymal component) (Fig. 3.48) is present as variably sized cellular nodules and frequently separated by hypocellular areas [58]. Stromal hyalinization and hyaline globules are nonspecific findings. Typical architectural patterns of SLCT can also be present in variable percentages (Fig. 3.49).
- The retiform component of an SLCT might be small or diffuse. The histological grade is intermediate or poorly differentiated [59].

3.12.1.2 Ancillary Studies

- Sex cord markers (inhibin, calretinin (Fig. 3.50), WT1 (Fig. 3.51), and CD56) and cytokeratin: positive.
- EMA: generally negative. In rare samples, the retiform component might be EMA positive (1 out of 19 cases) of SLCT [58].

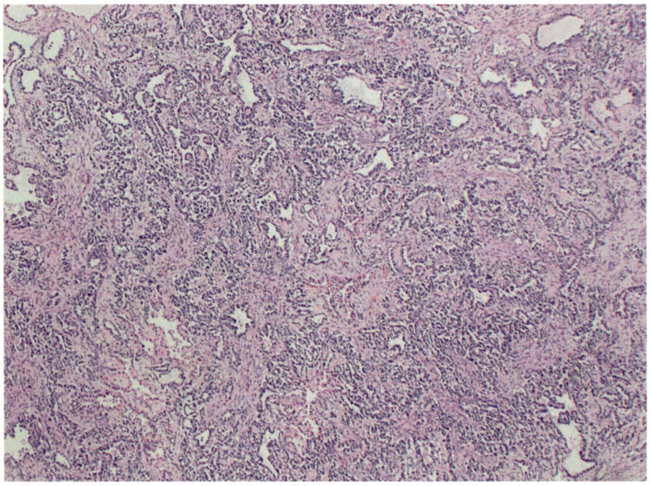

Fig. 3.43 A network of branching tubules with an admixture of slit-like lumens and dilated spaces (40×)

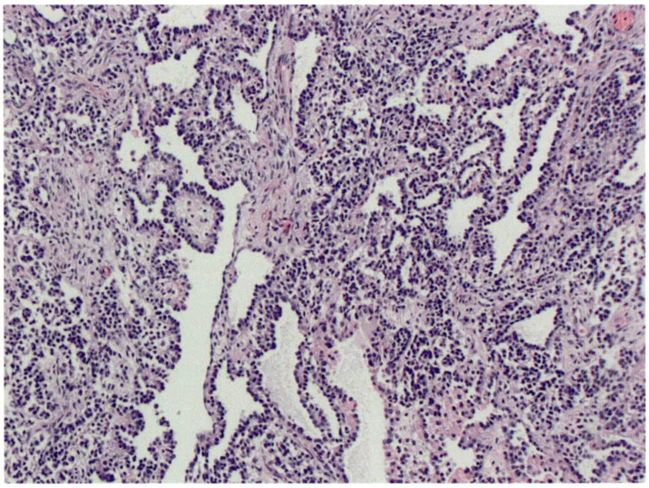

Fig. 3.44 The cuboidal-type epithelium lines the cystic spaces (100×)

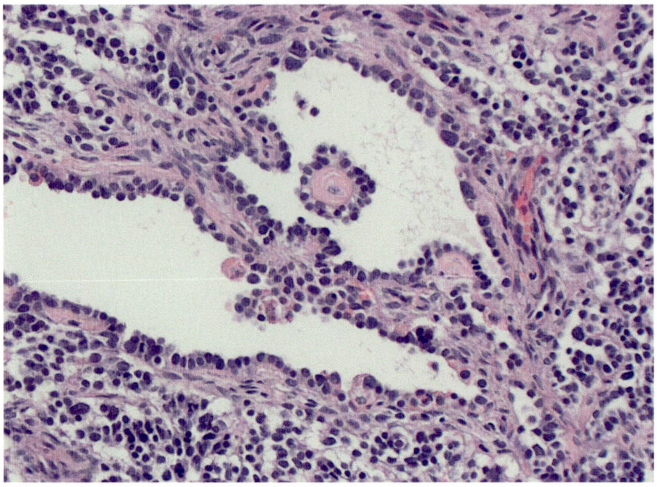

Fig. 3.45 Blunt rounded papillae with hyalinized cores (100×)

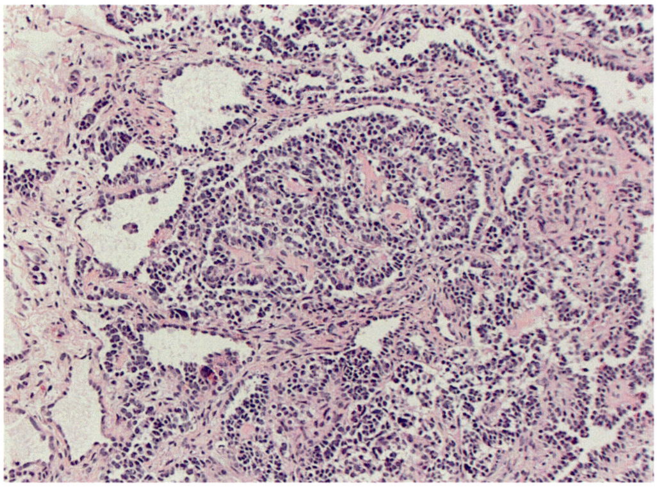

Fig. 3.46 The cystic space is filled with a large papillary structure (100×)

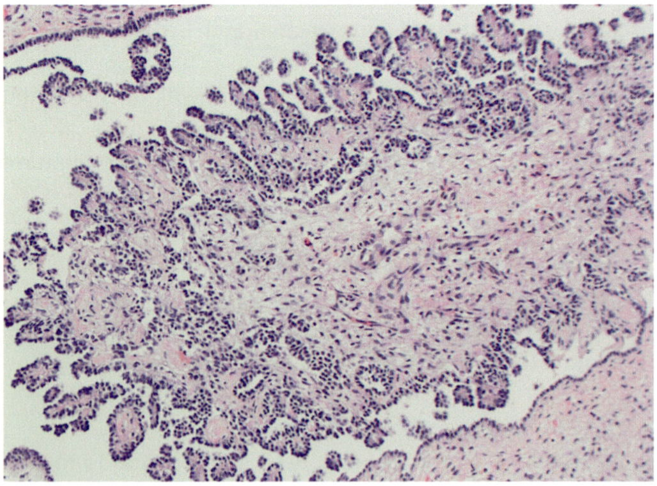

Fig. 3.47 Complex papillary pattern might mimic serous papillary carcinoma under lower power examination (200×)

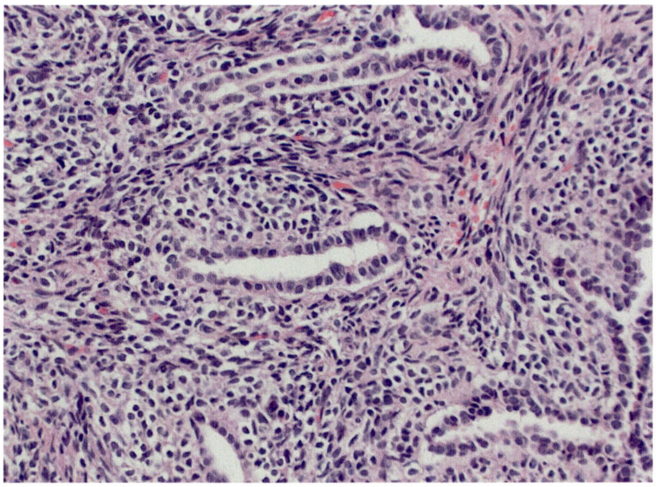

Fig. 3.48 Immature mesenchymal stroma between tubules (200×)

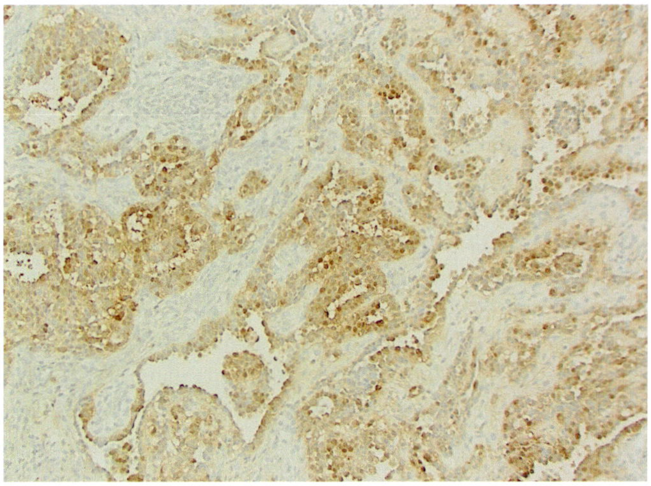

Fig. 3.50 Positive calretinin immunohistochemical stain in neoplastic cells (100×)

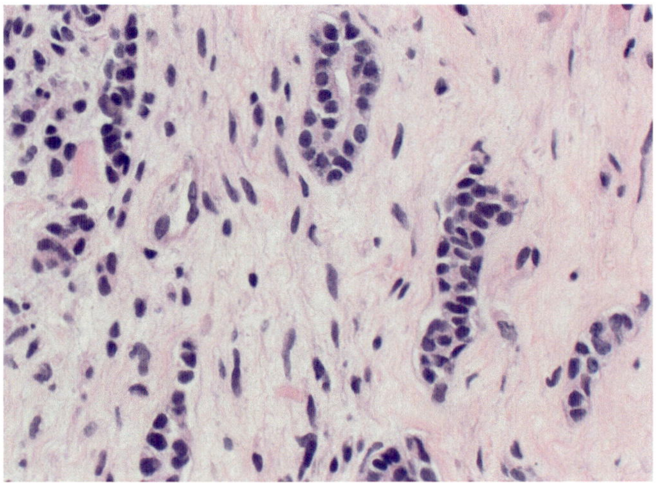

Fig. 3.49 Typical patterns of SLCT (cords and tubules) are at the periphery of the lesion (200×)

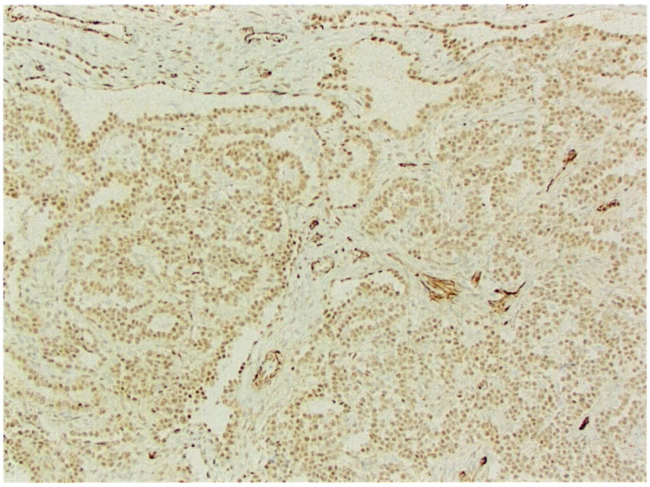

Fig. 3.51 WT1 nuclear positivity (100×)

3.12.1.3 Differential Diagnosis

- Yolk sac tumor (YSC)
  - Papillary structures in YST are lined by cells with abundant cytoplasm, but papillae in SLCT have single-layered cuboidal cells with scant cytoplasm.
  - Schiller Duval bodies: +/−.
  - Serum levels of AFP can rarely be increased in SLCT with retiform pattern. Heterologous mucinous elements can also be present in both YST and SLCT.
  - AFP positivity by immunohistochemistry supports the YST diagnosis.
- Serous carcinoma if the papillary architecture is prominent
  - The presence of focal typical SLCT architecture, androgenic manifestations, and young age is supportive of SLCT.
  - Inhibin and other sex cord markers are negative in serous carcinoma.
- Struma ovarii with papillary thyroid carcinoma
  - The presence of background teratoma elements supports struma ovarii.
  - Thyroglobulin and TSH are positive in struma ovarii and papillary thyroid carcinoma.

- Female adnexal tumor of probable Wolffian origin (FATWO)
  - The location of FATWO is at the broad ligament, ovarian hilum, fallopian tube, paravaginal area, and retroperitoneum [60]. FATWO usually has an admixture of architectural patterns, including solid, tubular, sieve-like, trabecular, and microcystic patterns. The stroma in FATWO varies from a delicate network of reticulin fibers separating the solid tubules to large areas of hyalinized collagen.
  - SF1 is negative in FATWO but positive in most sex cord-stromal tumors [61]. Inhibin is usually diffusely positive in sex cord-stromal tumors but focal or diffuse weak positive in FATWO [62].

3.12.1.4 Clinical Significance

- Retiform pattern is present in 10–15% of SLCT with a predilection in the younger age groups (average: 15 years). The androgenic manifestations are less commonly associated with the retiform pattern (25%) [63]. *DICER1* syndrome is an autosomal dominant disorder and is associated with multiple neoplasms, including pleuropulmonary blastoma, thyroid cancers, cystic nephroma, embryonal rhabdomyosarcoma of the uterine cervix, and ovarian SLCT [64]. SLCT with *DICER1* germline mutations are often intermediate to poorly differentiated tumors [65]. The diagnosis of SLCT in a young patient should lead to genetic consultation for *DICER1* syndrome.

References

1. Young RH. Ovarian sex cord-stromal tumours and their mimics. Pathology. 2018;50(1):5–15.
2. Irving JA, Alkushi A, Young RH, Clement PB. Cellular fibromas of the ovary: a study of 75 cases including 40 mitotically active tumors emphasizing their distinction from fibrosarcoma. Am J Surg Pathol. 2006;30(8):929–38.
3. Deavers MT, Malpica A, Liu J, Broaddus R, Silva EG. Ovarian sex cord-stromal tumors: an immunohistochemical study including a comparison of calretinin and inhibin. Mod Pathol. 2003;16(6):584–90.
4. Young RH, Prat J, Scully RE. Endometrioid stromal sarcomas of the ovary. A clinicopathologic analysis of 23 cases. Cancer. 1984;53(5):1143–55.
5. Young RH, Scully RE. Fibromatosis and massive edema of the ovary, possibly related entities: a report of 14 cases of fibromatosis and 11 cases of massive edema. Int J Gynecol Pathol. 1984;3(2):153–78.
6. Watkins JC, Young RH. Follicle cysts of the ovary: a report of 30 cases of a common benign lesion emphasizing its unusual clinical and pathologic aspects. Int J Gynecol Pathol. 2021;40(4):359–68.
7. Boyraz B, Watkins JC, Soubeyran I, Bonhomme B, Croce S, Oliva E, et al. Cystic granulosa cell tumors of the ovary: an analysis of 80 cases of an often diagnostically challenging entity. Arch Pathol Lab Med. 2022;146(12):1450–9.
8. McMullen ER, Huang T, Skala SL. Large ovarian follicle cyst: benign mimic of cystic adult granulosa cell tumor. Int J Gynecol Pathol. 2022;41(3):289–91.
9. Nakashima N, Young RH, Scully RE. Androgenic granulosa cell tumors of the ovary. A clinicopathologic analysis of 17 cases and review of the literature. Arch Pathol Lab Med. 1984;108(10):786–91.
10. Young RH, Prat J, Scully RE. Ovarian Sertoli-Leydig cell tumors with heterologous elements. I. Gastrointestinal epithelium and carcinoid: a clinicopathologic analysis of thirty-six cases. Cancer. 1982;50(11):2448–56.
11. Gui T, Cao D, Shen K, Yang J, Zhang Y, Yu Q, et al. A clinicopathological analysis of 40 cases of ovarian Sertoli-Leydig cell tumors. Gynecol Oncol. 2012;127(2):384–9.
12. Young RH, Scully RE. Ovarian Sertoli-Leydig cell tumors. A clinicopathological analysis of 207 cases. Am J Surg Pathol. 1985;9(8):543–69.
13. Prat J, Young RH, Scully RE. Ovarian Sertoli-Leydig cell tumors with heterologous elements. II. Cartilage and skeletal muscle: a clinicopathologic analysis of twelve cases. Cancer. 1982;50(11):2465–75.
14. Zhao C, Vinh TN, McManus K, Dabbs D, Barner R, Vang R. Identification of the most sensitive and robust immunohistochemical markers in different categories of ovarian sex cord-stromal tumors. Am J Surg Pathol. 2009;33(3):354–66.
15. Karnezis AN, Wang Y, Keul J, Tessier-Cloutier B, Magrill J, Kommoss S, et al. DICER1 and FOXL2 mutation status correlates with clinicopathologic features in ovarian sertoli-leydig cell tumors. Am J Surg Pathol. 2019;43(5):628–38.
16. Sigismondi C, Gadducci A, Lorusso D, Candiani M, Breda E, Raspagliesi F, et al. Ovarian Sertoli-Leydig cell tumors. a retrospective MITO study. Gynecol Oncol. 2012;125(3):673–6.
17. Young RH, Dickersin GR, Scully RE. Juvenile granulosa cell tumor of the ovary. A clinicopathological analysis of 125 cases. Am J Surg Pathol. 1984;8(8):575–96.
18. Al-Agha OM, Huwait HF, Chow C, Yang W, Senz J, Kalloger SE, et al. FOXL2 is a sensitive and specific marker for sex cord-stromal tumors of the ovary. Am J Surg Pathol. 2011;35(4):484–94.
19. Baillard P, Genestie C, Croce S, Descotes F, Rouleau E, Treilleux I, et al. Rare DICER1 and absent FOXL2 mutations characterize ovarian juvenile granulosa cell tumors. Am J Surg Pathol. 2021;45(2):223–9.
20. Young RH. Ovarian sex cord-stromal tumors: reflections on a 40-year experience with a fascinating group of tumors, including comments on the seminal observations of Robert E. Scully, MD. Arch Pathol Lab Med. 2018;142(12):1459–84.
21. Fuller PJ, Leung D, Chu S. Genetics and genomics of ovarian sex cord-stromal tumors. Clin Genet. 2017;91(2):285–91.
22. Irving JA, McCluggage WG. Ovarian spindle cell lesions: a review with emphasis on recent developments and differential diagnosis. Adv Anat Pathol. 2007;14(5):305–19.
23. Shah VI, Freites ON, Maxwell P, McCluggage WG. Inhibin is more specific than calretinin as an immunohistochemical marker for differentiating sarcomatoid granulosa cell tumour of the ovary from other spindle cell neoplasms. J Clin Pathol. 2003;56(3):221–4.
24. Susil BJ, Sumithran E. Sarcomatous change in granulosa cell tumor. Hum Pathol. 1987;18(4):397–9.
25. Wilson MK, Fong P, Mesnage S, Chrystal K, Shelling A, Payne K, et al. Stage I granulosa cell tumours: a management conundrum? Results of long-term follow up. Gynecol Oncol. 2015;138(2):285–91.
26. McConechy MK, Färkkilä A, Horlings HM, Talhouk A, Unkila-Kallio L, van Meurs HS, et al. Molecularly defined adult granulosa cell tumor of the ovary: the clinical phenotype. J Natl Cancer Inst. 2016;108(11):djw134.

27. Young RH, Oliva E, Scully RE. Luteinized adult granulosa cell tumors of the ovary: a report of four cases. Int J Gynecol Pathol. 1994;13(4):302–10.
28. Pelkey TJ, Frierson HF Jr, Mills SE, Stoler MH. The diagnostic utility of inhibin staining in ovarian neoplasms. Int J Gynecol Pathol. 1998;17(2):97–105.
29. Ganesan R, Hirschowitz L, Baltrušaitytė I, McCluggage WG. Luteinized adult granulosa cell tumor—a series of 9 cases: revisiting a rare variant of adult granulosa cell tumor. Int J Gynecol Pathol. 2011;30(5):452–9.
30. Guerrieri C, Anderson P, Hudacko R. Ciliated carcinoma of the endometrium. Int J Gynecol Pathol. 2021;40(2):141–7.
31. Meczekalski B, Szeliga A, Maciejewska-Jeske M, Podfigurna A, Cornetti P, Bala G, et al. Hyperthecosis: an underestimated nontumorous cause of hyperandrogenism. Gynecol Endocrinol. 2021;37(8):677–82.
32. Yamada S, Tanimoto A, Wang KY, Shimajiri S, Sasaguri Y. Stromal luteoma and nodular hyperthecosis of the bilateral ovaries associated with atypical endometrial hyperplasia of the uterus. Pathol Int. 2009;59(11):831–3.
33. Dunaif A, Hoffman AR, Scully RE, Flier JS, Longcope C, Levy LJ, et al. Clinical, biochemical, and ovarian morphologic features in women with acanthosis nigricans and masculinization. Obstet Gynecol. 1985;66(4):545–52.
34. Duun S. Bilateral virilizing hilus (Leydig) cell tumors of the ovary. Acta Obstet Gynecol Scand. 1994;73(1):76–7.
35. Malakzai HA, Abdul-Ghafar J, Ibrahimkhil AS, Haidary AM. A rare ovarian hilus cell tumour accompanying bilateral serous cystadenomas: report of a case. J Ovarian Res. 2021;14(1):81.
36. Jones MW, Harri R, Dabbs DJ, Carter GJ. Immunohistochemical profile of steroid cell tumor of the ovary: a study of 14 cases and a review of the literature. Int J Gynecol Pathol. 2010;29(4):315–20.
37. Kommoss F, Oliva E, Bhan AK, Young RH, Scully RE. Inhibin expression in ovarian tumors and tumor-like lesions: an immunohistochemical study. Mod Pathol. 1998;11(7):656–64.
38. Cao QJ, Jones JG, Li M. Expression of calretinin in human ovary, testis, and ovarian sex cord-stromal tumors. Int J Gynecol Pathol. 2001;20(4):346–52.
39. Paraskevas M, Scully RE. Hilus cell tumor of the ovary. A clinicopathological analysis of 12 Reinke crystal-positive and nine crystal-negative cases. Int J Gynecol Pathol. 1989;8(4):299–310.
40. Wong RW, McCluggage WG. Sex cord-stromal tumors with steroid cell tumor and fibroma components: report of 2 cases, including one of extraovarian origin. Int J Gynecol Pathol. 2019;38(2):151–6.
41. Deavers MT, Malpica A, Ordonez NG, Silva EG. Ovarian steroid cell tumors: an immunohistochemical study including a comparison of calretinin with inhibin. Int J Gynecol Pathol. 2003;22(2):162–7.
42. Clement PB, Young RH, Hanna W, Scully RE. Sclerosing peritonitis associated with luteinized thecomas of the ovary. A clinicopathological analysis of six cases. Am J Surg Pathol. 1994;18(1):1–13.
43. Hayes MC, Scully RE. Ovarian steroid cell tumors (not otherwise specified). A clinicopathological analysis of 63 cases. Am J Surg Pathol. 1987;11(11):835–45.
44. Irving JA, Young RH. Microcystic stromal tumor of the ovary: report of 16 cases of a hitherto uncharacterized distinctive ovarian neoplasm. Am J Surg Pathol. 2009;33(3):367–75.
45. McCluggage WG, Chong AS, Attygalle AD, Clarke BA, Chapman W, Rivera B, et al. Expanding the morphological spectrum of ovarian microcystic stromal tumour. Histopathology. 2019;74(3):443–51.
46. Irving JA, Lee CH, Yip S, Oliva E, McCluggage WG, Young RH. Microcystic stromal tumor: a distinctive ovarian sex cord-stromal neoplasm characterized by FOXL2, SF-1, WT-1, cyclin D1, and β-catenin nuclear expression and CTNNB1 mutations. Am J Surg Pathol. 2015;39(10):1420–6.
47. Singh K, Patel N, Patil P, Paquette C, Mathews CA, Lawrence WD. Primary ovarian solid pseudopapillary neoplasm with CTNNB1 c.98C>G (p.S33C) point mutation. Int J Gynecol Pathol. 2018;37(2):110–6.
48. Chen Q, Lu W, Lv W. Overlap of microcystic stromal tumor and primary solid pseudopapillary neoplasm of the ovary. Int J Clin Exp Pathol. 2015;8(9):11792–7.
49. Lee SH, Koh YW, Roh HJ, Cha HJ, Kwon YS. Ovarian microcystic stromal tumor: a novel extracolonic tumor in familial adenomatous polyposis. Genes Chromosomes Cancer. 2015;54(6):353–60.
50. McCluggage WG, Irving JA, Chong AS, Clarke BA, Young RH, Foulkes WD, et al. Ovarian microcystic stromal tumors are characterized by alterations in the beta-catenin-APC pathway and may be an extracolonic manifestation of familial adenomatous polyposis. Am J Surg Pathol. 2018;42(1):137–9.
51. Parra-Herran C. Endometrioid tubal intraepithelial neoplasia and bilateral ovarian microcystic stromal tumors harboring APC mutations: report of a case. Int J Gynecol Pathol. 2022;41(4):337–42.
52. Bi R, Bai QM, Yang F, Wu LJ, Cheng YF, Shen XX, et al. Microcystic stromal tumour of the ovary: frequent mutations of β-catenin (CTNNB1) in six cases. Histopathology. 2015;67(6):872–9.
53. Maeda D, Shibahara J, Sakuma T, Isobe M, Teshima S, Mori M, et al. β-catenin (CTNNB1) S33C mutation in ovarian microcystic stromal tumors. Am J Surg Pathol. 2011;35(10):1429–40.
54. Liu C, Gallagher RL, Price GR, Bolton E, Joy C, Harraway J, et al. Ovarian microcystic stromal tumor: a rare clinical manifestation of familial adenomatous polyposis. Int J Gynecol Pathol. 2016;35(6):561–5.
55. Young RH, Scully RE. Ovarian sex cord-stromal tumors: recent progress. Int J Gynecol Pathol. 1982;1(1):101–23.
56. Chivukula M, Hunt J, Carter G, Kelley J, Patel M, Kanbour-Shakir A. Recurrent gynandroblastoma of ovary—a case report: a molecular and immunohistochemical analysis. Int J Gynecol Pathol. 2007;26(1):30–3.
57. Wang Y, Karnezis AN, Magrill J, Tessier-Cloutier B, Lum A, Senz J, et al. DICER1 hot-spot mutations in ovarian gynandroblastoma. Histopathology. 2018;73(2):306–13.
58. Mooney EE, Nogales FF, Bergeron C, Tavassoli FA. Retiform Sertoli-Leydig cell tumours: clinical, morphological and immunohistochemical findings. Histopathology. 2002;41(2):110–7.
59. Young RH, Scully RE. Ovarian Sertoli-Leydig cell tumors with a retiform pattern: a problem in histopathologic diagnosis. A report of 25 cases. Am J Surg Pathol. 1983;7(8):755–71.
60. Shalaby A, Shenoy V. Female adnexal tumor of probable Wolffian origin: a review. Arch Pathol Lab Med. 2020;144(1):24–8.
61. Mirkovic J, Dong F, Sholl LM, Garcia E, Lindeman N, MacConaill L, et al. Targeted genomic profiling of female adnexal tumors of probable Wolffian origin (FATWO). Int J Gynecol Pathol. 2019;38(6):543–51.
62. Devouassoux-Shisheboran M, Silver SA, Tavassoli FA. Wolffian adnexal tumor, so-called female adnexal tumor of probable Wolffian origin (FATWO): immunohistochemical evidence in support of a Wolffian origin. Hum Pathol. 1999;30(7):856–63.
63. Young RH. Sertoli-Leydig cell tumors of the ovary: review with emphasis on historical aspects and unusual variants. Int J Gynecol Pathol. 1993;12(2):141–7.
64. Robertson JC, Jorcyk CL, Oxford JT. DICER1 syndrome: DICER1 mutations in rare cancers. Cancers (Basel). 2018;10(5):143.
65. de Kock L, Terzic T, McCluggage WG, Stewart CJR, Shaw P, Foulkes WD, et al. DICER1 mutations are consistently present in moderately and poorly differentiated sertoli-leydig cell tumors. Am J Surg Pathol. 2017;41(9):1178–87.

4 Germ Cell Tumors

4.1 Well-Differentiated Neuroendocrine Tumor (WNET-Carcinoid) in the Background of Teratoma

4.1.1 A 56-Year-Old Woman with Skin Flushing

4.1.1.1 Key Diagnostic Features

- The trabecular (Figs. 4.1 and 4.2) and insular (Fig. 4.3) patterns of the ovarian carcinoid tumors are associated equally with cystic teratomas.
- The size of the carcinoid is significantly smaller in carcinoids with cystic teratoma [1].
- The neoplastic cells form parallel ribbons and cords in a trabecular pattern. Insular carcinoid has a nested appearance with peripherally located acini. Centrally located nuclei have chromatin with salt and pepper appearance.
- WNET can also be associated with a spectrum of mucinous lesions of the ovaries (Fig. 4.4) in the background of mature cystic teratoma [2].

4.1.1.2 Ancillary Studies

- Synaptophysin, chromogranin, CD56, CDX2, and TTF1 are variably expressed in primary ovarian WNET (carcinoid) [3, 4].
- The median Ki67 index is 2.3% and 9.7% in primary and metastatic carcinoid tumors (WNET), respectively [5].

4.1.1.3 Differential Diagnosis

- Metastatic neuroendocrine tumor
  - The history of carcinoid tumor at other anatomic sites, bilateral tumors, multinodular growth pattern, extraovarian disease, and carcinoid syndrome persistence following the ovarian tumor's removal support a metastatic disease.

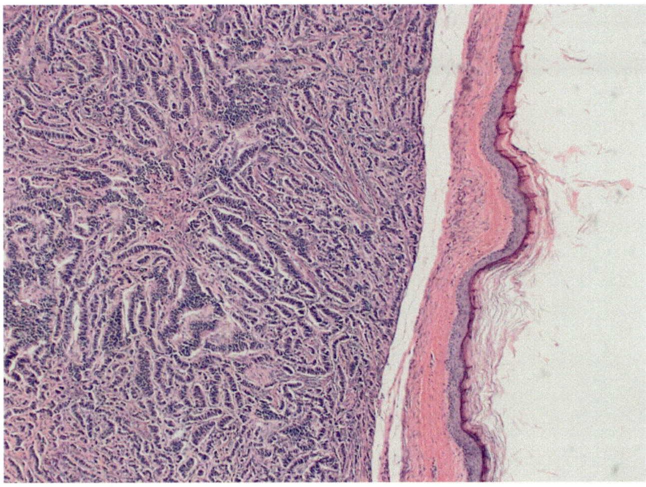

Fig. 4.1 Ectodermal elements (skin) of the teratoma (right) and WNET (left) (100×)

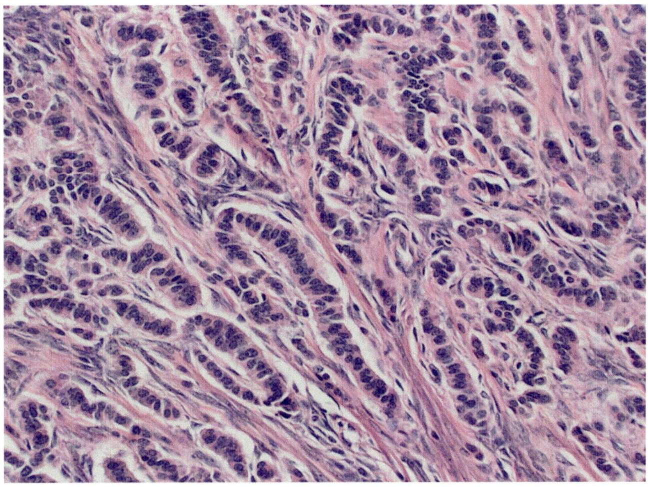

Fig. 4.2 Trabecular pattern of WNET in primary ovarian carcinoid tumor (200×)

O. Saglam, *Challenging Cases in Gynecologic Surgical Pathology*, https://doi.org/10.1007/978-3-031-51656-6_4

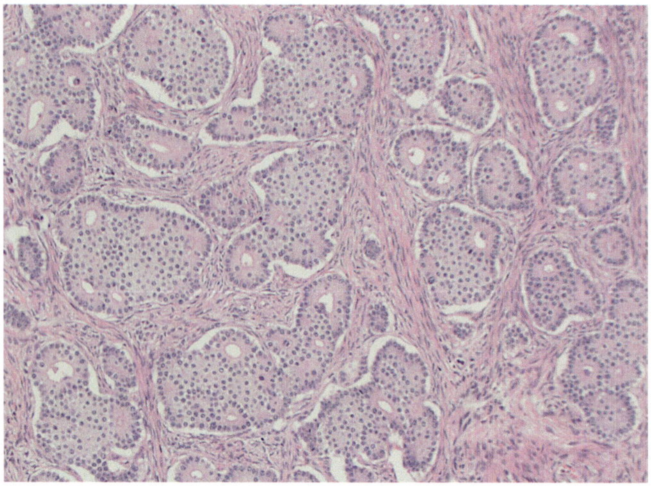

Fig. 4.3 Insular pattern of WNET in primary ovarian carcinoid tumor (100×)

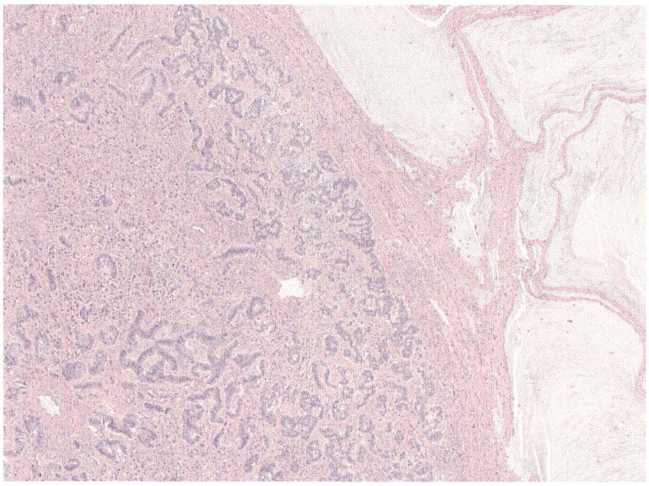

Fig. 4.4 Mucinous cystadenoma (right) and WNET (left) (40×)

  - The presence of an associated teratoma, Brenner tumor or sex cord-stromal tumor, and a unilateral tumor support an ovarian origin [6].
- Sertoli cell tumor
  - Multiple patterns, including hollow and solid tubules, trabeculae, diffuse, pseudopapillary, retiform, and spindled architectural patterns.
  - The Sertoli cells are cuboidal to columnar with pale cytoplasm.
  - Sex cord-stromal markers (inhibin, calretinin, SF1) are positive, and neuroendocrine markers except CD56 are negative.

4.1.1.4 Clinical Significance

- In small series, the prognosis of WNET associated with ovarian teratomas is good, with prolonged progression-free survival [7]. Ovarian carcinoid (WNET) can be a functional tumor and produce hormones that lead to carcinoid or Cushing's syndrome [8, 9]. The volume of carcinoid (WNET) in teratoma is positively associated with carcinoid syndrome.

4.2 Immature Teratoma with Embryoid Bodies (Malignant Mixed Germ Cell Tumor)

4.2.1 A 15-Year-Old Girl with an Ovarian Mass Lesion

4.2.1.1 Key Diagnostic Features

- Embryoid bodies are localized oval-to-round structures with a central germ disk composed of embryonal carcinoma-type epithelium underlain by thin yolk sac epithelium and associated with an amnion-like cavity (Fig. 4.5) [10]. These structures might be well-formed or fragmented. Embryoid bodies may fuse to form expansile aggregates (Fig. 4.6).
- The presence of embryoid bodies in immature teratoma samples is adequate for Malignant Mixed Germ Cell Tumor (MMGCT) diagnosis by some experts, and others consider embryoid bodies the most primitive formation

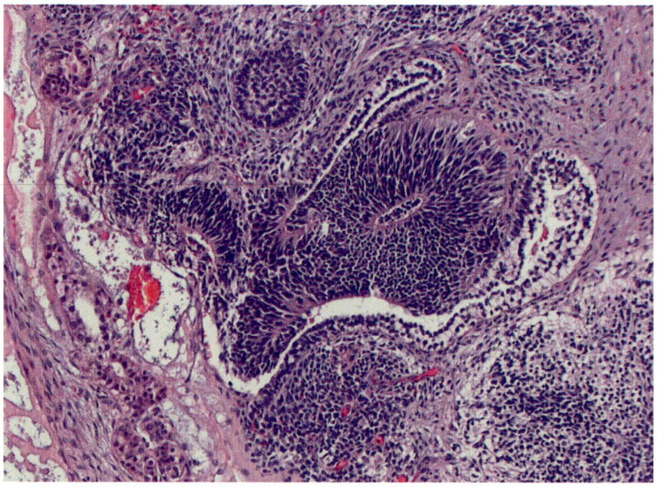

Fig. 4.5 Two embryoid bodies in an immature teratoma are partly fused. Darkly stained germ disk composed of embryonal carcinoma type epithelium and underlying thin yolk sac type epithelium has cytoplasmic vacuoles (periphery of the cystic cavity) (100×)

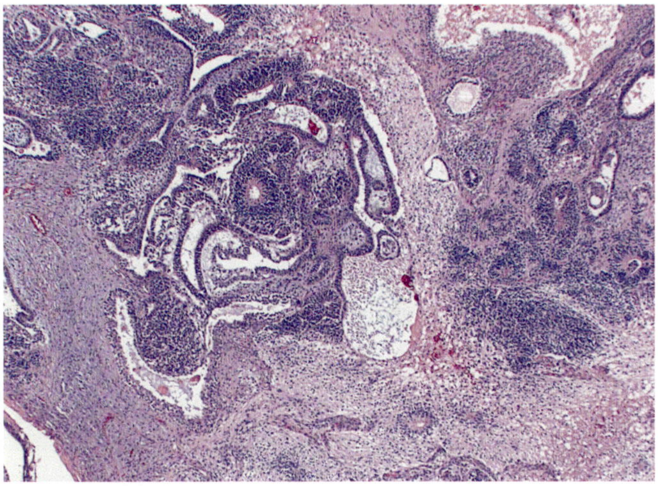

Fig. 4.6 Multiple embryoid bodies fuse to form expansile aggregate (left side) (40×)

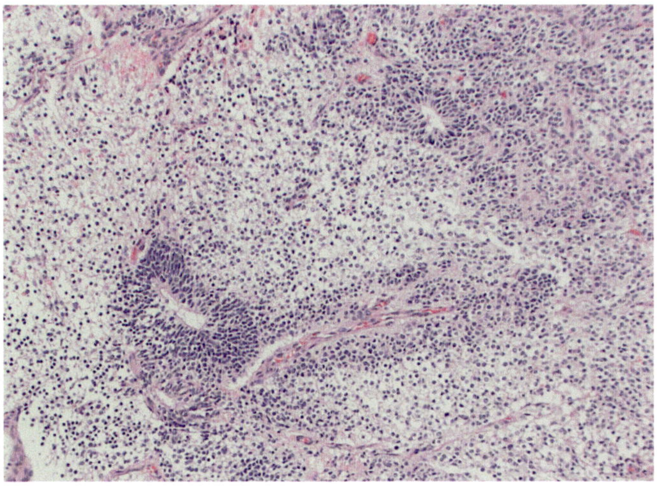

Fig. 4.7 Immature neuroectodermal elements (rosettes) in this section are from the same tumor (40×)

that may be present in an immature teratoma. Their presence should not dictate MMGCT diagnosis [10].

- Neuroectodermal tubules or rosettes in an immature teratoma are composed of small primitive cells with a high nuclear-to-cytoplasmic ratio arranged around an acinar space (Figs. 4.7 and 4.8).
- The grading of immature teratoma depends on the number of low-power microscopic fields containing aggregated amounts of immature neuroectoderm in one slide (grade 1: 1 field or less; grade 2: >1 up to 3; grade 3: >3 fields). The polyembryoma component is a primitive germ cell neoplasia. An isolated small focus of embryoid bodies is enough to grade teratoma as a high-grade neoplasia.

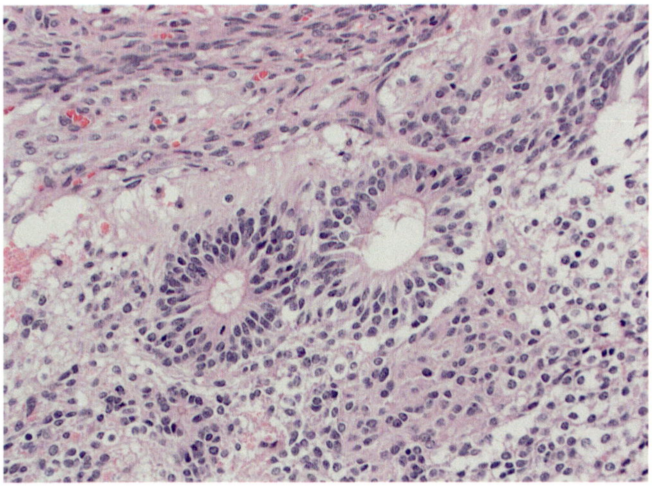

Fig. 4.8 Neuroectodermal elements are composed of small primitive mitotically active cells. The nuclear-cytoplasmic ratio is high. The primitive cells are polarized around rosette-like spaces (200×)

4.2.1.2 Ancillary Studies

- SALL4, glypican-3, and SOX-2 can be positive in immature neuroectodermal tissue [4, 11].
- Embryoid bodies are positive for AFP [12]. Immature gastrointestinal epithelium is also stained by AFP [13], and distinction is essential for tumor typing and grading.

4.2.1.3 Differential Diagnosis

- Yolk sac tumor (polyvesicular vitelline pattern)
  - Round to geographic-shaped cysts lined by flattened epithelium and smaller foci of nests and tubules in a background fibrous stroma.
  - The yolk sac vesicle of polyembryomas may become cystically dilated [14], but they preserve germ discs even in fragmented structures.
- Other patterns of yolk sac tumor or choriocarcinoma might co-exist with embryoid bodies [15].

4.2.1.4 Clinical Significance

- The presence of embryoid bodies in an immature teratoma might be the reason for the elevated serum AFP levels.
- The presence of embryoid bodies in an immature teratoma compels high-grade germ cell neoplasm.
- Correct tissue typing is essential for the identification of primary tumors at metastatic sites.

4.3 Struma Ovarii

4.3.1 A 32-Year-Old Woman with Cystic Ovarian Mass Lesion

4.3.1.1 Key Diagnostic Features

- The most common monodermal teratoma with thyroid tissue as a predominant (>50%) or sole component.
- The morphology is identical to normal thyroid tissue with diffuse, microfollicular, or tubular patterns [16]. Colloid fills variable-sized follicles lined by cuboidal or flat cells (Figs. 4.9 and 4.10).
- In cystic type, the paucity of thyroid follicles may lead to misdiagnosis of epithelial cysts [17]. The identification of thyroid tissue within the fibrous septa is the key to the correct diagnosis.

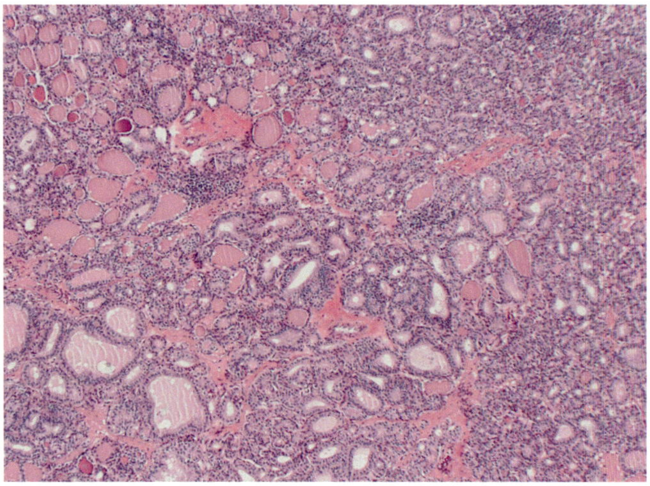

Fig. 4.9 Variable-sized follicles with luminal eosinophilic secretions (colloid) (100×)

- Benign changes such as papillary hyperplasia and adenomatous changes in the thyroid tissue or concurrent primary ovarian lesions, including serous and mucinous cystadenomas, Brenner tumor, thecoma, ovarian fibroma, and hilus cell hyperplasia, can be associated with struma ovarii [18, 19].
- Papillary, follicular, and anaplastic carcinomas of the thyroid tissue can arise in struma ovarii [18, 20–24].

4.3.1.2 Ancillary Studies

- Positive markers: PAX8, TTF1, and thyroglobulin.
- *KRAS* and *BRAF* mutations and PPARg-*PAX8* gene fusion can be detected in papillary and follicular carcinomas arising from struma ovarii [25, 26].

4.3.1.3 Differential Diagnosis

- Multilocular or unilocular epithelial cysts
  - Approximately one-third of struma ovarii cases are associated with serous or mucinous cystadenomas [17].
- Well-differentiated neuroendocrine tumor (NET)
  - NET of the ovaries can be seen in the background of teratoma (see Part I, Sect. 4.1).
  - Struma carcinoid is a mixed tumor with components of struma ovarii and carcinoid tumor in trabecular and insular patterns [27] (Figs. 4.11 and 4.12).
- Struma ovarii samples with microfollicular pattern versus adult granulosa cell tumor (AGCT)
  - AGCT usually has variable patterns.
  - The granulosa cells have pale nuclei with nuclear grooves.
  - Sex cord markers (inhibin, calretinin) are positive in AGCT.
  - See also Part I, Sects. 3.2 and 3.5,

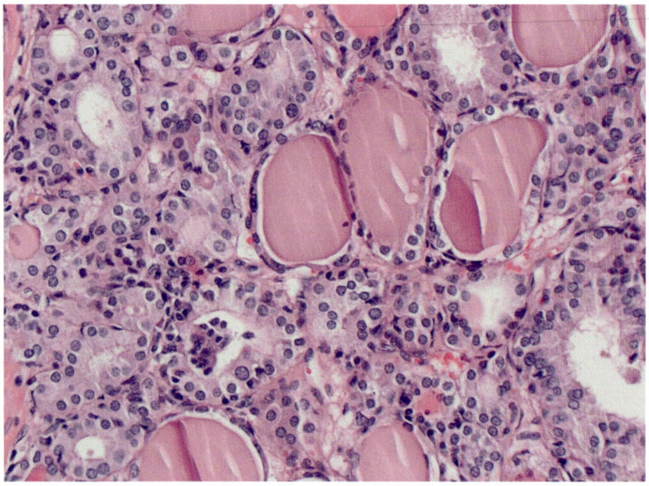

Fig. 4.10 Follicles are lined by cuboidal and flat monotonous cells with eosinophilic and clear cytoplasm (200×)

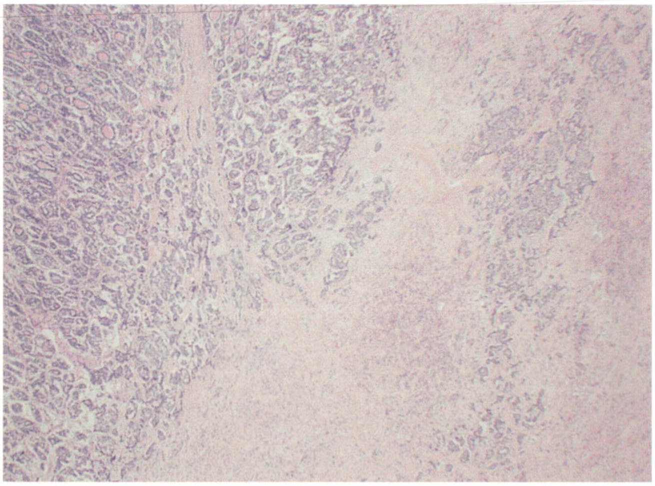

Fig. 4.11 Struma carcinoid is composed of thyroid tissue (left) and well-differentiated neuroendocrine tumor (right) (20×)

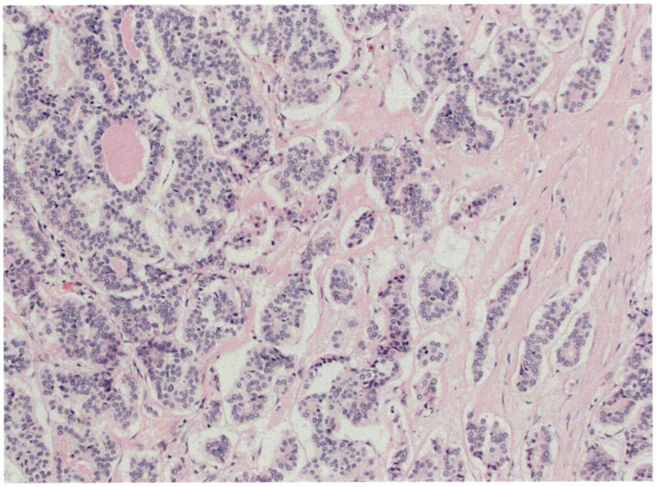

Fig. 4.12 The thyroid follicles with luminal colloid are next to NET with a trabecular architectural pattern in a hyalinized stroma (100×)

4.3.1.4 Clinical Significance

- The thyroid tissue within the struma ovarii can be hormonally active and clinically present with symptoms of hyperthyroidism [28].

References

1. Soga J, Osaka M, Yakuwa Y. Carcinoids of the ovary: an analysis of 329 reported cases. J Exp Clin Cancer Res. 2000;19(3):271–80.
2. Chatzipantelis P, Mavrogiorgis A, Kairi-Vassilatou E, Pafiti A. Ovarian neoplasm composed of an insular carcinoid tumor and a borderline mucinous cystadenoma arising in a mature cystic teratoma: a case report. Eur J Gynaecol Oncol. 2006;27(6):636–7.
3. Niu D, Li Z, Sun L, Cao D. Carcinoid arising from the teratomatous bronchial mucosa in a mature cystic teratoma of the ovary: a case report. Int J Gynecol Pathol. 2018;37(2):123–7.
4. Rabban JT, Zaloudek CJ. A practical approach to immunohistochemical diagnosis of ovarian germ cell tumours and sex cord-stromal tumours. Histopathology. 2013;62(1):71–88.
5. Zhang X, Jones A, Jenkins SM, Huang Y. Ki67 proliferative index in carcinoid tumors involving ovary. Endocr Pathol. 2018;29(1):43–8.
6. Baker PM, Oliva E, Young RH, Talerman A, Scully RE. Ovarian mucinous carcinoids including some with a carcinomatous component: a report of 17 cases. Am J Surg Pathol. 2001;25(5):557–68.
7. Opalińska M, Sowa-Staszczak A, Olearska H, Ulatowska-Bialas M, Gilis-Januszewska A, Hubalewska-Dydejczyk A. Clinical approach to neuroendocrine neoplasm associated with ovarian teratoma. Front Endocrinol (Lausanne). 2021;12:770266.
8. Huang B, Wu X, Zhou Q, Hu Y, Zhao H, Zhu H, et al. Cushing's syndrome secondary to ectopic ACTH secretion from carcinoid tumor within an ovarian mature teratoma: a case report and review of the literature. Gynecol Endocrinol. 2014;30(3):192–6.
9. Robboy SJ, Norris HJ, Scully RE. Insular carcinoid primary in the ovary. A clinicopathologic analysis of 48 cases. Cancer. 1975;36(2):404–18.
10. Safdar NS, Stall JN, Young RH. Malignant mixed germ cell tumors of the ovary: an analysis of 100 cases emphasizing the frequency and interrelationships of their tumor types. Am J Surg Pathol. 2021;45(6):727–41.
11. Cao D, Guo S, Allan RW, Molberg KH, Peng Y. SALL4 is a novel sensitive and specific marker of ovarian primitive germ cell tumors and is particularly useful in distinguishing yolk sac tumor from clear cell carcinoma. Am J Surg Pathol. 2009;33(6):894–904.
12. Nakashima N, Murakami S, Fukatsu T, Nagasaka T, Fukata S, Ohiwa N, et al. Characteristics of "embryoid body" in human gonadal germ cell tumors. Hum Pathol. 1988;19(10):1144–54.
13. WHO Classification of Tumours Editorial Board. Female genital tumours. Lyon (France): International Agency for Research on Cancer; 2020. (WHO Classification of tumours series, 5th ed.; vol4). https://publications.iarc.fr/592.
14. Young RH, Ulbright TM, Policarpio-Nicolas ML. Yolk sac tumor with a prominent polyvesicular vitelline pattern: a report of three cases. Am J Surg Pathol. 2013;37(3):393–8.
15. Jondle DM, Shahin MS, Sorosky J, Benda JA. Ovarian mixed germ cell tumor with predominance of polyembryoma: a case report with literature review. Int J Gynecol Pathol. 2002;21(1):78–81.
16. Szyfelbein WM, Young RH, Scully RE. Struma ovarii simulating ovarian tumors of other types. A report of 30 cases. Am J Surg Pathol. 1995;19(1):21–9.
17. Szyfelbein WM, Young RH, Scully RE. Cystic struma ovarii: a frequently unrecognized tumor. A report of 20 cases. Am J Surg Pathol. 1994;18(8):785–8.
18. Devaney K, Snyder R, Norris HJ, Tavassoli FA. Proliferative and histologically malignant struma ovarii: a clinicopathologic study of 54 cases. Int J Gynecol Pathol. 1993;12(4):333–43.
19. Wei S, Baloch ZW, LiVolsi VA. Pathology of struma ovarii: a report of 96 cases. Endocr Pathol. 2015;26(4):342–8.
20. Castillo Simón AG, Martínez Ramos CV, Rodríguez Morales VV, Núñez Arana B, Dominguez Prado I, Muñoz Iglesias JL. Follicular thyroid carcinoma arising in a struma ovarii and femoral metastasis. Rev Esp Med Nucl Imagen Mol (Engl Ed). 2022;41(5):325–6.
21. Barrera JR, Manalo LA, Ang FL. Papillary thyroid-type carcinoma arising from struma ovarii. BMJ Case Rep. 2012;2012.
22. Goffredo P, Sawka AM, Pura J, Adam MA, Roman SA, Sosa JA. Malignant struma ovarii: a population-level analysis of a large series of 68 patients. Thyroid. 2015;25(2):211–5.
23. Roth LM, Karseladze AI. Highly differentiated follicular carcinoma arising from struma ovarii: a report of 3 cases, a review of the literature, and a reassessment of so-called peritoneal strumosis. Int J Gynecol Pathol. 2008;27(2):213–22.
24. Fukunaga M, Ishibashi T, Koyama T, Onoue K, Kitai S, Tanaka K, et al. Malignant struma ovarii with a predominant component of anaplastic carcinoma. Int J Gynecol Pathol. 2016;35(4):357–61.
25. Tsukada T, Yoshida H, Ishikawa M, Asami Y, Shiraishi K, Kato T. Malignant struma ovarii presenting with follicular carcinoma: a case report with molecular analysis. Gynecol Oncol Rep. 2019;30:100498.
26. Tan A, Stewart CJ, Garrett KL, Rye M, Cohen PA. Novel BRAF and KRAS mutations in papillary thyroid carcinoma arising in struma ovarii. Endocr Pathol. 2015;26(4):296–301.
27. Roth LM, Talerman A. The enigma of struma ovarii. Pathology. 2007;39(1):139–46.
28. Podfigurna A, Szeliga A, Horwat P, Maciejewska-Jeske M, Meczekalski B. Hyperthyroidism associated with struma ovarii—a case report and review of literature. Gynecol Endocrinol. 2021;37(12):1143–50.

5 Miscellaneous Ovarian Lesions

5.1 Small Cell Carcinoma of the Ovary, Hypercalcemic Type (SCCOHT)

5.1.1 A 23-Year-Old Woman with Abdominal Swelling and Pain

5.1.1.1 Key Diagnostic Features

- The architectural growth patterns include sheets (77%) (Fig. 5.1), nests, cords, and trabeculae, and are mixed (23%) with scattered follicle-like spaces (80%) with secretions [1] (Fig. 5.2).
- Brisk mitotic activity (Fig. 5.3).
- The cell types are predominantly monomorphic, round, small cells with scant cytoplasm. Large cells or spindle cells might be present. The large cells in rhabdoid morphology might be predominant in rare cases (large cell variant) (Fig. 5.4).
- Mucinous cysts or signet ring-like cells are rare components (12%) (Fig. 5.5).

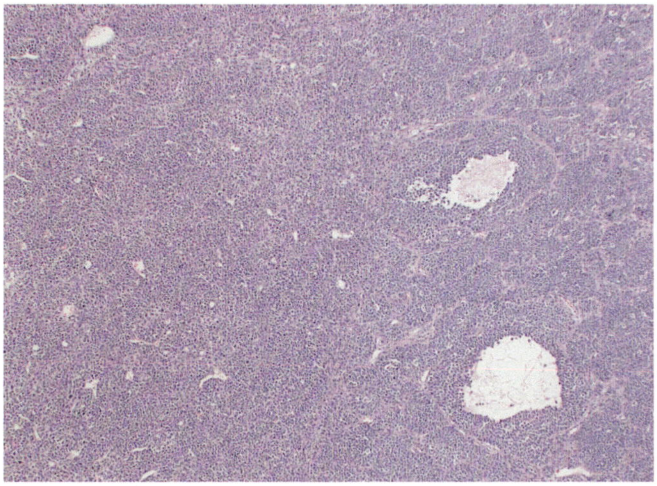

Fig. 5.1 Diffuse proliferation of small blue cells with areas of follicle-like spaces (20×)

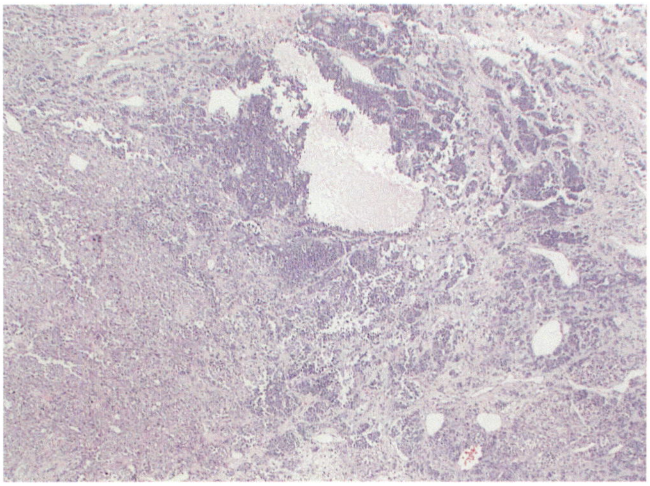

Fig. 5.2 There are two types of cells in this figure: The small blue cells around the follicle-like spaces and larger cells with a moderate amount of cytoplasm (20×)

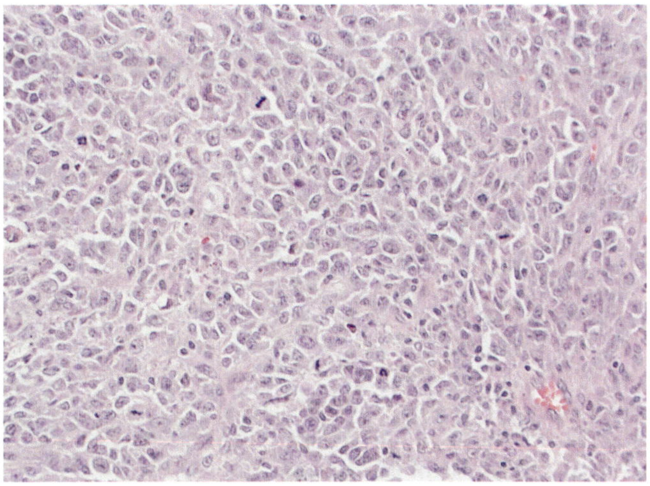

Fig. 5.3 The mitotic activity is high (200×)

O. Saglam, *Challenging Cases in Gynecologic Surgical Pathology*, https://doi.org/10.1007/978-3-031-51656-6_5

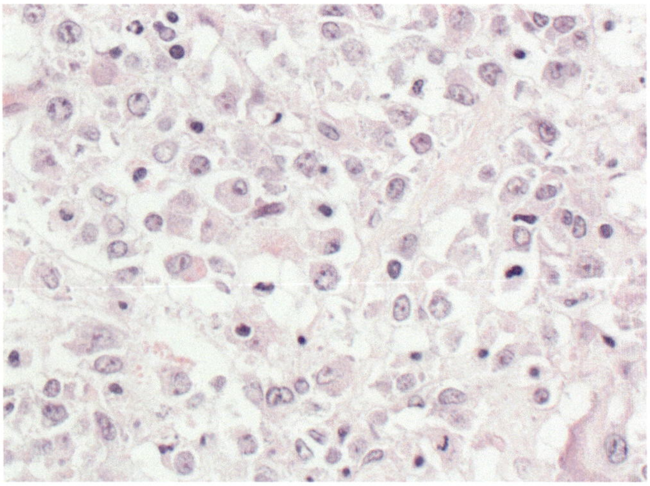

Fig. 5.4 The large cells have eccentric nuclei (rhabdoid) appearance (200×)

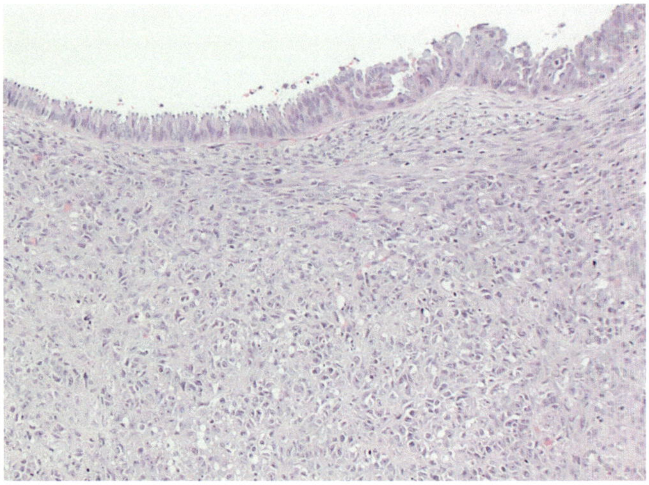

Fig. 5.5 A mucinous-type cystic lesion is present in proximity to the large cell component of SCCOHT (40×)

5.1.1.2 Ancillary Studies

- EMA, keratins, SALL4, CD10, calretinin, inhibin, neuroendocrine markers, WT1: variable expression [2]. p53 has a mutation pattern.
- Lack of expressions of BRG1 (*SMARCA4*) and BRM (*SMARCA2*) (94%) by immunohistochemistry [3].
- *SMARCA4* germline or somatic mutations in almost all cases [3, 4].

5.1.1.3 Differential Diagnosis

- Adult granulosa cell tumor (AGCT)
  - The patient's age is one of the key factors. AGCT has various morphological features. The diffuse pattern can be in the differential diagnosis of SCCOHT. The nuclei are pale with grooves, and mitotic activity is low in AGCT.
- Juvenile granulosa cell tumor (JGCT)
  - Overlapping features are the patient's age and follicle-like spaces in morphology. The majority of cells in JGCT have abundant eosinophilic cytoplasm. The majority of cells in SCCOHT are small cells with scant cytoplasm. Large cells in SCCOHT have a rhabdoid appearance with hyaline globules.
- Dysgerminoma
  - The polygonal cells have clear cytoplasm in the background of lymphocytic aggregates. There might be artifactual spaces mimicking follicular appearance.
  - Immunostains for OCT3/4, CD117, and PLAP are expressed in dysgerminoma.
- Lymphoma
  - Dyscohesive cells and lack of follicle-like space are supportive of lymphoma.
  - Lymphocyte common antigen expression confirms the diagnosis.
- Desmoplastic small round cell tumor
  - Well-circumscribed solid nodules of tumor cells within an abundant desmoplastic stroma.
  - Neoplastic cells are uniform with small hyperchromatic nuclei, inconspicuous nucleoli, and scant cytoplasm.
  - In large cell pattern, epithelioid cells with more significant pleomorphism can mimic carcinoma.
  - Positive staining with a variety of epithelial, neural, and mesenchymal markers.
- Ewing sarcoma group
  - The predominant component is small cells in sheets or nests. The neoplastic cells have round to ovoid hyperchromatic nuclei and scant cytoplasm. The mitotic activity is high. Homer Wright rosettes consisting of a central fibrillar core surrounded by concentrically arranged tumor cells may be present.
  - Immunohistochemical stains for CD99, FLI1, NKX2.2 [5], and ERG are variable positive.
  - Tumors in the Ewing family contain *EWSR1* and other variant chromosomal translocations [6].

5.1.1.4 Clinical Significance

- Favorable prognostic factors include age > 30, normal calcium levels, tumor size <10 cm, and absence of large cells for Stage IA disease [1]. Genetic counseling and mutational analysis of the *SMARCA4* gene might help to detect familial cases [7].

Endometrium

6

6.1 Corded and Hyalinized Endometrioid Carcinoma (CHEC)

6.1.1 A 59-Year-Old Woman with Postmenopausal Bleeding

6.1.1.1 Key Diagnostic Features

- Rare subtype of endometrioid adenocarcinoma with epithelioid and spindle cells.
- Epithelioid cells in cords or clusters are embedded in a hyalinized stroma [1] (Figs. 6.1 and 6.2).
- There might be osseous (24%) or chondroid metaplasia (4.5%), or a myxoid matrix (38.5%) [2, 3].
- Glandular, corded, and spindled components merge at some foci (Figs. 6.1 and 6.3).
- Usually associated with low-grade endometrioid carcinoma with squamous differentiation (Fig. 6.4).
- Histological grade depends on conventional endometrioid carcinoma component.

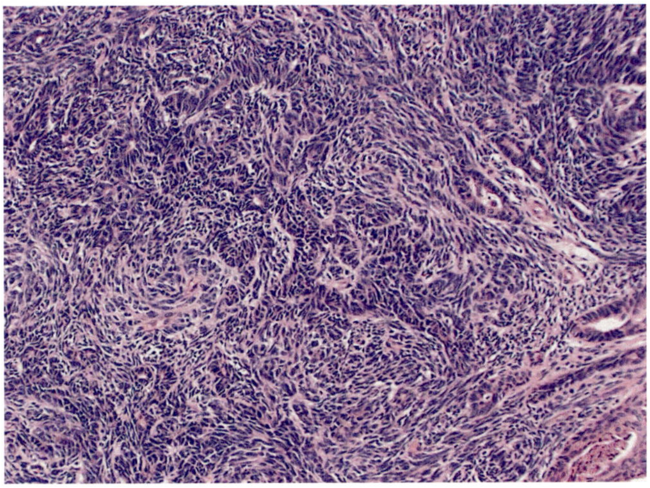

Fig. 6.2 Spindle cells form interlacing fascicles and merge with the glandular compoent in this field. No cytological atypia or mitotic activity is noticeable within the spindle cell component (100×)

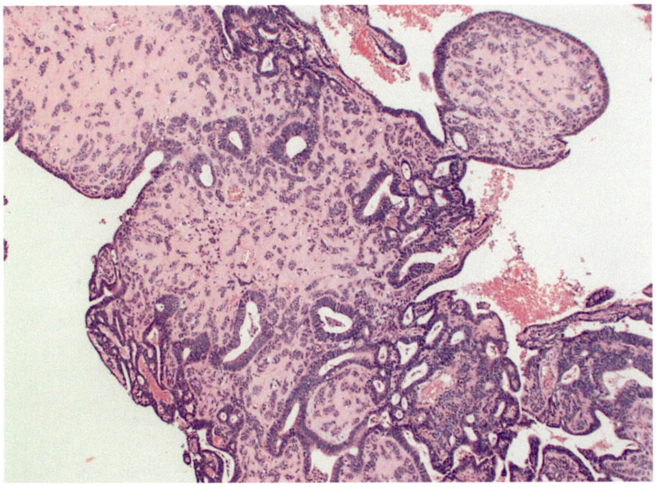

Fig. 6.1 Biphasic lesion with glandular and corded-hyalinized components. The epithelioid cells form small cords and trabeculae-like structures. They are in continuity with glandular epithelium in some foci (40×)

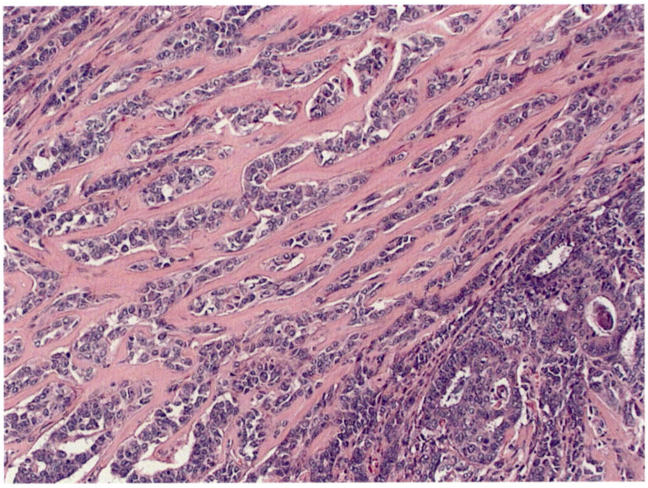

Fig. 6.3 Uniform epithelioid cells in a trabecular pattern embedded in a hyalinized stroma are next to the glandular component (right lower side). There is moderate cytological atypia (200×)

O. Saglam, *Challenging Cases in Gynecologic Surgical Pathology*, https://doi.org/10.1007/978-3-031-51656-6_6

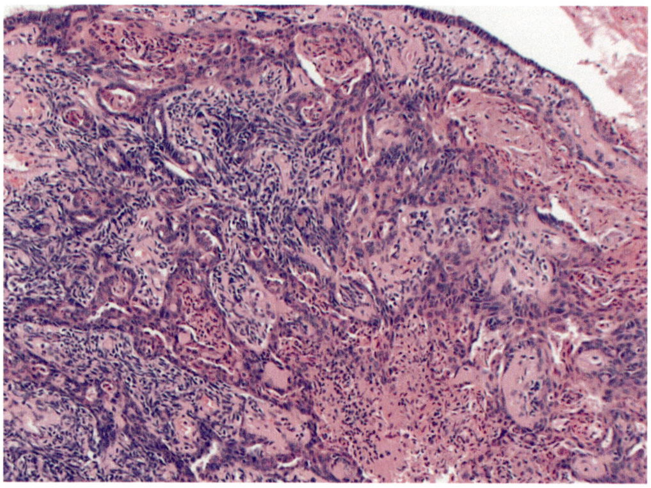

Fig. 6.4 Squamous differentiation is often prominent in the conventional adenocarcinoma component (100×). All figures are from the same biopsy sample

6.1.1.2 Ancillary Studies

- Cytokeratin and EMA are often weak to moderate intensity positive in the corded and spindled components [4].
- Beta-catenin nuclear expression in all components. Loss of E-cadherin expression in the spindle and corded epithelioid cells [5] suggests a process of epithelial-mesenchymal transition.
- p53 has a normal/wild-type expression pattern in the majority of cases (89%) [6].

6.1.1.3 Differential Diagnosis

- Carcinosarcoma
  - Usually diagnosed in postmenopausal women (mean age: 70 years) with extrauterine disease [7].
  - Spatially distinct high-grade carcinomatous and sarcomatous components.
  - *TP53* mutations are common.
- Uterine tumor resembling ovarian sex cord tumor
  - Well-circumscribed nodular lesions with morphological patterns resembling ovarian sex cord tumors.
  - See Part II, Sect. 8.1.
- Mesonephric-like adenocarcinoma with corded and hyalinized pattern (rare case report) [8]
  - Tumor cells in cords and trabeculae embedded in a hyalinized stroma with architectural features of mesonephric-like adenocarcinoma.
  - No squamous or mucinous differentiation.
  - See Part II, Sect. 6.11.
- Low-grade endometrial stromal sarcoma with sex cord-like differentiation
  - Small, monomorphic blue cells grow in sheets that focally whorl around delicate arteriole-like vessels.
  - In some foci, tumor cells arrange in cords, nests, and trabeculae, forming sex cord-like elements.
  - Associated with *PHF1* genetic rearrangements [9].

6.1.1.4 Clinical Significance

- CHEC is usually a low-grade carcinoma (FIGO grades 1&2). However, rare high-grade CHEC is reported in small series [6, 10]. *CTNNB1* (beta-catenin) mutations involving exon 3 are common in low-grade and high-grade CHEC [5, 10].

6.2 Metastatic Carcinoma Involving the Endometrium

6.2.1 A 45-Year-Old Woman Who Is on Tamoxifen

6.2.1.1 Key Diagnostic Features

- Diffuse infiltration of the endometrium by small neoplastic cells that spare the glands (Fig. 6.5). The myometrium can contain metastatic nodules.
- The neoplastic cells would have a plasmacytoid/signet ring cell appearance. Intracytoplasmic vacuoles or lumens are frequently identified (Fig. 6.6).
- Breast cancer is the most common extragenital tumor metastasizing to the endometrium [11]. In a case series, 64% of total metastatic carcinomas are lobular-type breast carcinoma, supporting the idea that Invasive Lobular Carcinoma is more likely to spread to the gynecologic organs [12].
- The most common primary genital site is the ovaries.

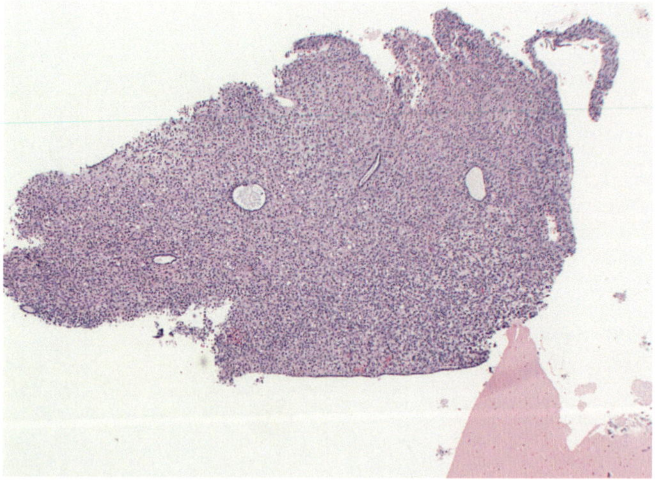

Fig. 6.5 Inactive glandular epithelium appears normal and undisturbed, and the stroma is slightly pinkish in low-power examination (40×)

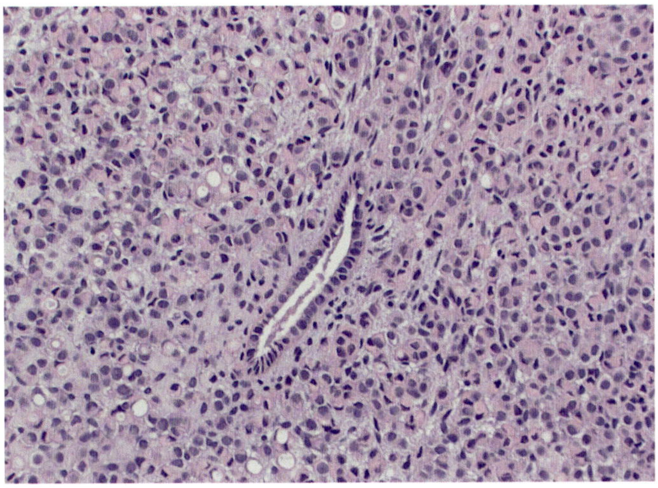

Fig. 6.6 The neoplastic cells have a diffuse growth pattern. The nuclei are eccentrically located and have a signet ring cell appearance. Intracytoplasmic lumen formation is present in several neoplastic cells (200×)

6.2.1.2 Ancillary Studies

- GATA3, CK7: positive
- Discordance of ER, PR, and HER2 expression between primary and metastatic breast cancers is 18%, 40%, and 13.6%, respectively [13]. The biomarker expression should be re-tested at metastatic anatomical sites

6.2.1.3 Differential Diagnosis

- Metastatic carcinoma with signet ring cell features such as primary gastric, colorectal, and lung primary cancers
  - Clinical history is the key to the diagnosis.
  - The frequency of GATA3 expression in adenocarcinomas of lung, stomach, and colon is less than 10% [14].
  - CD20 and CDX2 (colorectal cancer), TTF1, Napsin A (lung adenocarcinoma), Villin and CEA (gastric cancer) can be in the panel of immunohistochemical studies depending on clinical history.
- Metastatic goblet cell adenocarcinoma (AKA adenocarcinoma ex-goblet cell carcinoid of the appendix) in diffuse pattern [15, 16]
  - Peritoneal surfaces and ovaries are more commonly involved, and rare cases present with uterine metastasis.
  - Tumor cells with goblet cell morphology in small tubules, nests, clusters, or cords.
  - Expression of both epithelial (CK7, CK20) and neuroendocrine markers.

6.2.1.4 Clinical Significance

- Abnormal uterine bleeding is the most common symptom of metastatic lobular carcinoma to the endometrium. The neoplastic cells can be scant in the biopsy specimens and present as a component of endometrial polyps [17, 18].

6.3 Endometrioid Carcinoma with Mucinous Features

6.3.1 A 65-Year-Old Woman with Postmenopausal Bleeding

6.3.1.1 Key Diagnostic Features

- Endometrial adenocarcinoma is composed of varying amounts of mucin-secreting glandular epithelium (Fig. 6.7) and at least focal endometrioid-type adenocarcinoma or atypical endometrial hyperplasia (Endometrial Intraepithelial Neoplasia—EIN).
- There might be scattered goblet cells.
- Nuclei are usually low grade (FIGO grade 1 to 2) (Fig. 6.8).

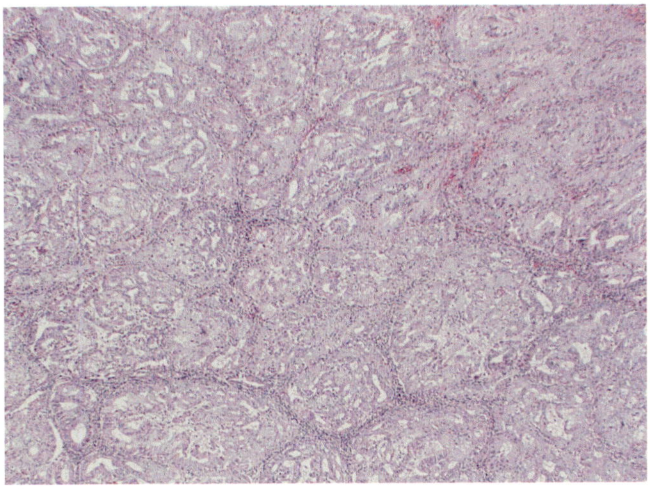

Fig. 6.7 The mucinous component of endometrioid adenocarcinoma (40×)

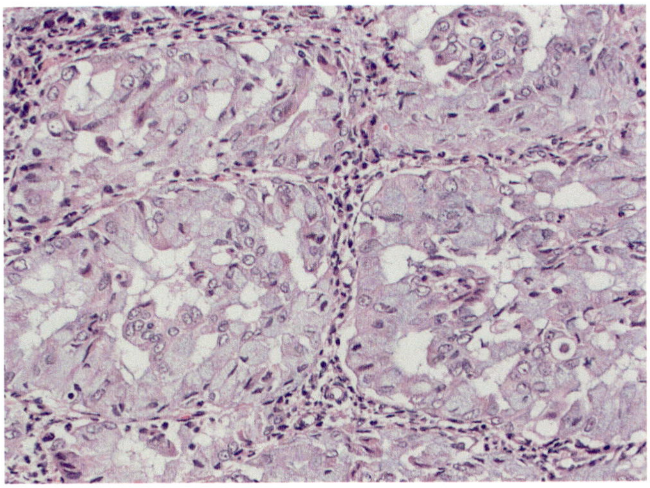

Fig. 6.8 Mucinous-type lining epithelium with low-grade nuclear features. Scattered goblet cells are also in the field (200×)

- Endometrioid adenocarcinoma or EIN can be focal, and adequate sampling is essential to rule out primary endometrial gastric/gastrointestinal type adenocarcinoma [19].

6.3.1.2 Ancillary Studies

- CK7: usually positive
- CK20, CEA, and CDX2: might be focal positive
- P16: negative or patchy positive

6.3.1.3 Differential Diagnosis

- Metastatic carcinoma from the gastrointestinal tract
  - Clinical correlation is contributory to the diagnosis.
  - The presence of background EIN and endometrioid-type cancer supports primary endometrial carcinoma.
  - The immunostaining profile might overlap with metastatic upper or lower gastrointestinal tract tumors.
- Metastatic HPV-dependent endocervical adenocarcinoma
  - Presence of endocervical adenocarcinoma in situ is supportive of primary endocervical adenocarcinoma.
  - P16 is diffusely positive in human papilloma virus (HPV)-dependent endocervical cancers.
  - In situ hybridization test for high-risk HPV is helpful in the diagnosis of primary endocervical adenocarcinoma in cases with equivocal p16 results.
- Primary gastric/gastrointestinal type endometrial carcinoma
  - Extremely rare and relatively new diagnostic entity, included in the latest edition of the WHO Blue Book for Female Genital Tumors.
  - For similar morphologic features to those of endocervical counterpart, see Part III, Sect. 9.4.

6.3.1.4 Clinical Significance

- Mucinous differentiation in endometrioid-type adenocarcinoma is more common in older patients and is associated with an increased likelihood of myometrial invasion. However, this finding does not affect the disease stage or risk of recurrence [20].

6.4 Low-Grade Endometrioid Carcinoma with Clear Cells

6.4.1 A 45-Year-Old Woman with Perimenopausal Bleeding

6.4.1.1 Key Diagnostic Features

- All subtypes of endometrial cancer might have focal cytoplasmic clearing [21, 22].
- Architectural patterns and the nuclear grade dictate the final histological subtype.
- Cytoplasmic clearing can be associated with the presence of squamous cells, intracytoplasmic glycogen, neoadjuvant therapy, or NOS (Fig. 6.9).
- In low-grade endometrioid adenocarcinoma (FIGO grades 1 and 2), the nuclei are uniformly low grade (Figs. 6.10 and 6.11).
- The secretary-type change presents with sub-or supranuclear vacuoles.

6.4.1.2 Ancillary Studies

- Immunophenotype is the same as the conventional-type low-grade endometrioid carcinoma.
- P16: patchy positive.
- P53: normal/wild-type staining.
- ER/PR: positive.

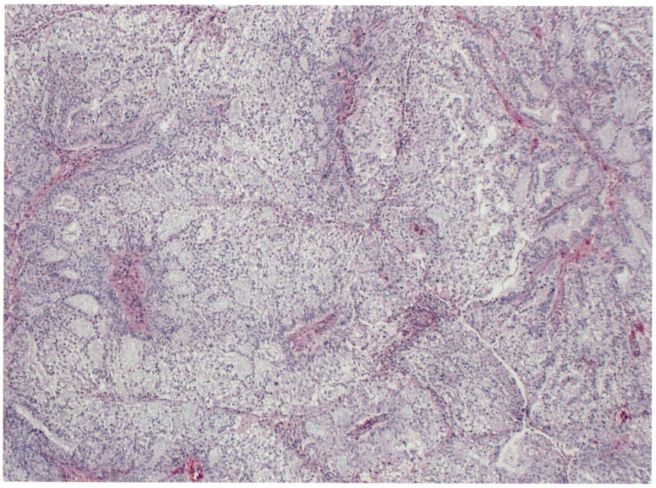

Fig. 6.9 Low-grade endometrioid adenocarcinoma with broad zones of clear cells (40×)

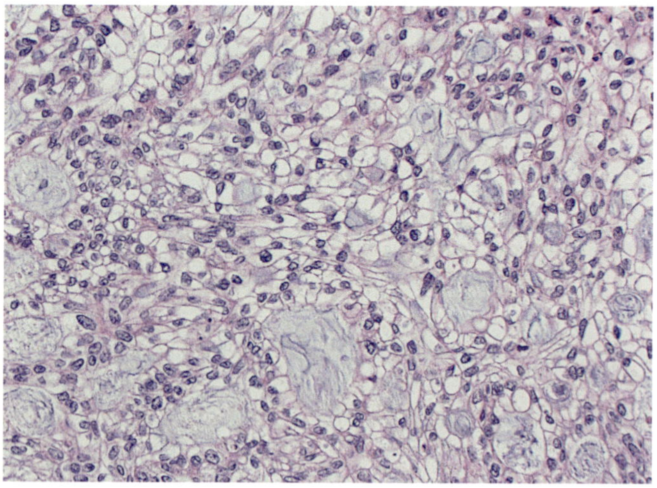

Fig. 6.10 Clear cells with mild nuclear atypia form acini and solid areas (100×)

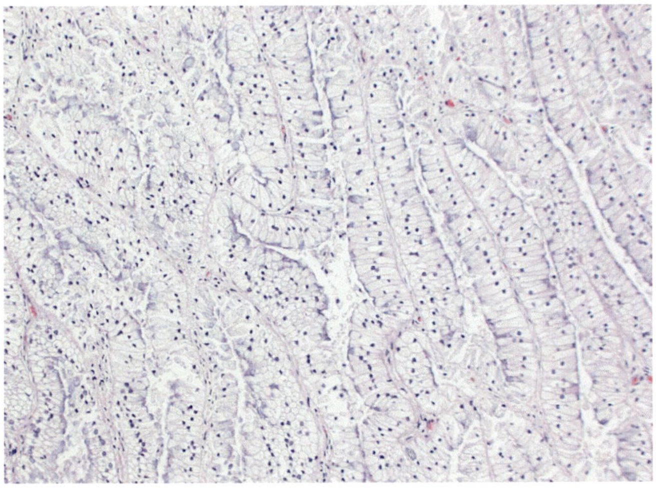

Fig. 6.11 Nuclei are small and uniform. The cell borders are distinct (40×)

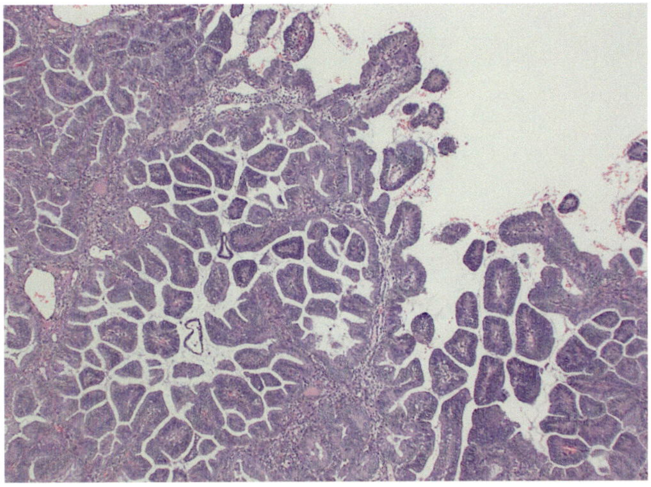

Fig. 6.12 Endometrioid adenocarcinoma with papillary pattern. The papillary structures with or without fibrovascular cores. Mucinous-type differentiation is focally present (40×)

6.4.1.3 Differential Diagnosis

- Yolk sac tumor of the endometrium (YSTE)
  - Rare malignancy of the endometrium in adult patients.
  - YSTE can be admixed with epithelial and other germ cell tumors.
  - See Part II, Sect. 6.15,
- Clear cell carcinoma
  - Architectural patterns include tubulocystic, papillary, and solid types.
  - Significant cytological atypia should be present, at least focally.
  - Various cell types, including low cuboidal, polyhedral, hobnail, signet-ring-like, mucinous, or flattened cells.
  - Napsin A, HNF-1ß, and AMACR: positive [23].
  - ER and PR: negative or focal weak positive.
- Advanced-stage cancers with neoadjuvant therapy
  - Clinical history, pretreatment biopsies, and immunohistochemistry contribute to correct histologic typing in small samples.

6.4.1.4 Clinical Significance

- Differentiating low-grade endometrioid adenocarcinoma with clear cells from high-grade cancers is significant for treatment and prognosis.

6.5 Low-Grade Endometrioid Carcinoma with Papillary Architecture

6.5.1 A 50-Year-Old Woman with Thickened Endometrial Strips by Imaging Studies

6.5.1.1 Key Diagnostic Features

- Predominantly papillary architecture. The glandular component can be sparse (Fig. 6.12).

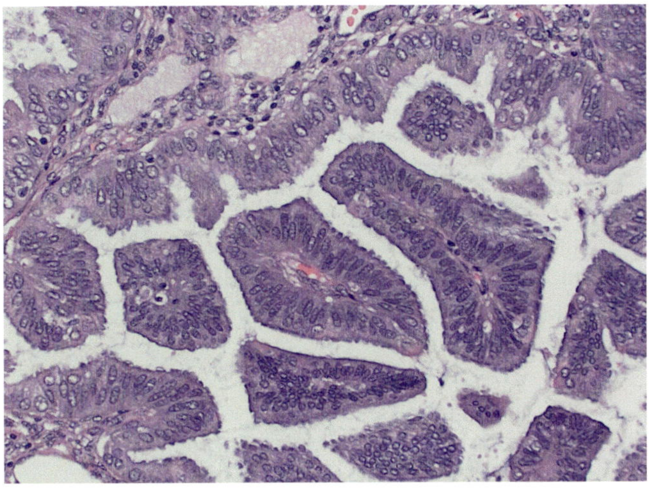

Fig. 6.13 The lining epithelium is columnar type without conspicuous nucleoli. Nuclei are vertically oriented to the basement membrane (200×)

- The nuclei are stratified, columnar, and vertically oriented to the basement membrane. Nucleoli are inconspicuous (Fig. 6.13).
- There might be mucinous metaplasia.
- Low-to-intermediate grade lesions [24].
- Well-differentiated endometrioid adenocarcinoma with long, slender, and finger-like papillae is called endometrioid adenocarcinoma with villoglandular pattern.

6.5.1.2 Ancillary Studies

- P53: normal/wild-type staining pattern
- ER/PR: diffusely positive
- p16: patchy positive

6.5.1.3 Differential Diagnosis

- Serous carcinoma

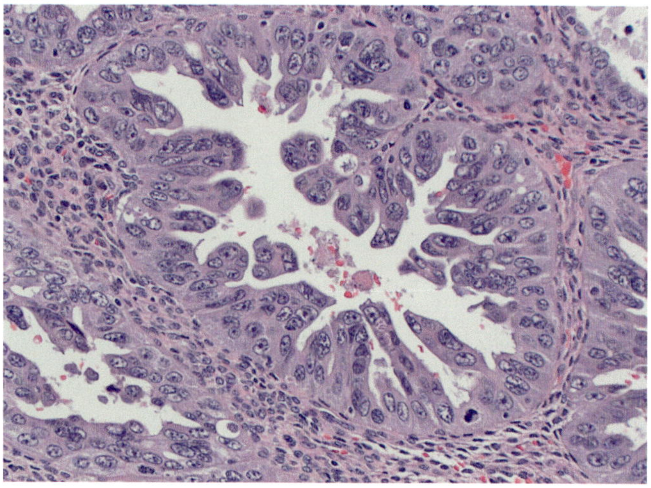

Fig. 6.14 Serous-type endometrial carcinoma. The neoplastic cells have round pleomorphic nuclei and prominent nucleoli (200×)

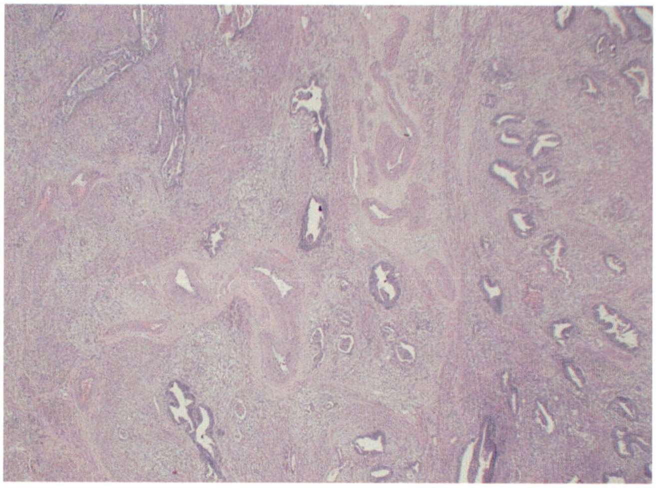

Fig. 6.15 Low-grade endometrioid adenocarcinoma with MELF pattern of myometrial invasion next to large vessels (40×)

- Marked nuclear pleomorphism, round nuclei with prominent eosinophilic nucleoli, numerous mitotic figures, and conspicuous apoptosis (Fig. 6.14)
- P53: mutation pattern
- P16: diffusely positive [25]

6.5.1.4 Clinical Significance

- Low-grade endometrioid adenocarcinoma with papillary architecture might be associated with microcytic elongated and fragmented (MELF) pattern of myometrial invasion and a higher frequency of lymphovascular invasion [26].

6.6 Endometrioid Carcinoma with Microcystic Elongated and Fragmented (MELF) Pattern of Myometrial Invasion

6.6.1 Small Cell Clusters with Abundant Eosinophilic or Vacuolated Cytoplasm Resembling Histiocytes in a Sentinel Lymph Node from a Patient with Endometrial Cancer

6.6.1.1 Key Diagnostic Features

- In the background of prominent fibromyxoid stromal reaction, elongation, and microcyst formation of neoplastic glands with outpouchings or fragmentation [27] (Figs. 6.15 and 6.16).
- The lining epithelium is flattened or might have eosinophilic cytoplasm (Fig. 6.17).
- The associated carcinoma is usually low-grade (FIGO grades 1 and 2) endometrioid type.

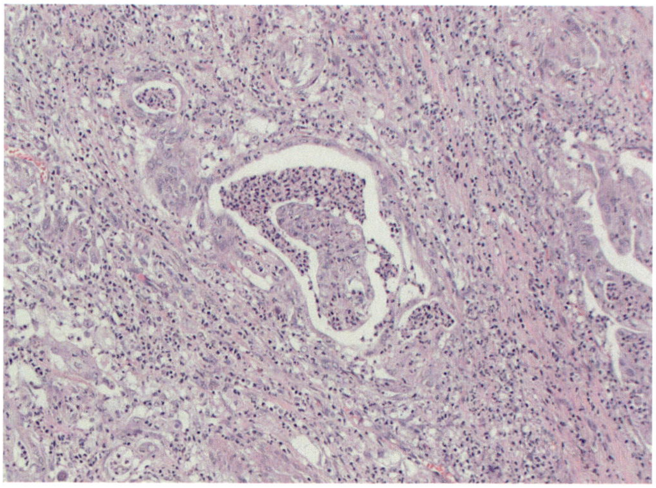

Fig. 6.16 In the background of myxoid stroma and surrounding inflammatory cells, the neoplastic glands form microcysts. The lining epithelium is flattened. There are intraluminal cells (200×)

- MELF pattern of myometrial invasion is associated with a larger tumor size, myometrial invasion of more than 50% of the uterine wall, lymphovascular invasion (Fig. 6.18), lymph node metastasis, papillary architecture, and mucinous differentiation [28].

6.6.1.2 Ancillary Studies

- MELF pattern is associated with a higher risk of isolated tumor cells (ITC) in sentinel lymph nodes of FIGO grade 1 endometrial carcinoma [29]. Cytokeratin facilitates ITC detection in lymph node evaluation.
- The neoplastic epithelium in MELF pattern is positive for p16 and p21 and negative for Ki-67 labeling suggesting growth arrest or cellular senescence [28].

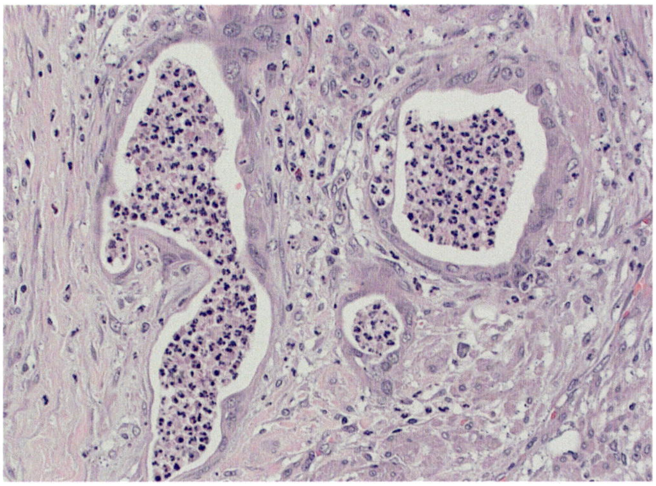

Fig. 6.17 The neoplastic glands are elongated with outpouchings. The lining epithelium is partly flattened or has an eosinophilic cytoplasm (200×)

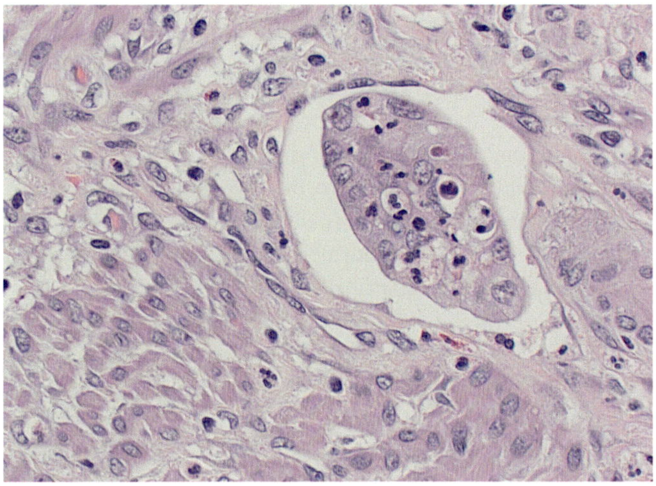

Fig. 6.18 Lymphovascular invasion in close proximity of neoplastic glands within the myometrium (400×)

6.6.1.3 Differential Diagnosis

- The neoplastic glands with flattened lining epithelium might be misinterpreted as lymphovascular space invasion under low-power examination.

6.6.1.4 Clinical Significance

- PORTEC-1 and PORTEC-2 clinical trials failed to show an independent impact of MELF pattern myometrial invasion on the risk of recurrence in patients with early-stage endometrial cancer [30].

6.7 Endometrioid Carcinoma with Progestin Treatment Effect

6.7.1 A 35-Year-Old Woman with FIGO Grade 1 Endometrioid Adenocarcinoma Treated with Progestins

6.7.1.1 Key Diagnostic Features

- Regressive changes in low-grade endometrioid adenocarcinoma (FIGO grade 1) with progesterone treatment effect are variable.
- Neoplastic glands display complex outlines and confluency (cribriform or papillary patterns) [31] (Figs. 6.19 and 6.20). The architectural abnormalities might be pronounced despite a loss of cytologic atypia.
- A decrease in mean gland cellularity, number of mitotic figures, frequency of nucleoli, high nuclear grade, and secretory change are present in post-treatment biopsies [32].
- Metaplasia is common after the hormonal treatment, including mucinous (Fig. 6.21), eosinophilic (Fig. 6.22), and squamous types.
- The morphological features of complete response to therapy include dilated, irregular glands lined by flattened inactive epithelium and decidualized stroma (Fig. 6.23).

6.7.1.2 Ancillary Studies

- Following medroxyprogesterone acetate therapy, ER, PR, Ki67, and Bcl-2 are significantly downregulated [32].

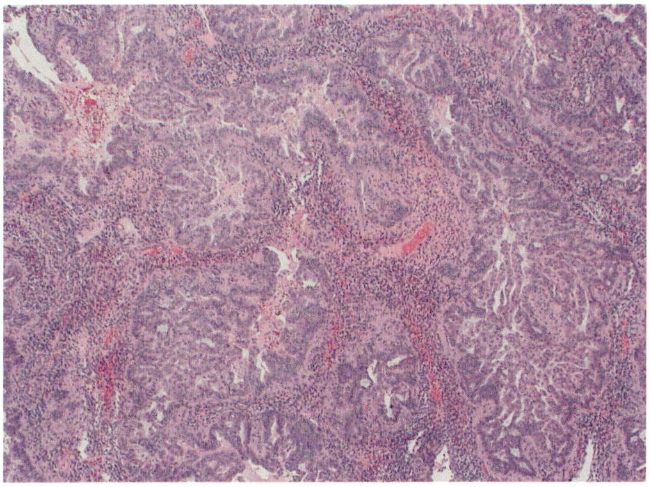

Fig. 6.19 Progestin-treated endometrioid adenocarcinoma with a confluent growth pattern (40×)

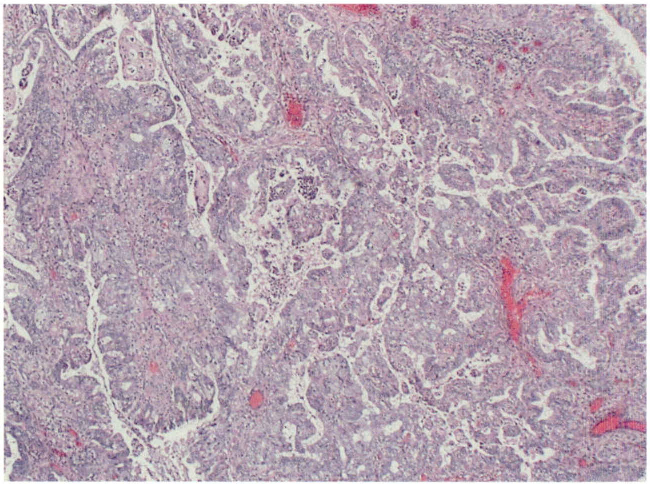

Fig. 6.20 Progestin-treated endometrioid adenocarcinoma with a papillary growth pattern (40×)

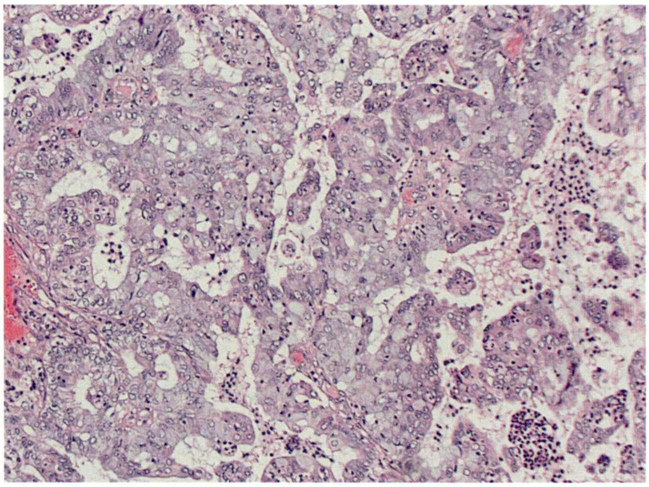

Fig. 6.21 Areas of mucinous metaplasia. Cytological atypia is minimal (200×)

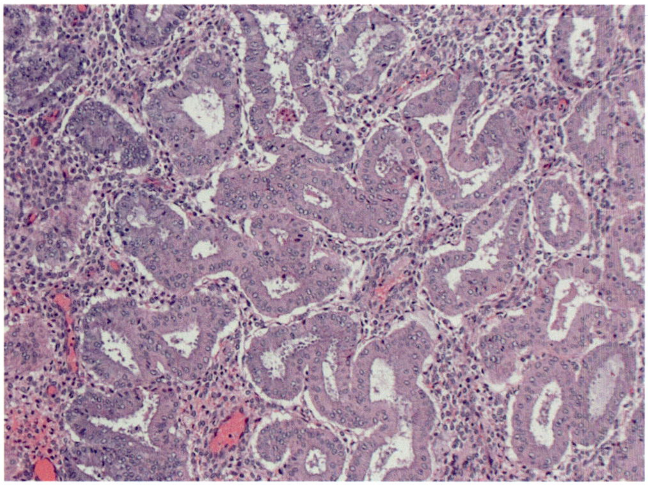

Fig. 6.22 Areas of oxyphilic/eosinophilic metaplasia (200×)

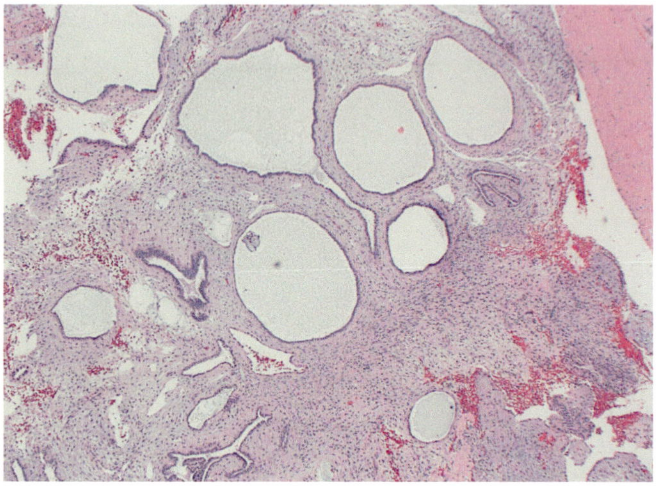

Fig. 6.23 Dilated irregular glands and decidualized endometrial stroma, complete response to therapy

Non-responders to progesterone have tumors with a high baseline proliferation rate with Ki67 [33].

6.7.1.3 Differential Diagnosis

- A review of the initial (untreated) biopsy is essential to evaluate the degree of histological changes.
- The predictors of failure to therapy are persistent cytologic atypia (presence of coarse nuclear chromatin and nucleoli) and architectural abnormalities (presence of glandular crowding, cribriform, and papillary patterns) after 6 months of treatment [31]. A discordant pattern of bland cytology with a confluent architecture is not indicative of a failed response to therapy.

6.7.1.4 Clinical Significance

- No response or partial response to therapy in biopsy specimens guides the treatment options.

6.8 Endometrial Mucinous Metaplasia with Complex Architecture

6.8.1 An Endometrial Biopsy from a 36-Year-Old Woman for Infertility Work-Up

6.8.1.1 Key Diagnostic Features

- Focal crowded and irregular glands with budding, tufting, or branching with a mucinous-type lining epithelium [34].
- Endometrial mucinous metaplasia is classified as A, B, and C subgroups depending on the complexity of proliferation. In type A metaplasia, mucinous epithelial cells present singly or in small tufts within architecturally benign glands and might involve endometrial surface epi-

thelium (Fig. 6.24). Type B proliferations are more complex and consist of mucin-containing epithelial cells forming small pseudoglands with rigid, punched-out spaces without supporting stroma (Figs. 6.25 and 6.26). A conspicuous cytologic atypia or architectural features such as a filiform growth pattern characterize type C alterations [35].

- The mucin-secreting cells can intermix with tubal-type cells, and the nuclear atypia varies from absent to mild.
- Complex mucinous metaplasia (types B and C) may occur in association with complex endometrial hyperplasia and well-differentiated carcinoma.
- Full intestinal-type differentiation is rare and can occur in the endometrial surface or polyps [36].

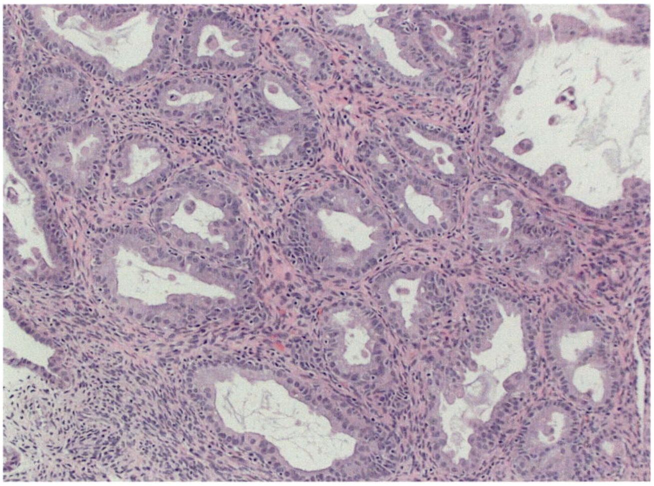

Fig. 6.24 Small micropapillary tufting is within the morphological spectrum of simple mucinous metaplasia (Type A) (100×)

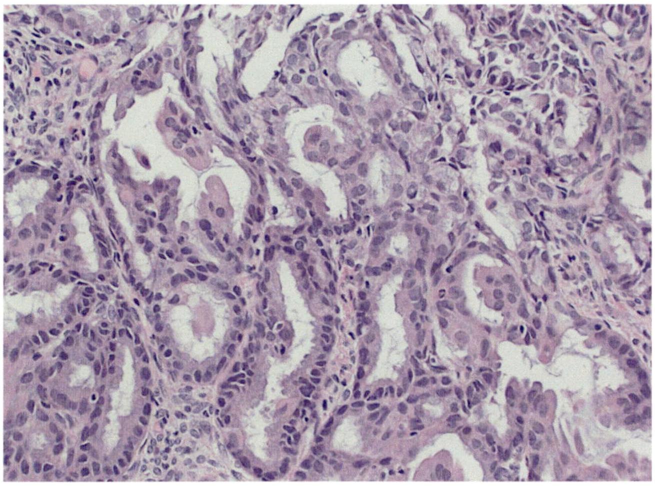

Fig. 6.25 This small mucinous lesion (around 1 mm) has microglandular architecture and micropapillary tufting (Type B). The cytological atypia is minimal (200×)

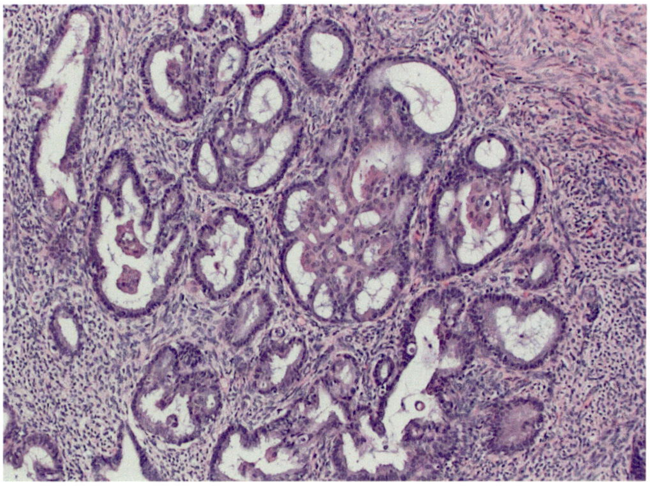

Fig. 6.26 Complex mucinous metaplasia with cribriform architecture in the background of simple mucinous metaplasia (100×)

6.8.1.2 Ancillary Studies

- Mutations in *KRAS* are identified in 89% of cases with papillary mucinous metaplasia, in contrast to a rate of 14% in simple mucinous metaplasia [37].
- Endometrial mucinous metaplasia can express vimentin and variable staining for estrogen and progesterone receptors. No immunoreactivity with carcinoembryonic antigen (CEA) and p53 is detected [38].

6.8.1.3 Differential Diagnosis

- Endocervical microglandular hyperplasia in biopsy/curetting specimens
  - The endocervical glands with a homogeneous architecture, prominent subnuclear vacuoles, minimal cytologic atypia or mitotic activity, and reserve-like subsurface epithelial populations are compatible with endocervical microglandular hyperplasia.
- Endometrioid carcinoma with mucinous features
  - Mucinous adenocarcinomas associated with a florid mucinous endometrial metaplasia can be cytologically bland with minimal mitotic activity. The lack of endometrial stromal cells between complex glands is diagnostic for carcinoma.
  - In addition to diffuse and more complex glandular architecture in carcinoma, squamous-type metaplasia can be present.
  - Mucinous metaplasia without an associated carcinoma or endometrial hyperplasia often exhibits small micropapillary projections with uniform nuclei and rare mitotic figures [39].

6.8.1.4 Clinical Significance

- Mucinous metaplasia is a reactive process in cervical stenosis or agenesis [34]. Architecturally complex mucinous metaplasia is associated with endometrial hyperplasia or mucinous-type endometrial carcinoma [35, 40].

- Mucinous changes occur as a spectrum of histological findings ranging from metaplasia to carcinoma, synchronously involving the cervix, uterine corpus, fallopian tubes, and ovaries in patients with *STK-11* gene mutations (Peutz-Jeghers syndrome) [41].

6.9 Polypoid Adenomyoma (PAM)

6.9.1 Imaging Studies Are Consistent with Submucosal Leiomyoma in a 40-Year-Old Woman

6.9.1.1 Key Diagnostic Features

- An adenomyoma is composed of endometrial glands and surrounding endometrial stroma within a leiomyomatous stroma. Adenomyomas can present as a polypoid lesion (PAM) of the endometrium or a nodular lesion within the uterine wall.
- The endometrial glands are generally spaced without back-to-back arrangements and range from small, simple glands to more irregularly shaped glands and large cysts (Fig. 6.27).
- The glandular epithelium is surrounded by endometrial stroma and smooth muscle fibers (Fig. 6.28).
- There might be sex cord-like elements and cells with bizarre nuclei within the stroma [42].
- The most common site is the uterine corpus, followed by the cervix and broad ligament [43].

6.9.1.2 Ancillary Studies

- N/A.

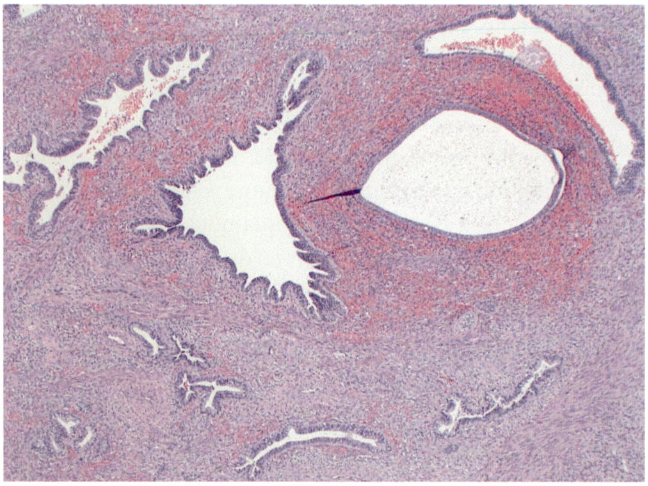

Fig. 6.27 Well-spaced, dilated endometrial glands and stroma within a leiomyomatous stroma of a polypoid lesion (40×)

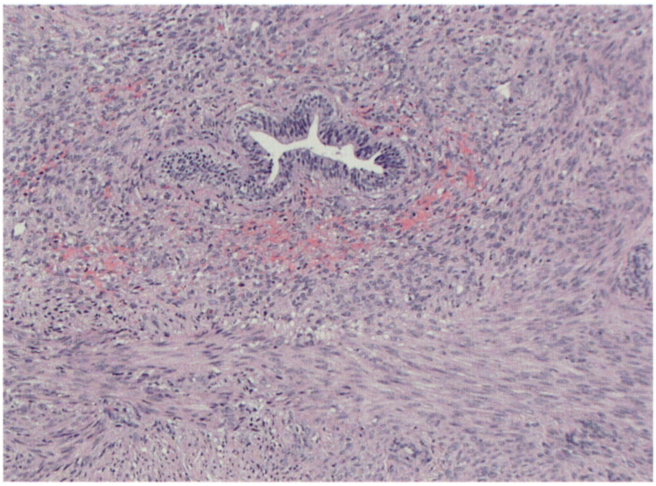

Fig. 6.28 Proliferative-type endometrial gland, stroma, and surrounding benign smooth muscle (100×)

6.9.1.3 Differential Diagnosis

- Atypical polypoid adenomyoma
  - Irregular, crowded endometrial glands with cytological atypia and squamous morules embedded in a cellular myofibroblastic stroma.
  - See Part II, Sect. 6.10.
- Mullerian Adenosarcoma
  - Broad papillary fronds are covered with epithelium projecting into cystic spaces lined by columnar or cuboidal endometrial-type epithelium.
  - See Part II, Sect. 7.13.

6.9.1.4 Clinical Significance

- PAM is a benign biphasic lesion of the gynecological tract.

6.10 Atypical Polypoid Adenomyoma (APA)

6.10.1 A 39-Year-Old Woman with Infertility

6.10.1.1 Key Diagnostic Features

- Common anatomical sites are the lower uterine segment and the cervix, followed by the uterine corpus.
- Sessile/flat or exophytic polyps.
- Irregular, crowded glands within a fibromyoblastic stroma. The stromal cells form short, interlacing fascicles (Figs. 6.29 and 6.30).
- Squamous morular metaplasia with or without necrosis is frequently associated with the glandular component (Fig. 6.31).
- The cytological atypia is mild to moderate in the glandular epithelium.

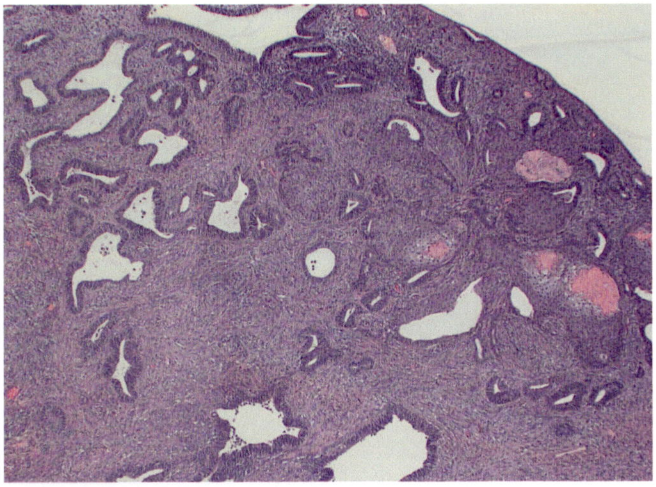

Fig. 6.29 The glandular crowding of APA within a myofibroblastic stroma (40×)

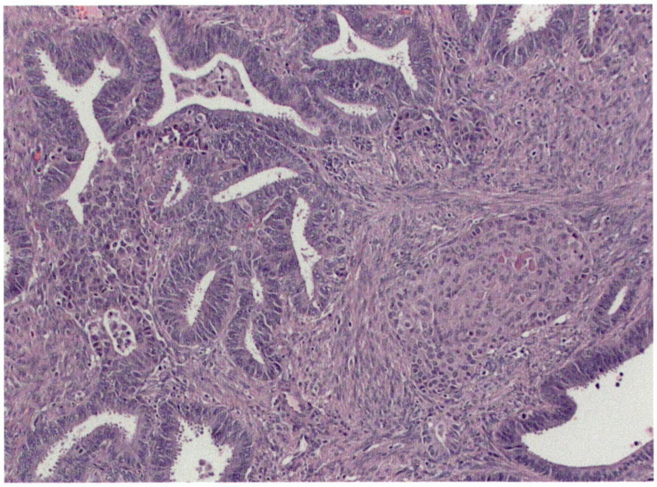

Fig. 6.30 The myofibroblastic stroma forms short fascicules. The glandular epithelium has mild to moderate cytological atypia (100×)

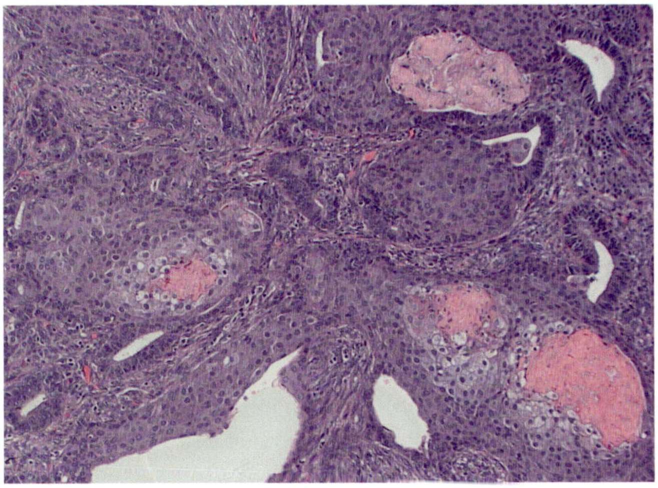

Fig. 6.31 The squamous morular epithelium is associated with glandular epithelium. There might be keratin or necrosis at the center of the squamous epithelium (100×)

6.10.1.2 Ancillary Studies: (Limited, Usually Not Required)

- The stromal p16 expression might be helpful in differential diagnosis from myoinvasive endometrial carcinoma. P16 is diffusely (10 out of 12 cases) expressed in the stroma of APA, and it is negative in the myoinvasive endometrial carcinoma [44]. SATB2 has diffuse nuclear immunoreactivity in stromal cells of APA in contrast to negative staining of endometrial polyp, adenomyoma, and adenosarcoma [45].

6.10.1.3 Differential Diagnosis

- Well-differentiated endometrioid adenocarcinoma with myometrial invasion and desmoplastic reaction (biopsy specimens)
  - The stromal component of APA has short fascicules. The normal myometrium has elongated smooth muscle fibers. Identifying tissue fragments of adenocarcinoma without myometrial invasion supports cancer diagnosis.
  - The myomatous stroma of APA is negative for caldesmon and positive for SMA and desmin [46].
- Adenomyomatous polyps/adenomyoma
  - See Part II, Sect. 6.9.

6.10.1.4 Clinical Significance

- In a recent metanalysis, overall risks of the recurrence and progression to cancer are 28.9% and 16.6%, respectively [47]. APA is associated with infertility due to the anatomic location [48].

6.11 Mesonephric-Like Adenocarcinoma

6.11.1 A 55-Year-Old Woman with Vaginal Discharge

6.11.1.1 Key Diagnostic Features

- Multiple architectural patterns, including tubular, glandular, retiform (Fig. 6.32), papillary (Fig. 6.33), solid, ductal, glomeruloid, and spindle-cell component, can be present in combinations [49].
- The lumens of glands/tubules are filled with dense eosinophilic secretions.
- The nuclei are often crowded, open, and vesicular and resemble those of papillary thyroid carcinoma with pseudo-inclusions and grooves (Fig. 6.34).
- Mitotic activity is variable.
- No mucinous or squamous differentiation.
- No histologic grading system.
- Might be diagnosed in the endometrium or uterine wall (Fig. 6.35).

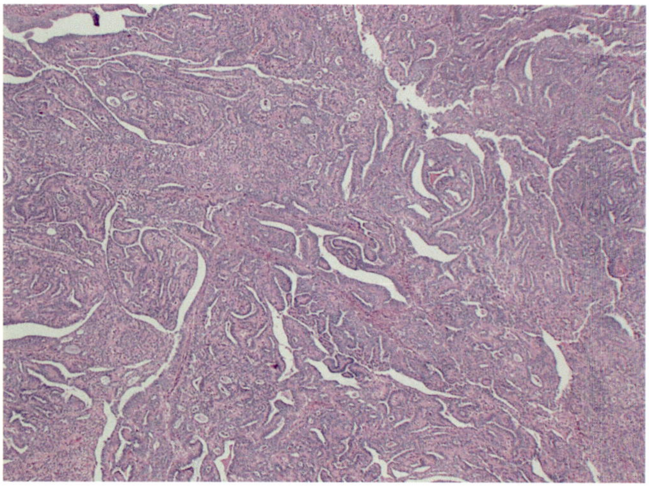

Fig. 6.32 The architectural patterns are tubular, solid, and reticular (slit-like space). Dense eosinophilic secretions are present in lumens of tubules (40×)

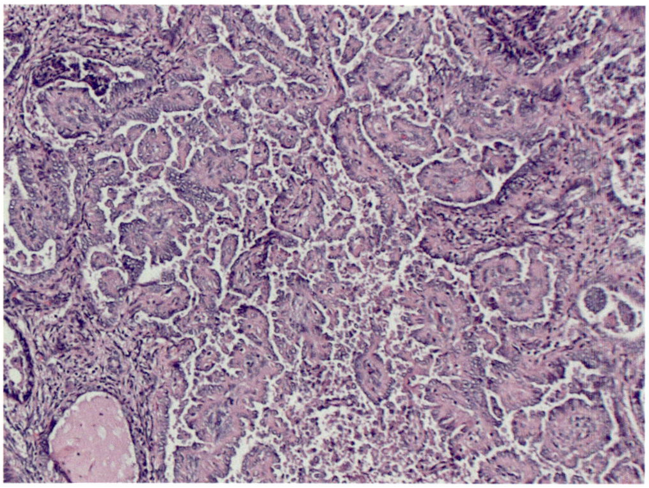

Fig. 6.33 Papillary/micropapillary architecture of mesonephric-like carcinoma of the endometrium (100×)

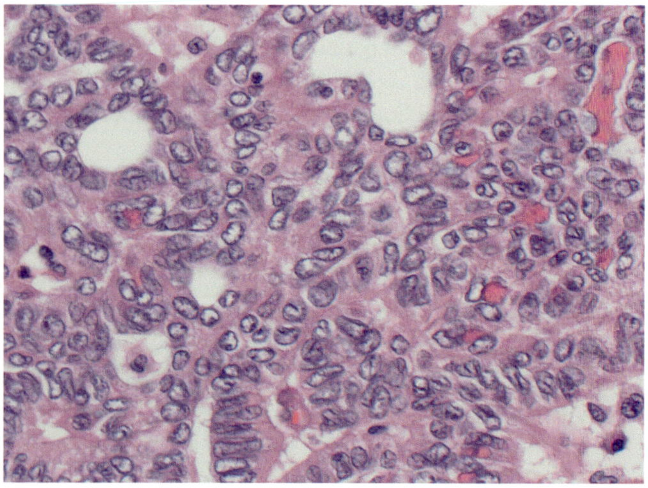

Fig. 6.34 Nuclei are crowded and vesicular with a coffee-bean appearance and rare pseudo-inclusions

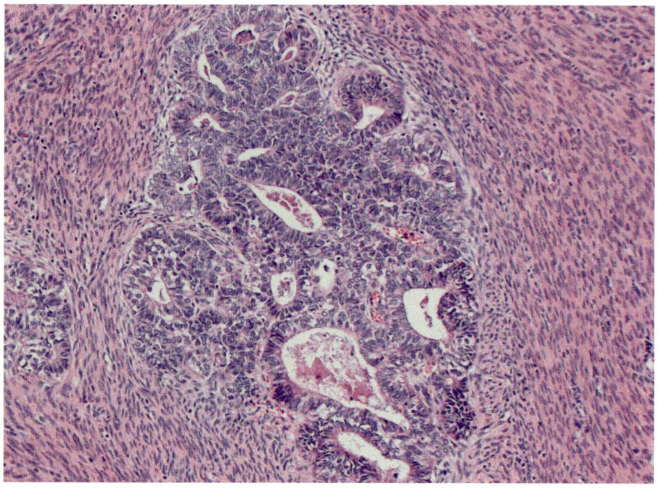

Fig. 6.35 This lesion is at the uterine wall in a postmenopausal woman (100×). The endometrium is benign with atrophic changes

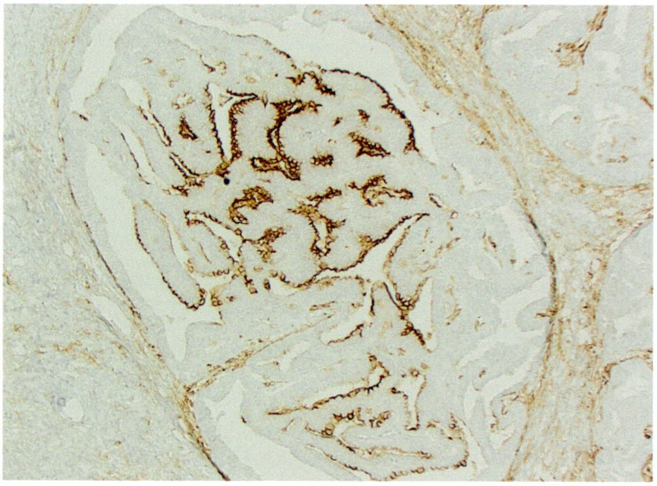

Fig. 6.36 CD10 has a patchy luminal staining pattern (200×)

6.11.1.2 Ancillary Studies

- Positive stains: GATA3, PAX8, CD10 (luminal) (Fig. 6.36), TTF1, calretinin, and AR [50]
- P53: normal/wild-type staining
- Negative stains: ER, Napsin A, and AMACR
- Somatic *KRAS* mutations, *BRAF* hotspot mutations, *PIK3CA,* and *PTEN* mutations [51]

6.11.1.3 Differential Diagnosis

- Endometrioid adenocarcinoma
  - Overlapping glandular and papillary (villoglandular) architectural patterns.
  - The nuclei in low-grade endometrioid adenocarcinoma are pseudostratified and columnar cell type.
  - Squamous or mucinous differentiation might be present in endometrioid adenocarcinoma.
  - ER/PR: positive; p16: patchy positive.

- Clear cell carcinoma
  - Tubulocystic, papillary, and solid architectural patterns
  - At least focal significant cytological atypia
  - Various cell types, including low cuboidal, polyhedral, hobnail, and flattened cells
  - Napsin A and AMACR: Positive
  - GATA3, CD10: negative

6.11.1.4 Clinical Significance

- Limited experience due to rare incidence. Small case series support clinically aggressive behavior. Diagnosis is usually at an advanced disease stage. Recurrences can occur at local or distant sites with a predilection of pulmonary metastasis [52].

6.12 Undifferentiated/Dedifferentiated Carcinoma

6.12.1 A 60-Year-Old Woman with Postmenopausal Bleeding

6.12.1.1 Key Diagnostic Features

- Monomorphic neoplasm composed of small- to intermediate-sized dyscohesive cells arranged in sheets without any apparent glandular differentiation (undifferentiated carcinoma).
- Undifferentiated carcinoma lacks morphological features of any epithelial differentiation.
- A component of FIGO grade 1 or 2 endometrioid carcinoma is present in 40% of undifferentiated carcinoma [53] (dedifferentiated carcinoma).
- When the differentiated component is available, there is a sharp separation from the undifferentiated component (Fig. 6.37).

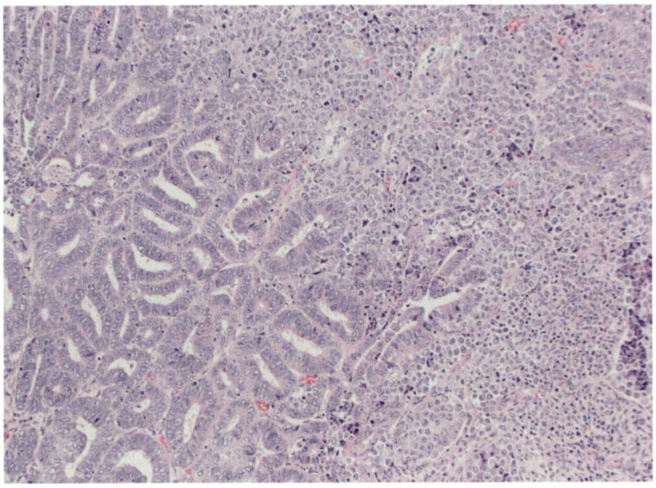

Fig. 6.37 Abrupt transition between differentiated and undifferentiated components of dedifferentiated endometrial carcinoma (100×)

- There might be focal marked nuclear pleomorphism, broad zones of necrosis (Fig. 6.38), dyscohesive cells (Fig. 6.39), rhabdoid-cell morphology (Fig. 6.40), multinucleation, spindling, and abrupt keratinization within the undifferentiated component.

6.12.1.2 Ancillary Studies

- Focal or diffuse EMA and cytokeratin expression in 80% of cases.
- Focal neuroendocrine marker expression (less than 10% of the lesion by definition).
- Lack of PAX8 expression in 83% of cases [54].
- The majority of samples (69%) from undifferentiated/dedifferentiated carcinomas have abnormal mismatch repair protein (MMR) testing results [55].
- Loss of BRG-1 (*SMARCA4*), INI-1 (*SMARCB1*), and *ARID1A* might be detected by immunohistochemistry [56].

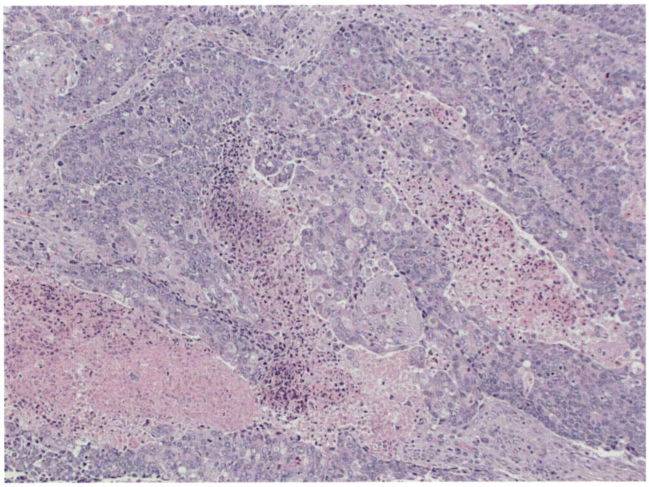

Fig. 6.38 The neoplastic cells are separated by large zones of necrosis (100×)

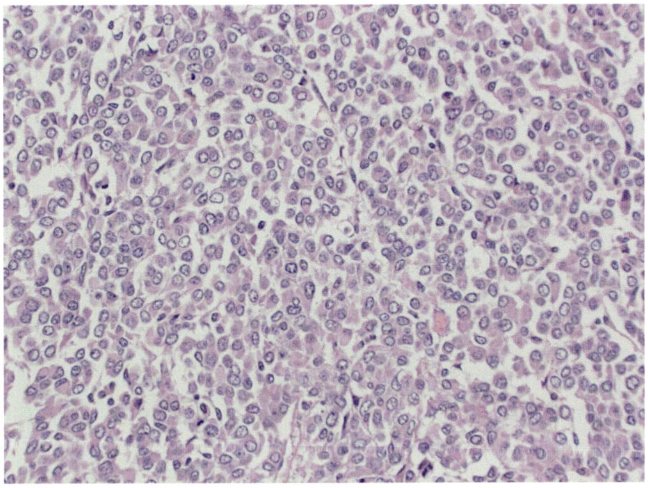

Fig. 6.39 Relatively monomorphic and dyscohesive cells (200×)

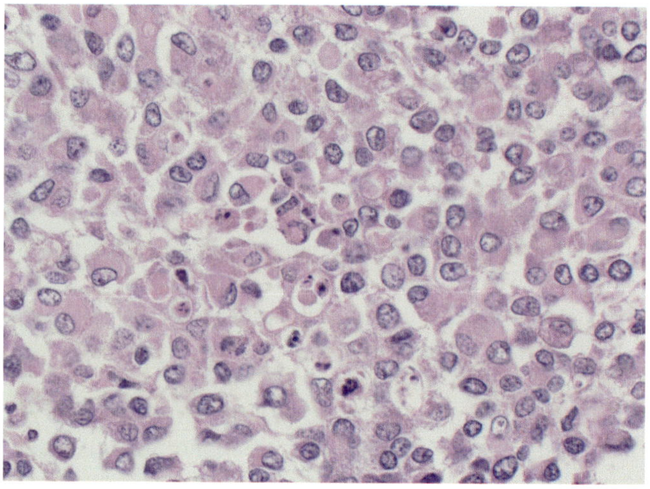

Fig. 6.40 Rhabdoid cell morphology (400×)

6.12.1.3 Differential Diagnosis

- FIGO grade 3 endometrioid adenocarcinoma
  - Cohesive cells with at least focal glandular formation or squamous differentiation.
  - PAX8 expression is usually retained.
- Lymphoma and plasmacytoma versus undifferentiated carcinoma
  - Diffuse sheets of atypical, dyscohesive cells with or without necrosis.
  - CD45 (lymphoma) and CD138 (plasmacytoma) are positive.
- *SMARCA4*-deficient uterine sarcoma
  - Younger age (median 24 years).
  - The morphology might be indistinguishable alone [57]. The presence of focal and vague phyllodiform architecture and stromal hyalinization favors the diagnosis of SMARCA4-deficient sarcoma.
  - Microsatellite instability is not detected [57].

6.12.1.4 Clinical Significance

- The 5-year overall survival is worse than FIGO grade 3 endometrioid adenocarcinoma (84% for stage I/II, 38% for stage III, and 12% for stage IV disease) [55].

6.13 Clear Cell Carcinoma (CCC), Oxyphilic Type

6.13.1 A 70-Year-Old Woman with Vaginal Spotting

6.13.1.1 Key Diagnostic Features

- Tubules, cysts, or solid areas lined by cuboidal cells with abundant oxyphilic (eosinophilic) cytoplasm and well-defined cell borders. Scattered eosinophilic globules are nonspecific findings (Fig. 6.41).
- The signet ring-type cells might be present (Fig. 6.42) in addition to mucinous, hobnail, and attenuated cells.
- In most cases, at least a focal typical CCC component is identified with adequate sampling (Fig. 6.43).
- More frequently reported as a component of ovarian CCC [58].

6.13.1.2 Ancillary Studies

- Reactive with Napsin A and HNF-beta
- Negative or weak ER and PR expression

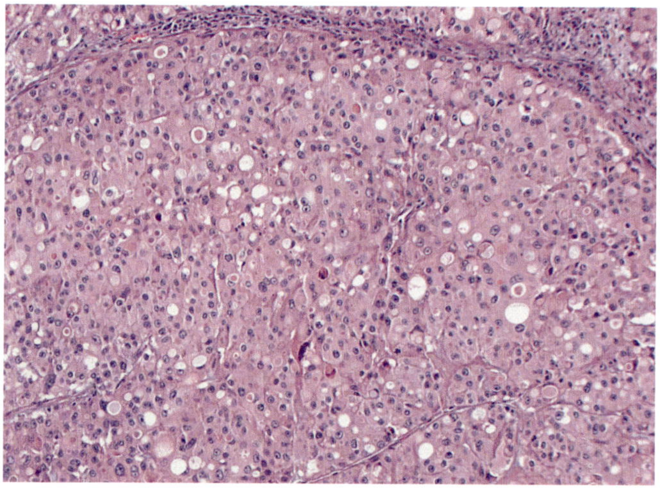

Fig. 6.41 The architectural pattern is solid in this area. The neoplastic cells are large, round to polygonal, with well-defined cell borders. The cytoplasm is abundant and eosinophilic. Nuclei are vesicular and pleomorphic with prominent nucleoli. Scattered hyaline globules are in the field (100×)

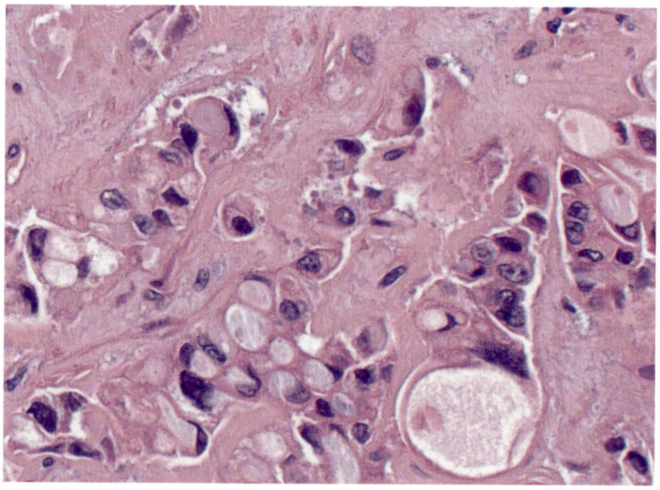

Fig. 6.42 Signet ring-type cells within the hyalinized stroma (200×)

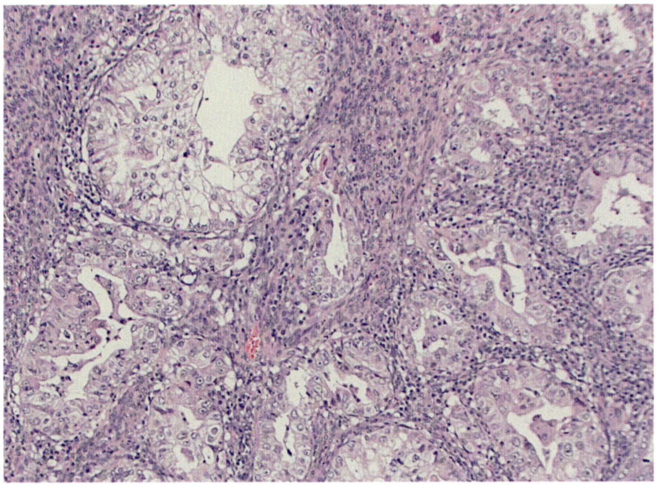

Fig. 6.43 Typical minor clear cell carcinoma component is focally present (100×)

6.13.1.3 Differential Diagnosis

- Yolk sac tumor (YST)
  - Rare tumor of the endometrium in adult patients.
  - YST can be mixed tumors with other epithelial or germ cell tumor components.
  - All patterns of YST described in the ovaries can be a component of the lesion
  - See Part II, Sect. 6.15.
- Metastatic renal cell carcinoma or hepatocellular carcinoma to the endometrium
  - Extremely rare, clinical correlation is required.
  - AMACR, vimentin, and CD10 are positive in the oncocytic variant of renal cell carcinoma.
  - HepPar1, pCEA, and CD10 are positive in hepatocellular carcinoma.

6.13.1.4 Clinical Significance

- Presence of oxyphilic cells in the ovarian CCC is not associated with clinical prognosis [59]

6.14 Mixed Neuroendocrine and Endometrioid Carcinoma (NEEC)

6.14.1 A 65-Year-Old Woman with Endometrial Thickening by Imaging Studies

6.14.1.1 Key Diagnostic Features

- The morphological features of endometrial neuroendocrine carcinoma (NEC) are similar to those of NEC at other anatomical sites.
- The majority of NEC in the endometrium are admixed with other carcinoma types, more commonly endometrioid type (Fig. 6.44) [60, 61]. The pathology report should include individual tumor types and their approximate percentages.
- The small cell NEC is characterized by a high nuclear to cytoplasmic ratio, nuclear hyperchromasia, molding, and crush artifact. There might be focal spindling of the nuclei. The large cell NEC has appreciable cytoplasm and coarse nuclear chromatin, often with prominent nucleoli (Fig. 6.45). The architectural patterns include insular/nested, trabecular, pseudoglandular, and solid types.
- Broad zones of necrosis (Fig. 6.46) and high mitotic activity are common findings in small- and large-cell NEC.

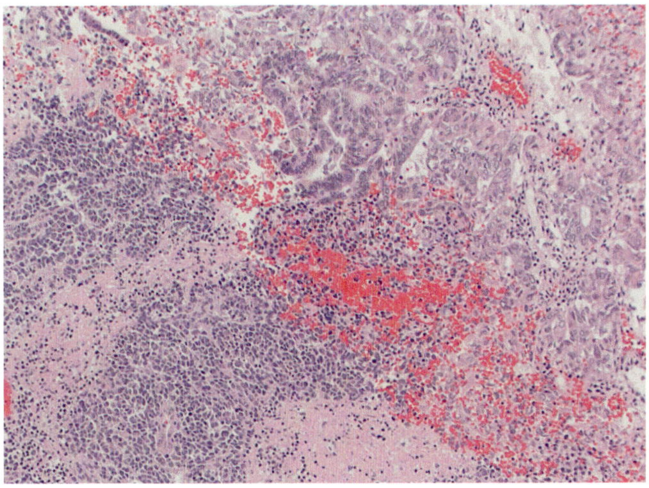

Fig. 6.44 The area of sharp demarcation between neuroendocrine carcinoma and adenocarcinoma (100×)

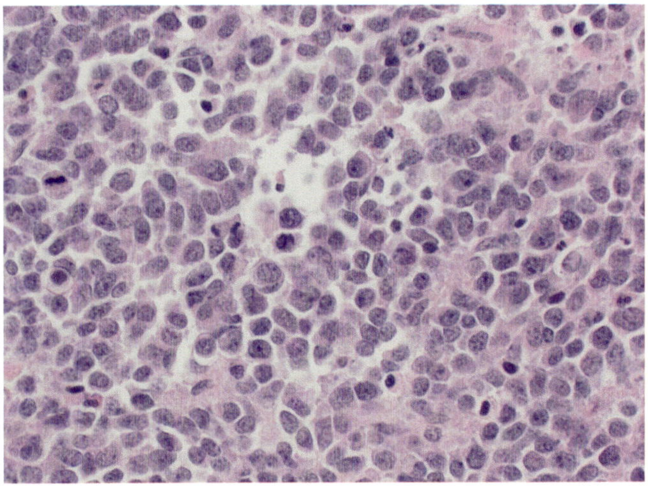

Fig. 6.45 The neoplastic cells have typical nuclear features, including salt and pepper chromatin and prominent nucleoli. The mitotic figures are frequent (200×)

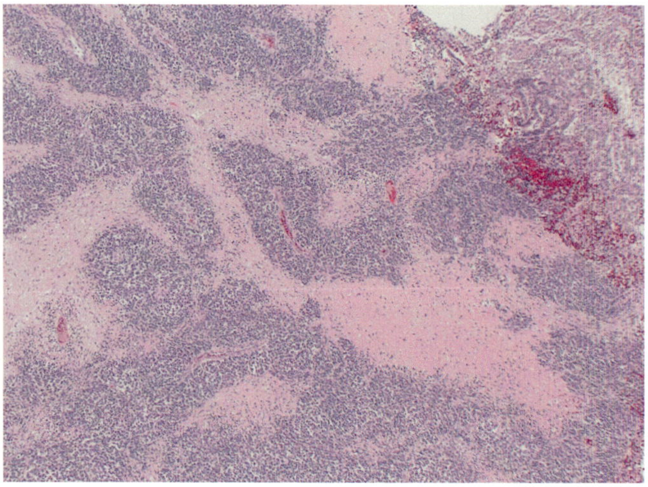

Fig. 6.46 Broad zones of necrosis are scattered among small blue cells (40×)

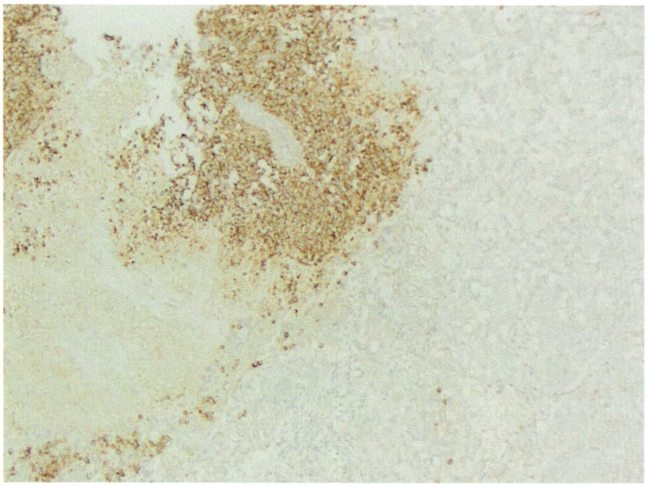

Fig. 6.47 Synaptophysin highlights the NEC component, but it is not reactive in adenocarcinoma (40×)

6.14.1.2 Ancillary Studies

- One or more neuroendocrine markers (synaptophysin, chromogranin, CD56, and INSM1) are positive (Fig. 6.47).
- NEC of the endometrium might rarely be TTF1 positive (1 sample out of 18).
- NEC of the endometrium is associated with microsatellite instability (8 samples out of 18) [62].
- NEC of the endometrium is molecularly heterogeneous and might fall into all four subgroups of The Cancer Genome Atlas (TCGA) molecular classification [63].

6.14.1.3 Differential Diagnosis

- Dedifferentiated/undifferentiated carcinoma
  - Solid pattern with dyscohesive cells.
  - Neuroendocrine maker expression is limited to less than 10% of the lesion by definition.
  - See Part II, Sect. 6.12.
- FIGO grade 3 endometrioid carcinoma
  - Focal gland/acini formation
  - Squamous or mucinous differentiation

6.14.1.4 Clinical Significance

- The 5-year survival is 38% for NEC and 68.8% for FIGO grade 3 endometrioid carcinoma [64]. Compared to patients with endometrioid adenocarcinoma, patients with NEC present with a later disease stage and have decreased survival. Patients with pure NEC have a significantly worse prognosis compared to mixed cell types [65].

6.15 Yolk Sac Tumor (YST) of the Endometrium

6.15.1 A 68-Year-Old Female Presented with Intermittent Vaginal Spotting for 9 Months

6.15.1.1 Key Diagnostic Features

- The histologic patterns include microcystic/reticular, glandular, solid, papillary, and hepatoid types. An admixture of histologic patterns is frequently observed (Figs. 6.48 and 6.49).
- Around 45% of uterine YST is associated with somatic components (epithelial carcinoma) and 15% with a second germ cell component. Schiller-Duval bodies can be present in around 23% of cases [66].

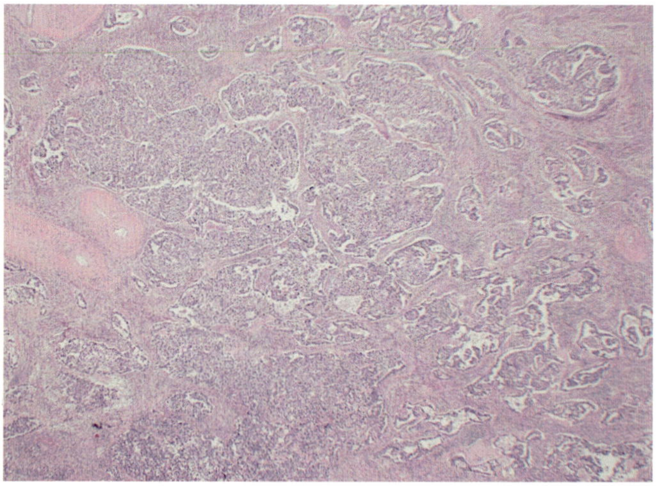

Fig. 6.48 YST invading myometrium (40×)

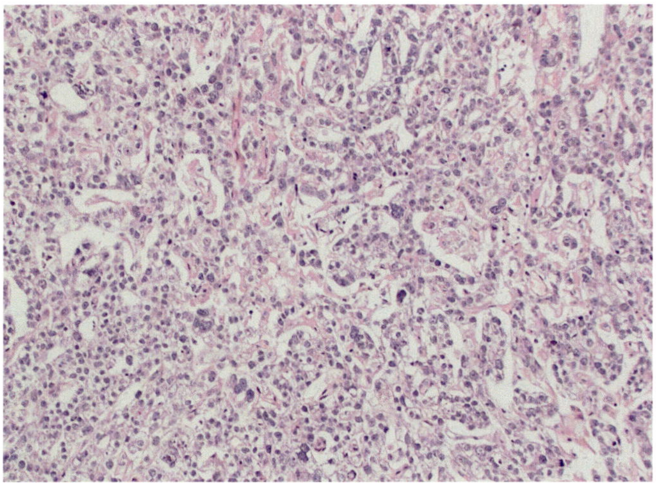

Fig. 6.49 Microcytic and solid patterns of YST (100×)

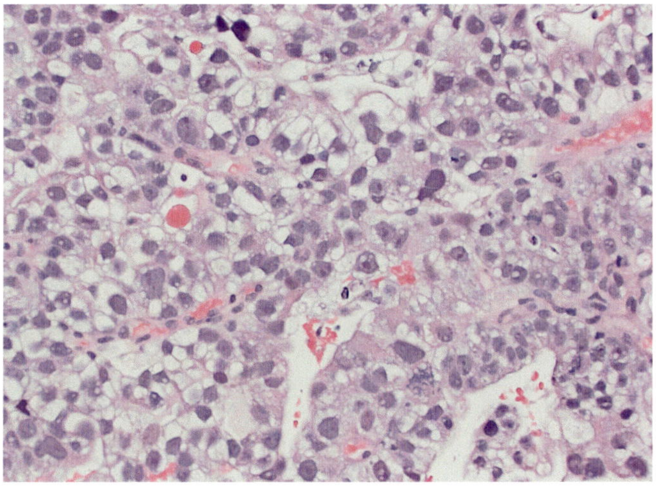

Fig. 6.50 The nuclear grade is high, and there is cytoplasmic clearing. The hyaline bodies are in the field (200×)

- Marked cytological atypia (Fig. 6.50) and easily identifiable mitotic figures are typical findings. The cytoplasm might be scant to abundant and either clear or eosinophilic. The subnuclear or supranuclear cytoplasmic vacuolation might be prominent or a focal feature.
- Eosinophil hyaline globules are nonspecific findings.

6.15.1.2 Ancillary Studies

- Polyphenotypic marker expression (epithelial and germ cell markers).
- Alpha-fetoprotein (AFP): a specific marker of YST.
- SALL4 (Fig. 6.51), glypican-3, cytokeratin 7 and 20, CDX2, Villin, and PAX8: variable expression
- EMA: −/+ [67]
- GATA3: expressed in primitive patterns of YST (reticular/microcystic, polyvesicular, and polyembryoma) but not in differentiated forms (glandular and hepatoid) [68]

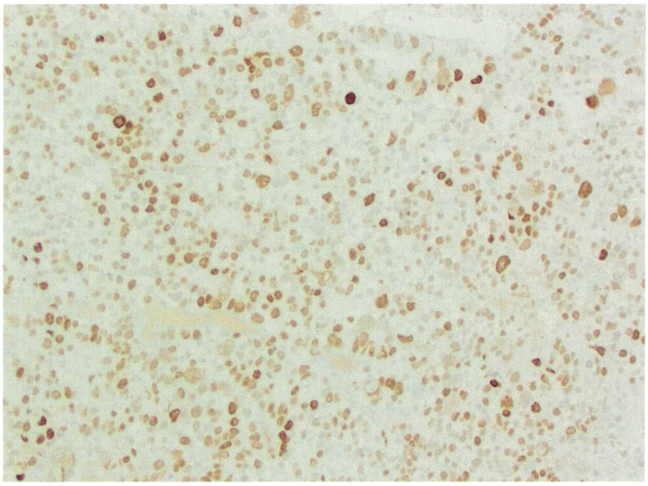

Fig. 6.51 Germ cell marker (SALL4) nuclear expression (100×)

6.15.1.3 Differential Diagnosis (Depends on Prominent Architectural Pattern)

- Clear cell carcinoma
  - The architectural patterns are solid, papillary, and tubular.
  - Hobnail, clear, eosinophilic, mucinous, signet ring, and attenuated cells.
  - Napsin A and PAX8: Positive.
  - SALL4, Villin, and AFP: Negative.
- Metastatic colon cancer (glandular/intestinal architectural patterns of YST)
  - Presence of "dirty" central necrosis
  - Lack of cytoplasmic clearing or vacuoles
  - Lack of germ cell marker expression

6.15.1.4 Clinical Significance

- The benefit of germ cell-appropriate chemotherapy in somatically derived YST is not clear for postmenopausal women.

References

1. Clement PB, Young RH. Endometrioid carcinoma of the uterine corpus: a review of its pathology with emphasis on recent advances and problematic aspects. Adv Anat Pathol. 2002;9(3):145–84.
2. Murray SK, Clement PB, Young RH. Endometrioid carcinomas of the uterine corpus with sex cord-like formations, hyalinization, and other unusual morphologic features: a report of 31 cases of a neoplasm that may be confused with carcinosarcoma and other uterine neoplasms. Am J Surg Pathol. 2005;29(2):157–66.
3. Travaglino A, Arciuolo D, Santoro A, Raffone A, Raimondo D, Casadio P, et al. Corded and hyalinized endometrioid carcinoma: summary of clinical, histological, immunohistochemical and molecular data. Pathol Res Pract. 2023;247:154515.
4. Rabban JT, Gilks CB, Malpica A, Matias-Guiu X, Mittal K, Mutter GL, et al. Issues in the differential diagnosis of uterine low-grade endometrioid carcinoma, including mixed endometrial carcinomas:

recommendations from the International Society of Gynecological Pathologists. Int J Gynecol Pathol. 2019;38 Suppl 1(Iss 1 Suppl 1):S25–39.
5. Wani Y, Saegusa M, Notohara K. Aberrant nuclear beta-catenin expression in the spindle or corded cells in so-called corded and hyalinized endometrioid carcinomas. Another critical role of the unique morphological feature. Histol Histopathol. 2009;24(2):149–55.
6. Safdar NS, Thompson EF, Gilks CB, Isacson C, Bennett JA, Clarke B, et al. Corded and hyalinized and spindled endometrioid endometrial carcinoma: a clinicopathologic and molecular analysis of 9 tumors based on the TCGA classifier. Am J Surg Pathol. 2021;45(8):1038–46.
7. Cantrell LA, Blank SV, Duska LR. Uterine carcinosarcoma: a review of the literature. Gynecol Oncol. 2015;137(3):581–8.
8. Patel V, Kipp B, Schoolmeester JK. Corded and hyalinized mesonephric-like adenocarcinoma of the uterine corpus: report of a case mimicking endometrioid carcinoma. Hum Pathol. 2019;86:243–8.
9. D'Angelo E, Ali RH, Espinosa I, Lee CH, Huntsman DG, Gilks B, et al. Endometrial stromal sarcomas with sex cord differentiation are associated with PHF1 rearrangement. Am J Surg Pathol. 2013;37(4):514–21.
10. Ladwig NR, Umetsu SE, Zaloudek C, Rabban J, Garg K. Corded and hyalinized endometrioid adenocarcinoma (CHEC) of the uterine corpus are characterized by CTNNB1 mutations and can show adverse clinical outcomes. Int J Gynecol Pathol. 2021;40(2):103–15.
11. Kumar NB, Hart WR. Metastases to the uterine corpus from extragenital cancers. A clinicopathologic study of 63 cases. Cancer. 1982;50(10):2163–9.
12. Braun A, Reddy S, Cheng L, Gattuso P, Yan L. Clinicopathologic review of metastatic breast cancer to the gynecologic tract. Int J Gynecol Pathol. 2023;42(4):414–20.
13. Liedtke C, Broglio K, Moulder S, Hsu L, Kau SW, Symmans WF, et al. Prognostic impact of discordance between triple-receptor measurements in primary and recurrent breast cancer. Ann Oncol. 2009;20(12):1953–8.
14. Miettinen M, McCue PA, Sarlomo-Rikala M, Rys J, Czapiewski P, Wazny K, et al. GATA3: a multispecific but potentially useful marker in surgical pathology: a systematic analysis of 2500 epithelial and nonepithelial tumors. Am J Surg Pathol. 2014;38(1):13–22.
15. Lowenthal BM, Lin GY, Tipps AMP, Hosseini M. Adenocarcinoma ex-goblet cell carcinoid of the appendix with metastatic peritoneal spread to Meckel's diverticulum and endometriosis. Int J Surg Pathol. 2017;25(7):623–8.
16. Reid MD, Basturk O, Shaib WL, Xue Y, Balci S, Choi HJ, et al. Adenocarcinoma ex-goblet cell carcinoid (appendiceal-type crypt cell adenocarcinoma) is a morphologically distinct entity with highly aggressive behavior and frequent association with peritoneal/intra-abdominal dissemination: an analysis of 77 cases. Mod Pathol. 2016;29(10):1243–53.
17. Arif SH, Mohammed AA, Mohammed FR. Metastatic invasive lobular carcinoma of the breast to the endometrium presenting with abnormal uterine bleeding; Case report. Ann Med Surg (Lond). 2020;51:41–3.
18. Briki R, Cherif O, Bannour B, Hidar S, Boughizane S, Khairi H. Uncommon metastases of invasive lobular breast cancer to the endometrium: a report of two cases and review of the literature. Pan Afr Med J. 2018;30:268.
19. Wong RW, Ralte A, Grondin K, Talia KL, McCluggage WG. Endometrial gastric (gastrointestinal)-type mucinous lesions: report of a series illustrating the spectrum of benign and malignant lesions. Am J Surg Pathol. 2020;44(3):406–19.
20. Worley MJ Jr, Davis M, Berhie SH, Muto MG, Feltmate CM, Berkowitz RS, et al. Mucinous differentiation does not impact stage or risk of recurrence among patients with grade 1, endometrioid type, endometrial carcinoma. Gynecol Oncol. 2014;135(1):54–7.
21. Hariri N, Qarmali M, Fadare O. Endometrial serous carcinoma with clear-cell change: frequency and immunohistochemical analysis. Int J Surg Pathol. 2018;26(2):126–34.
22. Silva EG, Young RH. Endometrioid neoplasms with clear cells: a report of 21 cases in which the alteration is not of typical secretory type. Am J Surg Pathol. 2007;31(8):1203–8.
23. Hoang LN, Han G, McConechy M, Lau S, Chow C, Gilks CB, et al. Immunohistochemical characterization of prototypical endometrial clear cell carcinoma—diagnostic utility of HNF-1β and oestrogen receptor. Histopathology. 2014;64(4):585–96.
24. Malpica A. How to approach the many faces of endometrioid carcinoma. Mod Pathol. 2016;29(Suppl 1):S29–44.
25. Yemelyanova A, Ji H, Shih Ie M, Wang TL, Wu LS, Ronnett BM. Utility of p16 expression for distinction of uterine serous carcinomas from endometrial endometrioid and endocervical adenocarcinomas: immunohistochemical analysis of 201 cases. Am J Surg Pathol. 2009;33(10):1504–14.
26. Ambros RA, Ballouk F, Malfetano JH, Ross JS. Significance of papillary (villoglandular) differentiation in endometrioid carcinoma of the uterus. Am J Surg Pathol. 1994;18(6):569–75.
27. Murray SK, Young RH, Scully RE. Unusual epithelial and stromal changes in myoinvasive endometrioid adenocarcinoma: a study of their frequency, associated diagnostic problems, and prognostic significance. Int J Gynecol Pathol. 2003;22(4):324–33.
28. Kihara A, Yoshida H, Watanabe R, Takahashi K, Kato T, Ino Y, et al. Clinicopathologic association and prognostic value of microcystic, elongated, and fragmented (MELF) pattern in endometrial endometrioid carcinoma. Am J Surg Pathol. 2017;41(7):896–905.
29. Pelletier MP, Trinh VQ, Stephenson P, Mes-Masson AM, Samouelian V, Provencher DM, et al. Microcystic, elongated, and fragmented pattern invasion is mainly associated with isolated tumor cell pattern metastases in International Federation of Gynecology and Obstetrics grade I endometrioid endometrial cancer. Hum Pathol. 2017;62:33–9.
30. van den Heerik A, Aiyer KTS, Stelloo E, Jürgenliemk-Schulz IM, Lutgens L, Jobsen JJ, et al. Microcystic elongated and fragmented (MELF) pattern of invasion: molecular features and prognostic significance in the PORTEC-1 and -2 trials. Gynecol Oncol. 2022;166(3):530–7.
31. Wheeler DT, Bristow RE, Kurman RJ. Histologic alterations in endometrial hyperplasia and well-differentiated carcinoma treated with progestins. Am J Surg Pathol. 2007;31(7):988–98.
32. Zaino RJ, Brady WE, Todd W, Leslie K, Fischer EG, Horowitz NS, et al. Histologic effects of medroxyprogesterone acetate on endometrioid endometrial adenocarcinoma: a Gynecologic Oncology Group study. Int J Gynecol Pathol. 2014;33(6):543–53.
33. Westin SN, Fellman B, Sun CC, Broaddus RR, Woodall ML, Pal N, et al. Prospective phase II trial of levonorgestrel intrauterine device: nonsurgical approach for complex atypical hyperplasia and early-stage endometrial cancer. Am J Obstet Gynecol. 2021;224(2):191.e1–191.e15.
34. Nicolae A, Preda O, Nogales FF. Endometrial metaplasias and reactive changes: a spectrum of altered differentiation. J Clin Pathol. 2011;64(2):97–106.
35. Nucci MR, Prasad CJ, Crum CP, Mutter GL. Mucinous endometrial epithelial proliferations: a morphologic spectrum of changes with diverse clinical significance. Mod Pathol. 1999;12(12):1137–42.
36. Wells M, Tiltman A. Intestinal metaplasia of the endometrium. Histopathology. 1989;15(4):431–3.
37. Yoo SH, Park BH, Choi J, Yoo J, Lee SW, Kim YM, et al. Papillary mucinous metaplasia of the endometrium as a possible precursor of endometrial mucinous adenocarcinoma. Mod Pathol. 2012;25(11):1496–507.
38. Qiu W, Mittal K. Comparison of morphologic and immunohistochemical features of cervical microglandular hyperplasia with

low-grade mucinous adenocarcinoma of the endometrium. Int J Gynecol Pathol. 2003;22(3):261–5.
39. Vang R, Tavassoli FA. Proliferative mucinous lesions of the endometrium: analysis of existing criteria for diagnosing carcinoma in biopsies and curettings. Int J Surg Pathol. 2003;11(4):261–70.
40. Sung JY, Jung YY, Kim HS. Clinicopathological characteristics and KRAS mutation status of endometrial mucinous metaplasia and carcinoma. Anticancer Res. 2018;38(5):2779–86.
41. Mangili G, Taccagni G, Garavaglia E, Carnelli M, Montoli S. An unusual admixture of neoplastic and metaplastic lesions of the female genital tract in the Peutz-Jeghers Syndrome. Gynecol Oncol. 2004;92(1):337–42.
42. Gilks CB, Clement PB, Hart WR, Young RH. Uterine adenomyomas excluding atypical polypoid adenomyomas and adenomyomas of endocervical type: a clinicopathologic study of 30 cases of an underemphasized lesion that may cause diagnostic problems with brief consideration of adenomyomas of other female genital tract sites. Int J Gynecol Pathol. 2000;19(3):195–205.
43. Tahlan A, Nanda A, Mohan H. Uterine adenomyoma: a clinicopathologic review of 26 cases and a review of the literature. Int J Gynecol Pathol. 2006;25(4):361–5.
44. Kihara A, Amano Y, Yoshimoto T, Matsubara D, Fukushima N, Fujiwara H, et al. Stromal p16 expression helps distinguish atypical polypoid adenomyoma from myoinvasive endometrioid carcinoma of the uterus. Am J Surg Pathol. 2019;43(11):1526–35.
45. McCluggage WG, Van de Vijver K. SATB2 is consistently expressed in squamous morules associated with endometrioid proliferative lesions and in the stroma of atypical polypoid adenomyoma. Int J Gynecol Pathol. 2019;38(5):397–403.
46. Strickland KC, Yuan L, Quade BJ, Nucci MR, Howitt BE. Clinicopathological and immunohistochemical features of uterine adenomyomatous polyps. Hum Pathol. 2019;84:239–45.
47. Raffone A, Travaglino A, Saccone G, Alviggi C, Mascolo M, De Placido G, et al. Management of women with atypical polypoid adenomyoma of the uterus: a quantitative systematic review. Acta Obstet Gynecol Scand. 2019;98(7):842–55.
48. Biasioli A, Londero AP, Orsaria M, Scrimin F, Mangino FP, Bertozzi S, et al. Atypical polypoid adenomyoma follow-up and management: systematic review of case reports and series and meta-analysis. Medicine (Baltimore). 2020;99(26):e20491.
49. Howitt BE, Nucci MR. Mesonephric proliferations of the female genital tract. Pathology. 2018;50(2):141–50.
50. Euscher ED, Bassett R, Duose DY, Lan C, Wistuba I, Ramondetta L, et al. Mesonephric-like carcinoma of the endometrium: a subset of endometrial carcinoma with an aggressive behavior. Am J Surg Pathol. 2020;44(4):429–43.
51. da Silva EM, Fix DJ, Sebastiao APM, Selenica P, Ferrando L, Kim SH, et al. Mesonephric and mesonephric-like carcinomas of the female genital tract: molecular characterization including cases with mixed histology and matched metastases. Mod Pathol. 2021;34(8):1570–87.
52. Pors J, Segura S, Chiu DS, Almadani N, Ren H, Fix DJ, et al. Clinicopathologic characteristics of mesonephric adenocarcinomas and mesonephric-like adenocarcinomas in the gynecologic tract: a multi-institutional study. Am J Surg Pathol. 2021;45(4):498–506.
53. Murali R, Davidson B, Fadare O, Carlson JA, Crum CP, Gilks CB, et al. High-grade endometrial carcinomas: morphologic and immunohistochemical features, diagnostic challenges and recommendations. Int J Gynecol Pathol. 2019;38 Suppl 1(Iss 1 Suppl 1):S40–63.
54. Ramalingam P, Masand RP, Euscher ED, Malpica A. Undifferentiated carcinoma of the endometrium: an expanded immunohistochemical analysis including PAX-8 and basal-like carcinoma surrogate markers. Int J Gynecol Pathol. 2016;35(5):410–8.
55. Hamilton SN, Tinker AV, Kwon J, Lim P, Kong I, Sihra S, et al. Treatment and outcomes in undifferentiated and dedifferentiated endometrial carcinoma. J Gynecol Oncol. 2022;33(3):e25.
56. Stewart CJ, Crook ML. SWI/SNF complex deficiency and mismatch repair protein expression in undifferentiated and dedifferentiated endometrial carcinoma. Pathology. 2015;47(5):439–45.
57. Kolin DL, Quick CM, Dong F, Fletcher CDM, Stewart CJR, Soma A, et al. SMARCA4-deficient uterine sarcoma and undifferentiated endometrial carcinoma are distinct clinicopathologic entities. Am J Surg Pathol. 2020;44(2):263–70.
58. Young RH, Scully RE. Oxyphilic clear cell carcinoma of the ovary. A report of nine cases. Am J Surg Pathol. 1987;11(9):661–7.
59. Bennett JA, Dong F, Young RH, Oliva E. Clear cell carcinoma of the ovary: evaluation of prognostic parameters based on a clinicopathological analysis of 100 cases. Histopathology. 2015;66(6):808–15.
60. Ariura M, Kasajima R, Miyagi Y, Ishidera Y, Sugo Y, Oi Y, et al. Combined large cell neuroendocrine carcinoma and endometrioid carcinoma of the endometrium: a shared gene mutation signature between the two histological components. Int Cancer Conf J. 2017;6(1):11–5.
61. Matsumoto H, Nasu K, Kai K, Nishida M, Narahara H, Nishida H. Combined large-cell neuroendocrine carcinoma and endometrioid adenocarcinoma of the endometrium: a case report and survey of related literature. J Obstet Gynaecol Res. 2016;42(2):206–10.
62. Pocrnich CE, Ramalingam P, Euscher ED, Malpica A. Neuroendocrine carcinoma of the endometrium: a clinicopathologic study of 25 cases. Am J Surg Pathol. 2016;40(5):577–86.
63. Howitt BE, Dong F, Vivero M, Shah V, Lindeman N, Schoolmeester JK, et al. Molecular characterization of neuroendocrine carcinomas of the endometrium: representation in all 4 TCGA groups. Am J Surg Pathol. 2020;44(11):1541–8.
64. Schlechtweg K, Chen L, St Clair CM, Tergas AI, Khoury-Collado F, Hou JY, et al. Neuroendocrine carcinoma of the endometrium: disease course, treatment, and outcomes. Gynecol Oncol. 2019;155(2):254–61.
65. Matsumoto H, Shimokawa M, Nasu K, Shikama A, Shiozaki T, Futagami M, et al. Clinicopathologic features, treatment, prognosis and prognostic factors of neuroendocrine carcinoma of the endometrium: a retrospective analysis of 42 cases from the Kansai Clinical Oncology Group/Intergroup study in Japan. J Gynecol Oncol. 2019;30(6):e103.
66. Ravishankar S, Malpica A, Ramalingam P, Euscher ED. Yolk sac tumor in extragonadal pelvic sites: still a diagnostic challenge. Am J Surg Pathol. 2017;41(1):1–11.
67. Nogales FF, Prat J, Schuldt M, Cruz-Viruel N, Kaur B, D'Angelo E, et al. Germ cell tumour growth patterns originating from clear cell carcinomas of the ovary and endometrium: a comparative immunohistochemical study favouring their origin from somatic stem cells. Histopathology. 2018;72(4):634–47.
68. Schuldt M, Rubio A, Preda O, Nogales FF. GATA binding protein 3 expression is present in primitive patterns of yolk sac tumours but is not expressed by differentiated variants. Histopathology. 2016;68(4):613–5.

Mesenchymal Lesions of the Uterus

7

7.1 Leiomyoma with Hydropic Change

7.1.1 Key Diagnostic Features

- Accumulation of abundant edema fluid within the tumor or adjacent myometrium (Fig. 7.1).
- Hydropic changes might be confined to the periphery of the tumor, or edematous connective tissue might divide the smooth muscle lesion into smaller nodules (Fig. 7.2) (perinodular hydropic degeneration) [1].
- The hydropic areas consist of scant fibroblasts, rounded clumps of collagen, and rarely proteinaceous material (Fig. 7.3).
- Cords of smooth muscle cells are present around the numerous blood vessels (varying sizes of capillaries and thick-walled hyalinized arteries) (Fig. 7.4).

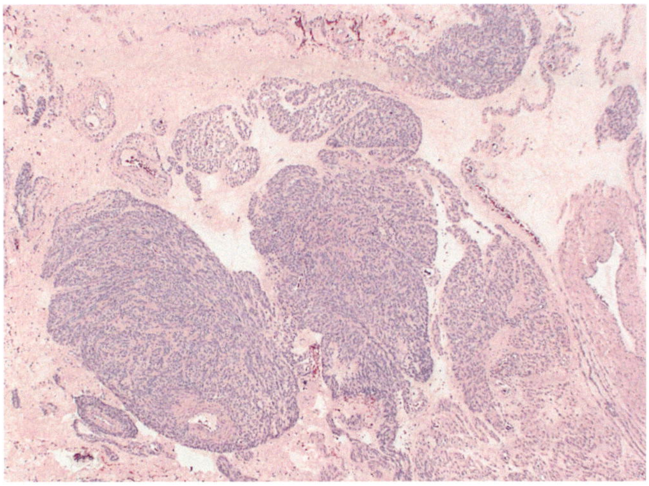

Fig. 7.2 A section with perinodular hydropic change. The smooth muscle nodules are free-floating in an edematous stroma (40×)

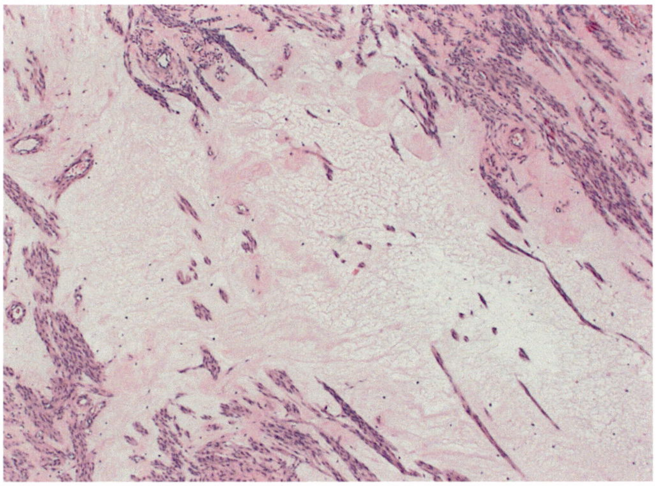

Fig. 7.1 Areas of hydropic change are composed of rare fibroblasts, straps of smooth muscle fibers, and occasional small blood vessels (40×)

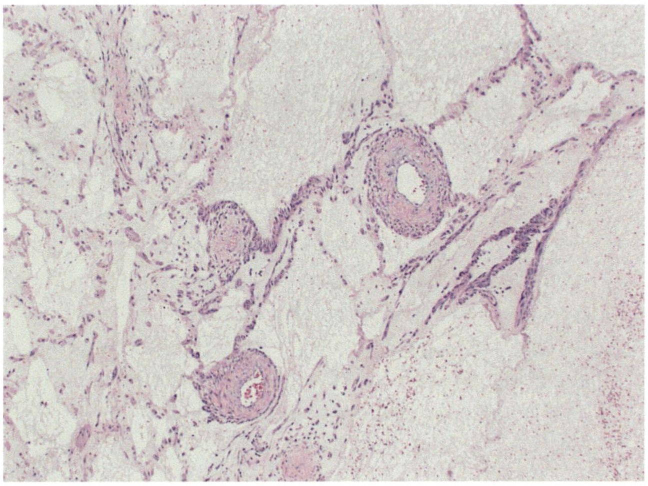

Fig. 7.3 Scant fibroblasts and proteinaceous material among the blood vessels (40×)

O. Saglam, *Challenging Cases in Gynecologic Surgical Pathology*, https://doi.org/10.1007/978-3-031-51656-6_7

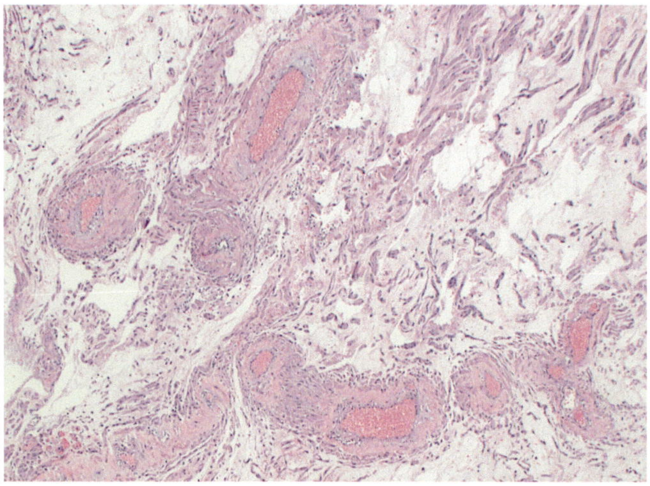

Fig. 7.4 Thick-walled blood vessels and cords of residual smooth muscle bundles (40×)

7.1.2 Ancillary Studies

- Alcian blue: negative in hydropic zones in contrast to positive staining in smooth muscle tumors with myxoid changes

7.1.3 Differential Diagnosis

- Intravenous leiomyomatosis
  - In samples with perinodular hydropic degeneration, there might be foci without hydropic tissue surrounding smooth muscle nodules. These might falsely give the impression of vascular spaces, and the lesion can be diagnosed as an intravenous leiomyoma.
  - Intravenous leiomyomatosis grossly appears as worm-like plugs.
  - See Part II, Sect. 7.3.
- Myxoid leiomyosarcoma
  - In rare leiomyomas with hydropic change, the lesion's borders are infiltrative into the myometrium or endometrium for a few millimeters, and the smooth muscle fibers of the myometrium might be separated by the edematous tissue [1], giving the false impression of invasion into the surrounding tissues.
  - Myxoid leiomyosarcoma in the gross examination is diffusely gelatinous and might have infiltrative borders in microscopic examination.
  - See Part II, Sect. 7.9.

7.1.4 Clinical Significance

- Hydropic change has no clinical significance.

7.2 Epithelioid Leiomyoma

7.2.1 A 53-Year-Old Postmenopausal Woman Presents to the Emergency Department with Vaginal Bleeding and Pelvic Pain

7.2.1.1 Key Diagnostic Features

- Round, polygonal cells with eosinophilic, granular, or clear cytoplasm in architectural patterns of diffuse sheets (Fig. 7.5), cords, trabeculae, or nests.
- No cytological atypia.
- In epithelioid smooth muscle tumors of the uterus, the grade 1 nuclei are bland with inconspicuous nucleoli and evenly distributed chromatin (Fig. 7.6). The grade 3

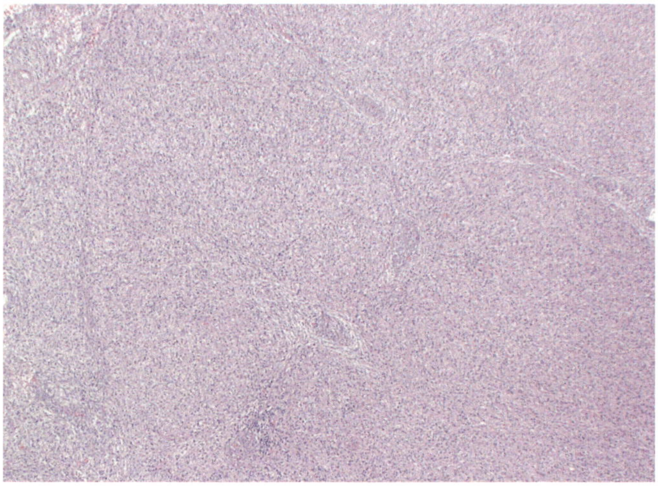

Fig. 7.5 Diffuse growth of epithelioid cells (40×)

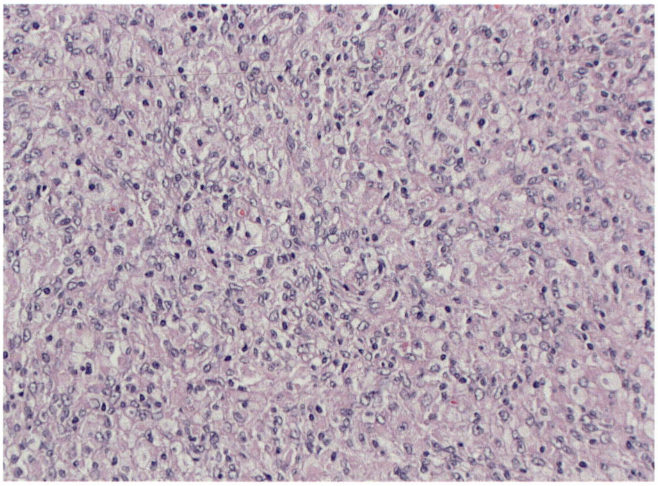

Fig. 7.6 Epithelioid cells with clear to eosinophilic cytoplasm. They do not display cytological atypia or mitotic activity (100×)

nuclei are markedly hyperchromatic with coarse, unevenly distributed chromatin and have prominent macronucleoli. A small nucleolus and an intermediate degree of atypia are features of grade 2 nuclei [2].

- The mitotic rate is less than 2 mitoses per 10 high-power fields.
- Smaller lesions (less than 1 cm) in plexiform growth pattern are referred to as "plexiform tumorlet" (Fig. 7.7). Tumorlets have round to polygonal cells with eosinophilic cytoplasm (Fig. 7.8). They might be solitary or multiple within the endometrium (Fig. 7.9), in the endomyometrial junction or uterine wall [3].

7.2.1.2 Ancillary Studies

- Smooth muscle markers (Desmin, h-caldesmon, SMA) are positive.

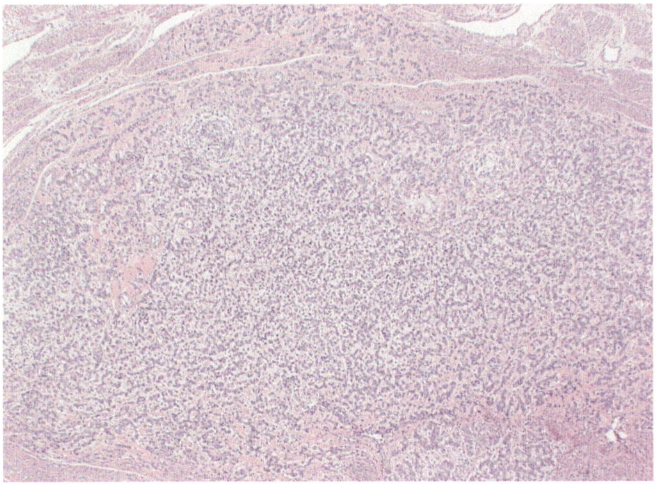

Fig. 7.7 Plexiform tumorlet in a corded pattern within the myometrium (40×)

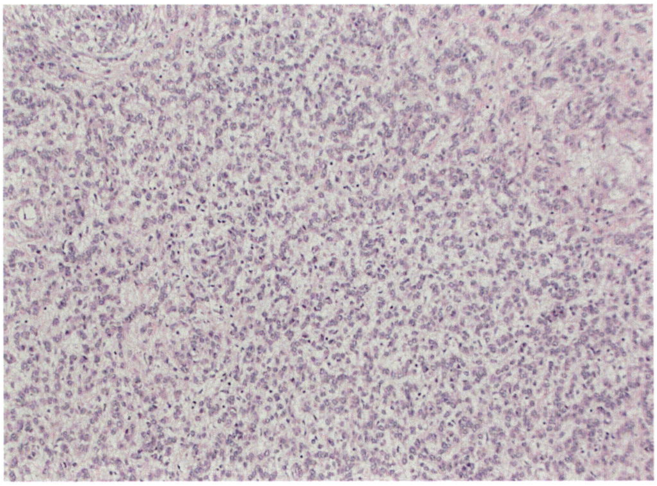

Fig. 7.8 The epithelioid cells of plexiform tumorlet have small round nuclei and eosinophilic to clear cytoplasm (200×)

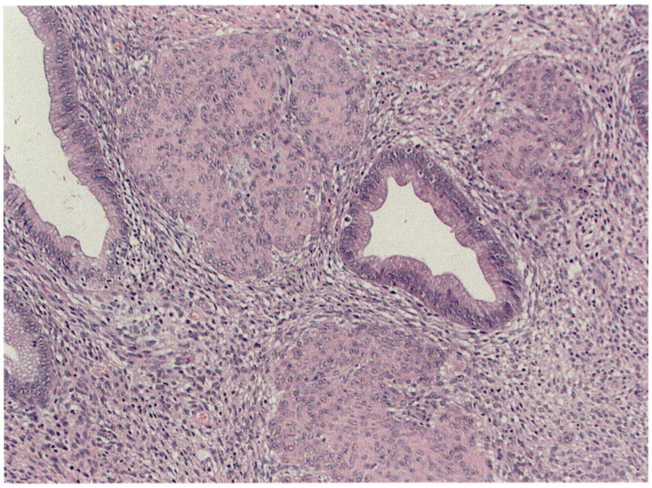

Fig. 7.9 Multiple plexiform tumorlets within the endometrium (200×)

7.2.1.3 Differential Diagnosis

- Epithelioid leiomyosarcoma
  - Moderate to severe cytological atypia.
  - Tumor cell necrosis.
  - Four or more mitotic figures per 10 high-power fields.
  - See Part II, Sect. 7.8.
- Perivascular epithelioid cell tumors (PEComa)
  - Proliferation of epithelioid and spindle cells in nested or diffuse patterns.
  - Nuclear atypia and mitotic activity are variable. Macronucleoli, multinucleated giant cells, intranuclear pseudoinclusions, spider-like giant cells, and melanin pigment can be present.
  - Positive for melanocytic and smooth muscle markers.
  - See Part II, Sect. 7.10.

7.2.1.4 Clinical Significance

- Criteria for smooth muscle tumors with uncertain malignant potential (STUMP) or sarcoma are not the same as conventional (spindle cell) smooth muscle lesions. An epithelioid smooth muscle tumor with a mitotic rate of 2 to 3 per 10 high power field and short of criteria for epithelioid leiomyosarcoma falls in the category of the STUMP.

7.3 Intravenous Leiomyomatosis (IVL)

7.3.1 A 32-Year-Old-Woman with a Pelvic Mass

7.3.1.1 Key Diagnostic Features

- Intravascular growth of benign smooth muscle cells in the absence of uterine leiomyoma or beyond the confines of uterine leiomyoma (Figs. 7.10 and 7.11).

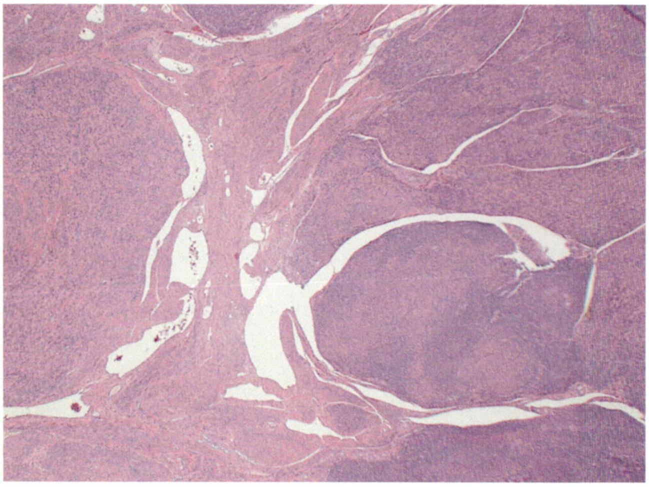

Fig. 7.10 A smooth muscle nodule is extending into the vascular space. Others are compressing large vessels (40×)

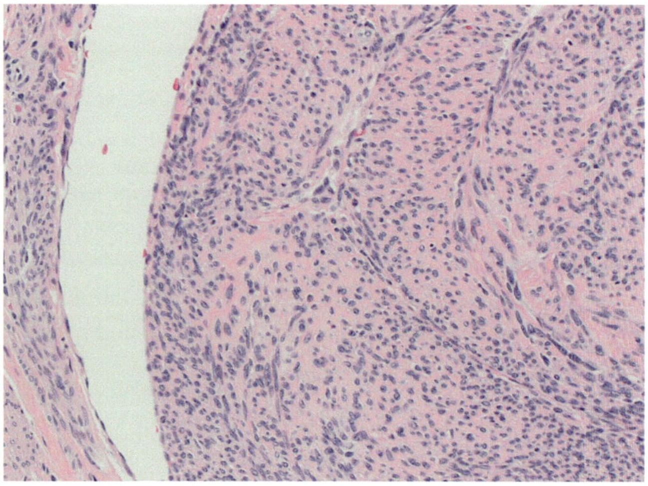

Fig. 7.11 Benign nodular smooth muscle proliferation and endothelial lining (100×)

- Multiple myometrial masses are typically associated with worm-like plugs within parametrial vessels. There may be a pelvic or extrapelvic extension [4].
- All of the morphological variants of leiomyoma, including leiomyoma with hydropic change, leiomyoma with hyalinization, cellular leiomyoma (Fig. 7.12), and leiomyoma with benign endometrial glands (intravascular adenomyomatosis), can be associated with IVL [5].

7.3.1.2 Ancillary Studies

- Overexpression of the *High Mobility Group AT-Hook 2 (HMGA-2)* is identified in subsets of IVL [6], but no *mediator complex subunit 12 (MED12)* oncogenic mutations [7].
- Smooth muscle markers are positive in IVL.

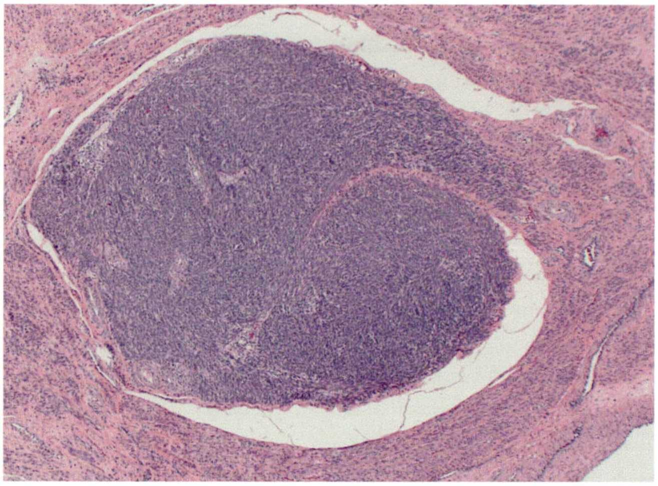

Fig. 7.12 Extension of cellular smooth muscle proliferation into the vascular space within the myometrium (40×)

7.3.1.3 Differential Diagnosis

- Cellular form of IVL versus endometrial stromal sarcoma (ESS)
  - ESS exhibits endometrial involvement and myometrial permeation. In contrast, cellular IVL involves the myometrium.
  - ESS with vascular involvement is a single nodule. IVL usually has multiple nodules with clefted contours.
  - ESS has a diffuse network of small arterioles. IVL has thick-walled blood vessels
  - Low-grade ESS has a diffuse expression of CD10.
- Cellular form of IVL versus diffuse leiomyomatosis of the uterus
  - Multiple confluent cellular leiomyomatous nodules replace myometrium in diffuse leiomyomatosis. The vascular spaces might be compressed, but there is no vascular involvement in diffuse leiomyomatosis.
- Mitotically active IVL versus leiomyosarcoma
  - Vascular involvement of leiomyosarcoma is not grossly visible. The cytological atypia is severe, and tumor cell necrosis can be identified in most cases.
- Epithelioid form of IVL versus epithelioid leiomyosarcoma
  - The presence of one or more of the following can fulfill the essential diagnostic criteria for epithelioid leiomyosarcoma: (1) Moderate to severe cytological atypia. (2) Tumor cell necrosis. (3) Four or more mitotic figures per 10 high-power fields.
- IVL with bizarre nuclei versus leiomyosarcoma
  - Increased number of mitotic figures and tumor cell necrosis are not present in IVL with bizarre nuclei.
- Intravenous lipoleiomyomatosis versus liposarcoma
  - The lack of mitotic figures and cytological atypia is consistent with the diagnosis of intravenous lipoleiomyomatosis.

7.3.1.4 Clinical Significance

- Complications of IVL include sudden death if there is an intracardiac extension [8].

7.4 Disseminated Peritoneal Leiomyomatosis (DPL)

7.4.1 Multiple Peritoneal Nodules Sampled in the Laparoscopic Surgery of a 26-Year-Old Woman

7.4.1.1 Key Diagnostic Features

- The presence of multiple benign smooth muscle nodules in peritoneal surfaces (Fig. 7.13).
- Smooth muscle cells might be admixed with myofibroblasts (Fig. 7.14).
- Usually associated with pregnancy and usage of oral contraceptives. Clusters of decidualized cells can be present within the nodules in pregnant patients [9].
- Association with endometriosis [10] and sex cord-like pattern [11] are described.

7.4.1.2 Ancillary Studies

- Strongly positive for desmin, caldesmon, ER, PR, and SMA [12]

7.4.1.3 Differential Diagnosis

- Benign metastasizing leiomyoma
  - Extrauterine (most commonly in the lung) well-circumscribed nodular proliferation of benign-appearing smooth muscle.
  - The history of uterine leiomyoma(s).

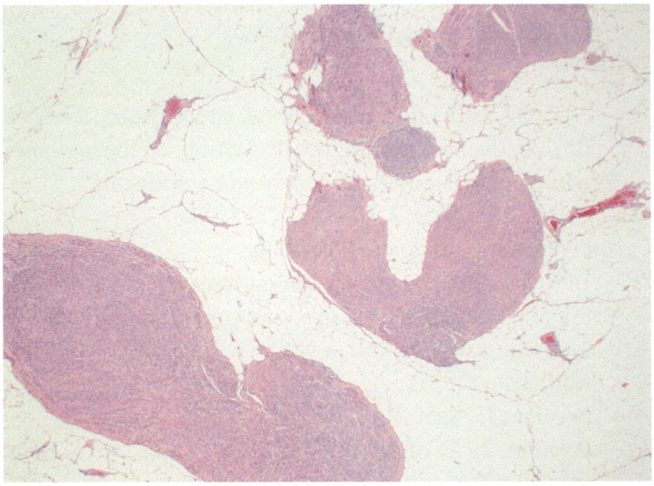

Fig. 7.13 Islands of benign-appearing smooth muscle nodules within the adipose tissue. There is no desmoplastic reaction (20×)

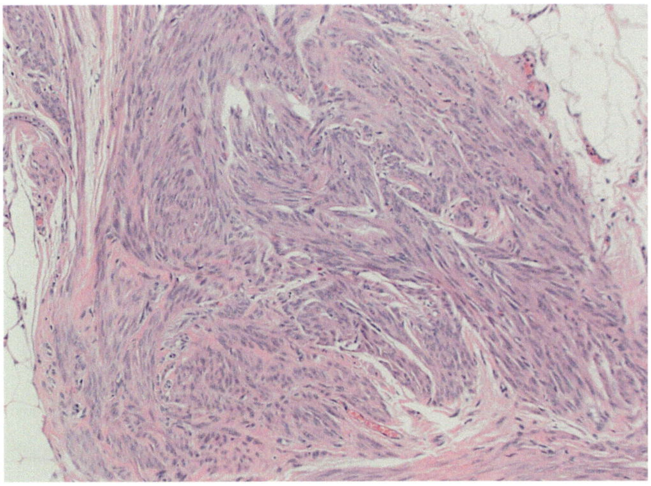

Fig. 7.14 Bland smooth muscle fibers with no mitotic figures or cytological atypia (100×)

  - Leiomyoma might be cellular or admixed with adipose tissue.
  - Benign metastasizing leiomyoma is clonally derived from uterine leiomyoma [13].
- Low-grade smooth muscle tumor with probable multicentric origin [14]
  - Peritoneal tumors with bland cytology and an increased number of mitoses do not fulfill the criteria for leiomyosarcoma.
  - Bland smooth muscle tumors are present in the uterus synchronously or asynchronously.

7.4.1.4 Clinical Significance

- Recurrence after surgery or malignant transformation occurs, especially after incomplete resections [15, 16].
- Laparoscopic myomectomy with uncontained morcellation might result in iatrogenic DPL [12].

7.5 Cotyledonoid Dissecting Leiomyoma (CDLM)

7.5.1 A Large Multinodular Tumor Adhering to the Right Posterolateral Wall of the Uterus and Extending into the Broad Ligament Was Resected at Hysterectomy for Uterine Prolapse

7.5.1.1 Key Diagnostic Features

- Disorganized swirled fascicules of smooth muscle form multiple irregular nodules and tongue-like structures within the myometrium (dissecting leiomyoma) (Figs. 7.15 and 7.16) or sometimes have an extrauterine extension (Cotyledonoid DissectingLeiomyoma) [17].

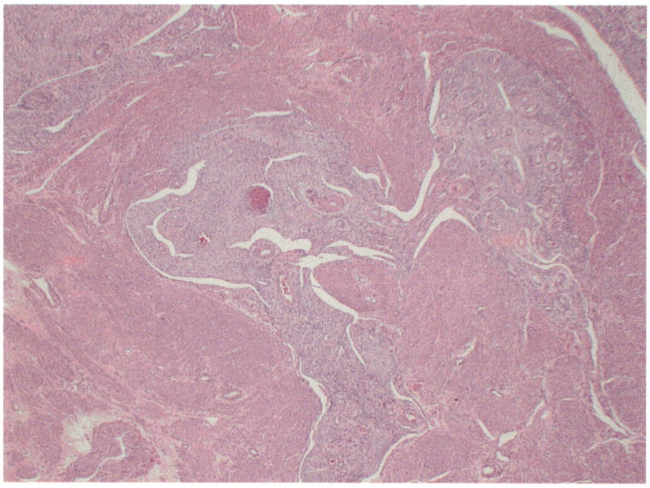

Fig. 7.15 Fascicules of smooth muscle cells form disorganized, irregular nodular structures within the myometrium (40×)

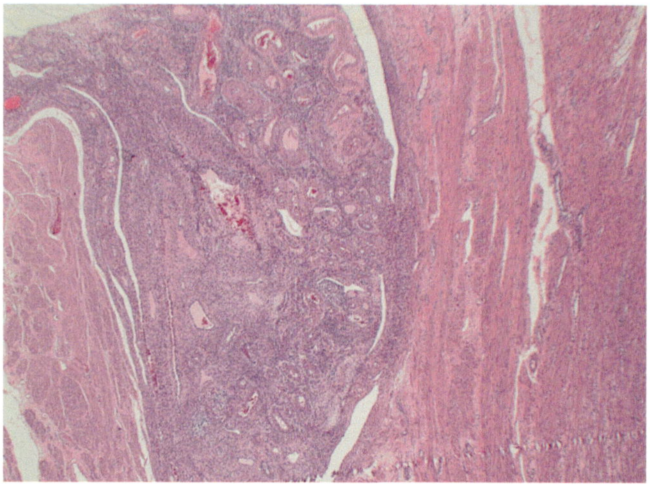

Fig. 7.16 Rounded tongues of smooth muscle islands dissect the myometrium (40×)

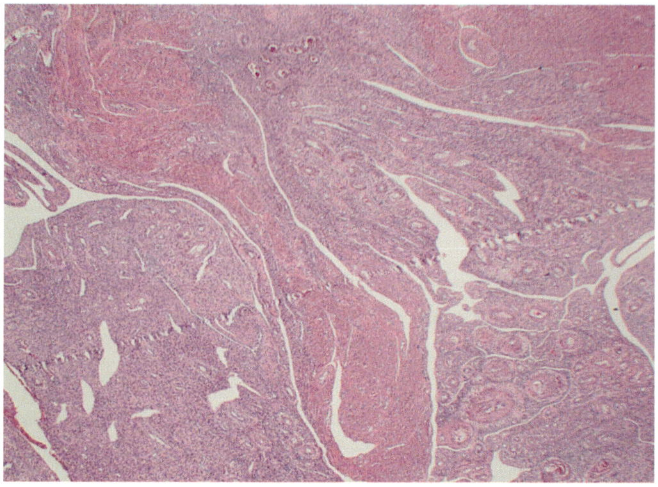

Fig. 7.17 There is a separation artifact and fibroconnective tissue between smooth muscle proliferation and myometrium (40×)

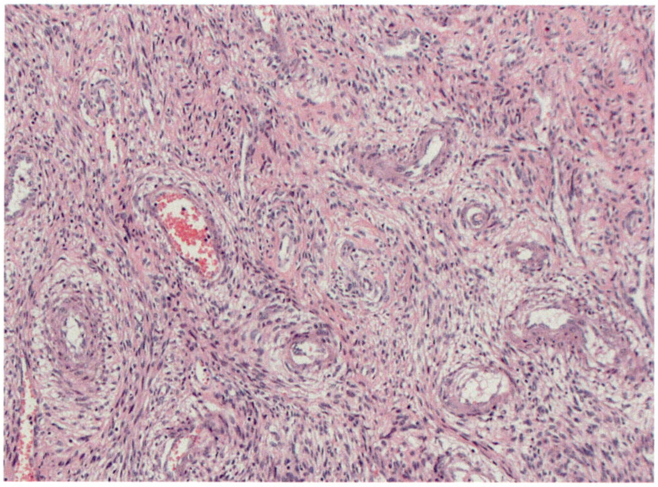

Fig. 7.18 The smooth muscle cells have bland nuclei and no mitotic activity. Multiple thick-walled vessels without an organizational pattern are among the smooth muscle fibers (100×)

- Fascicles of smooth muscle are separated by a hyalinized to hydropic connective tissue matrix in the myometrium.
- The smooth muscle fascicles in aggregate and fibrous connective tissue produce a multinodular growth pattern (Fig. 7.17).
- There might be an intravenous extension [18].
- The smooth muscle cells have bland cytological features, and there is no mitotic activity (Fig. 7.18).

7.5.1.2 Ancillary Studies

- CDLM expresses smooth muscle markers [19].

7.5.1.3 Differential Diagnosis

- Leiomyoma with perinodular hydropic change
  - Accumulation of intercellular fluid that may cause cystic degeneration in leiomyoma with hydropic changes. Nodules are well-circumscribed, and hydropic changes do not display intramural dissection of the myometrium or extramural cotyledonoid components.
  - See Part II, Sect. 7.1.
- Intravenous leiomyomatosis (IVL)
  - Intravascular growth of benign smooth muscle cells outside the confines of an index smooth muscle lesion.
  - Nodular lesions within a vascular space with a separation artifact.
  - See Part II, Sect. 7.3.
  - Around 20% of reported CDLM cases have some intravascular growth [19].
- Low-grade endometrial stromal sarcoma (LGESS)
  - The neoplastic cells of LGESS are oval to fusiform and have a diffuse growth pattern with numerous thin-

walled arterioles. CDLM might also have numerous blood vessels, which are thick-walled and less uniformly distributed. CD10 is positive, and desmin and h-caldesmon are negative in LGESS.

7.5.1.4 Clinical Significance

- Recurrences of CDLM after myomectomy are reported [20].

7.6 Fumarate Hydratase-Deficient Leiomyoma (FH-Deficient Leiomyoma)

7.6.1 A 36-Year-Old Woman with Cutaneous Leiomyoma(s) and Pelvic Mass

7.6.1.1 Key Diagnostic Features

- Alternating hypercellular and hypocellular areas with alveolar-type edema [21] (Fig. 7.19).
- Staghorn-pattern vasculature (Fig. 7.20).
- Scattered bizarre/atypical epithelioid cells with eosinophilic nucleoli and perinucleolar halo. Nuclei might be arranged in chains (Figs. 7.21 and 7.22).
- Fibrillary cytoplasm.
- Eosinophilic cytoplasmic globules might be associated with rhabdoid cell morphology (Fig. 7.23).

7.6.1.2 Ancillary Studies

- Immunohistochemical staining for S-2-succino-cysteine (2SC) has a diffuse granular cytoplasmic pattern, and fumarate hydratase (FH) expression is lost. 2SC positivity or loss of FH expression is not specific for germline mutations and can be associated with somatic FH mutations in leiomyoma(s) with bizarre nuclei. Both stains can serve as a screening tool [22].
- Smooth muscle markers are positive.

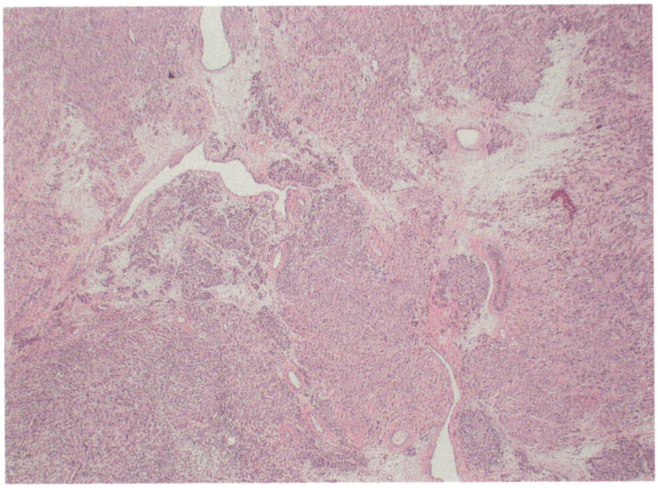

Fig. 7.19 Areas of alveolar-type edema alternate with smooth muscle proliferation. The vessels are thin-walled and sharply branched (20×)

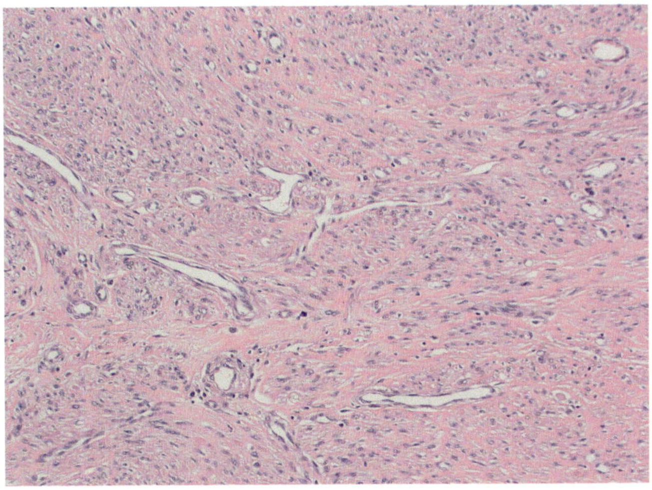

Fig. 7.20 Staghorn-pattern vasculature (40×)

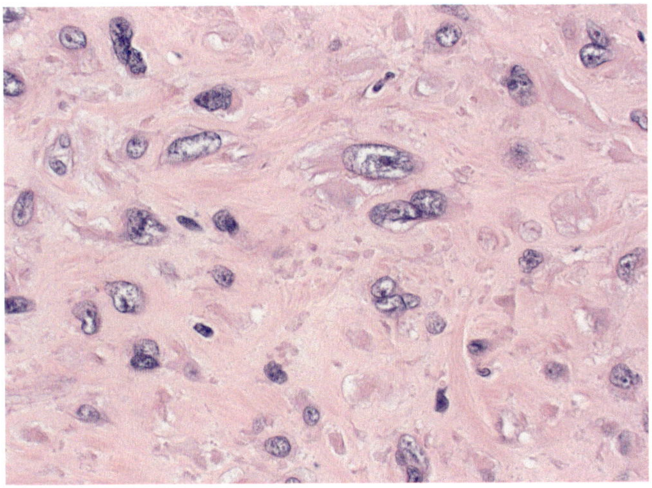

Fig. 7.21 Scattered enlarged epithelioid cells with optical clearing of nuclei and cherry-red eosinophilic nucleoli (400×)

7.6.1.3 Differential Diagnosis

- Epithelioid leiomyoma
  - Round, polygonal, and epithelioid cells with cytoplasmic clearing.
  - Lack of typical vasculature, eosinophilic cytoplasmic globules, and nuclear inclusions.
  - See Part II, Sect. 7.2.
- Leiomyosarcoma
  - Increased mitotic activity and tumor cell necrosis are not present in FH-deficient leiomyoma.
- Perivascular epithelioid cell neoplasm (PEComa)
  - Epithelioid cells with clear or granular cytoplasm.

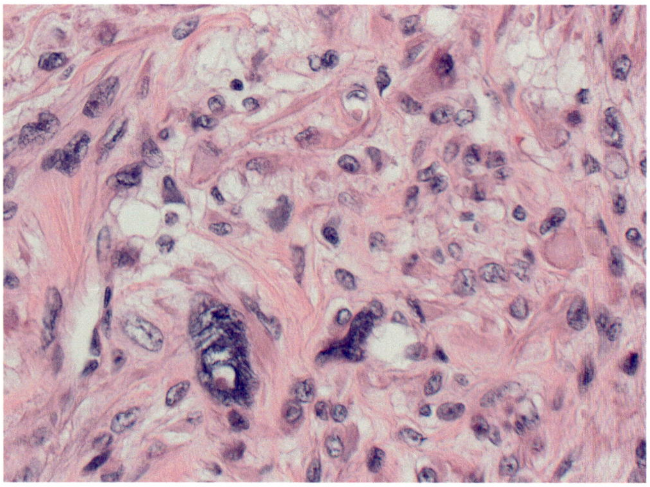

Fig. 7.22 The neoplastic cells have fibrillary cytoplasm. The epithelioid cell with bizarre nuclei has prominent red nucleoli and perinucleolar halo. A pink globule is present at the right side of the image (400×)

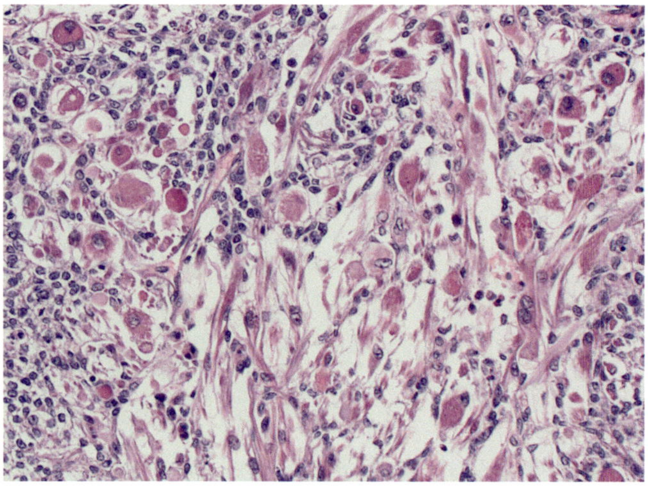

Fig. 7.23 The neoplastic cells have eccentric nuclei and abundant cytoplasm containing globular eosinophilic inclusions in this field (400×)

- Spindle and rhabdoid cells: +/− (usually minor component).
- The neoplastic cells are radially arranged around blood vessels in some samples.
- Positive for melanocytic and smooth muscle markers.
- See Part II, Sect. 7.10.

7.6.1.4 Clinical Significance

- Hereditary Leiomyomatosis and Renal Cell Carcinoma Syndrome (HLRCCS) is an autosomal dominant familial syndrome resulting from a germline mutation in the *FH* gene. HLRCC is associated with an increased incidence of smooth muscle tumors of the uterus and skin. The morphology is not specific for FH-germline mutation. Clinical correlation and genetic consultation might facilitate the identification of high-risk patients [23].

7.7 Leiomyoma with Bizarre Nuclei (Symplastic Leiomyoma)

7.7.1 A 49-Year-Old-Woman with Perimenopausal Bleeding

7.7.1.1 Key Diagnostic Features

- Large atypical multinucleated or mononucleated cells in diffuse sheet-like growth or localized proliferation in a regular leiomyoma (Fig. 7.24).
- Prominent nuclear pseudoinclusions (Figs. 7.25 and 7.26) or degenerating karyorrhectic nuclei. Karyorrhectic nuclei might be interpreted as atypical mitoses in the absence of typical mitotic figures [24].
- There might be rhabdoid cell morphology.
- Average mitotic count is 1–2 per 10 high-power fields.
- Tumor cell necrosis is not present.
- Vascular changes include fibrinoid necrosis of vessel walls, complete obliteration, and perivascular lymphocytic infiltrates [25].

7.7.1.2 Ancillary Studies

- The proliferative index by Ki67 might be high (>25%) [26], and 7% of leiomyomas with bizarre nuclei have a strong and diffuse expression of p16 and p53 [27].
- PHH3 might be useful in the assessment of mitotic counts [28].

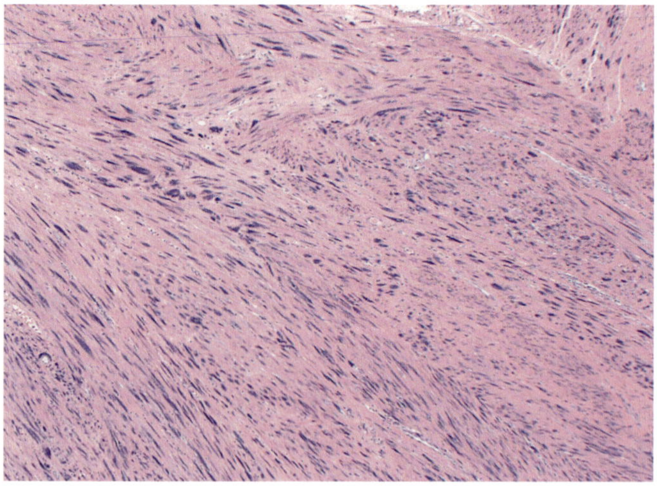

Fig. 7.24 Atypical smooth muscle cells in fascicular pattern (40×)

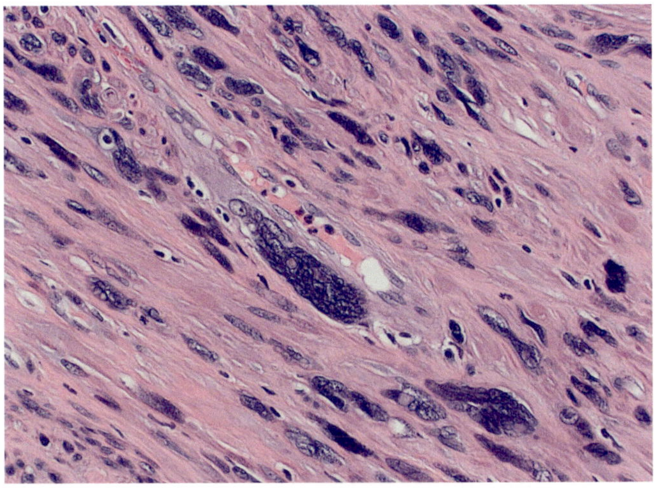

Fig. 7.25 Scattered multinucleated cells with prominent eosinophilic nucleoli (200×)

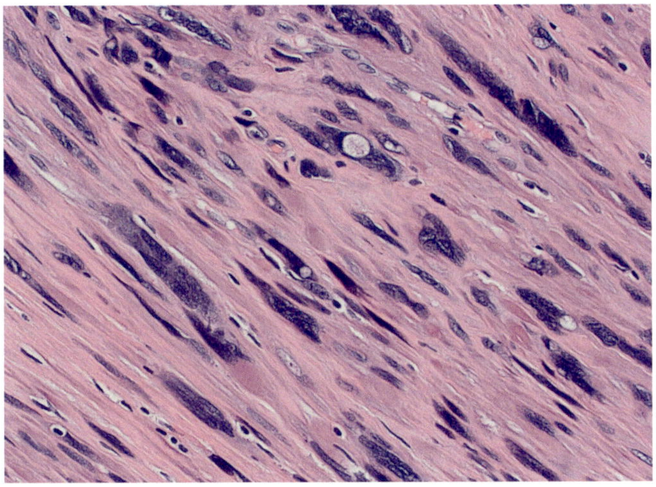

Fig. 7.26 Nuclear pseudoinclusions (200×)

7.7.1.3 Differential Diagnosis

- Leiomyosarcoma
  - Tumor cell necrosis or high mitotic activity should be present for diagnosis.
- Undifferentiated uterine sarcoma
  - In addition to significant cytological atypia, there is brisk mitotic activity and tumor cell necrosis. Nuclear karyorrhexis or pseudoinclusions are not present.
- Endometrial adenocarcinoma with a component of giant cell carcinoma
  - Endometrial cancer might have giant cells in poorly cohesive sheets and nests with marked inflammatory infiltrate [29]. Identification of focal usual epithelial types is diagnostic.

7.7.1.4 Clinical Significance

- Benign tumors.
- There are genetic similarities between leiomyoma(s) with bizarre nuclei and leiomyosarcomas [30]. Progressing from preexisting leiomyoma with bizarre nuclei to leiomyosarcoma might be one of the pathogenetic pathways for uterine leiomyosarcomas [31].

7.8 Epithelioid Leiomyosarcoma (ELMS)

7.8.1 A 68-Year-Old Woman with Postmenopausal Bleeding

7.8.1.1 Key Diagnostic Features

- More than 50% of the lesion has epithelioid cell morphology by definition.
- Cells are round with eosinophilic or clear cytoplasm arranged in diffuse, nested, or nodular patterns (Figs. 7.27 and 7.28).
- Epithelioid cells with one or more of the following criteria are considered as malignant epithelioid leiomyosarcoma per 2020 classification of female genital tract tumors (WHO, Blue Book):
  - Cytological atypia is moderate to severe (Fig. 7.29).
  - Tumor cell necrosis (Fig. 7.30).
  - Four or more mitosis per 10 high-power fields [32].

7.8.1.2 Ancillary Studies

- Desmin (Fig. 7.31), h-caldesmon, SMA: Positive
- HMB45: might be focaland weakly positive [33]

7.8.1.3 Differential Diagnosis

- Perivascular epithelioid cell tumor (PEComa)
  - Epithelioid cells with clear or granular cytoplasm.
  - Spindle and rhabdoid cells +/− (usually minor component).

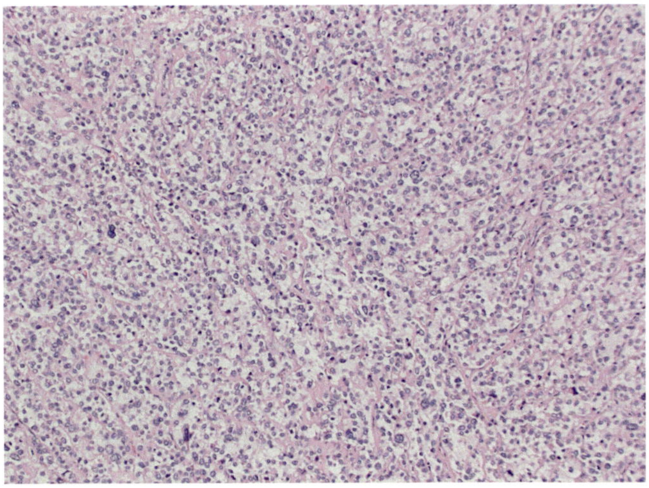

Fig. 7.27 The epithelioid cells have a diffuse and nested growth pattern (40×)

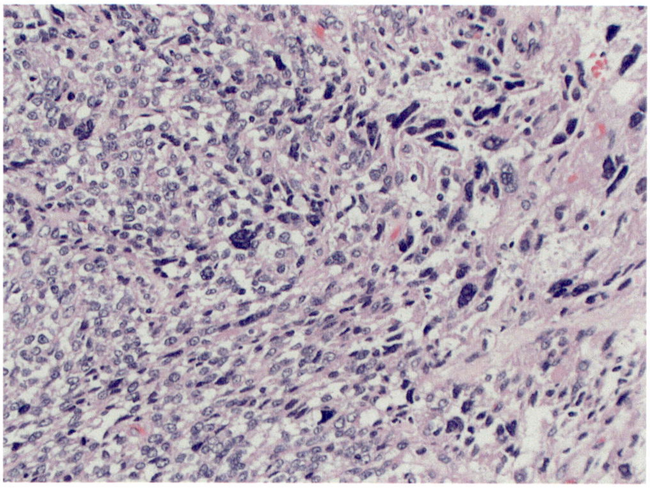

Fig. 7.28 Merging of epithelioid and spindle cells with significant cytological atypia (100×)

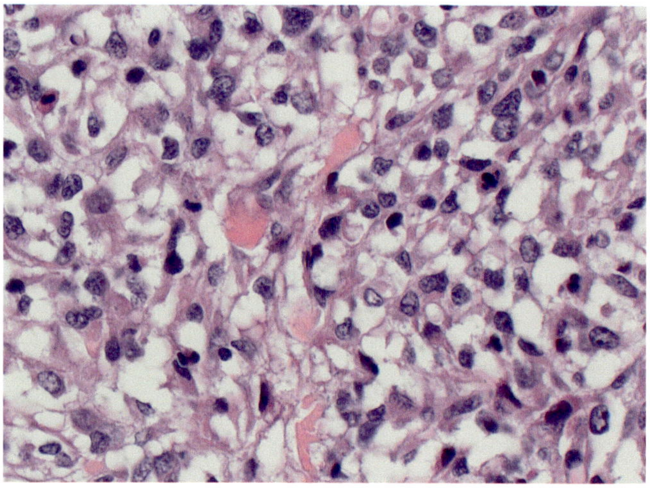

Fig. 7.29 The neoplastic cells have clear cytoplasm and moderate to severe cytological atypia (200×)

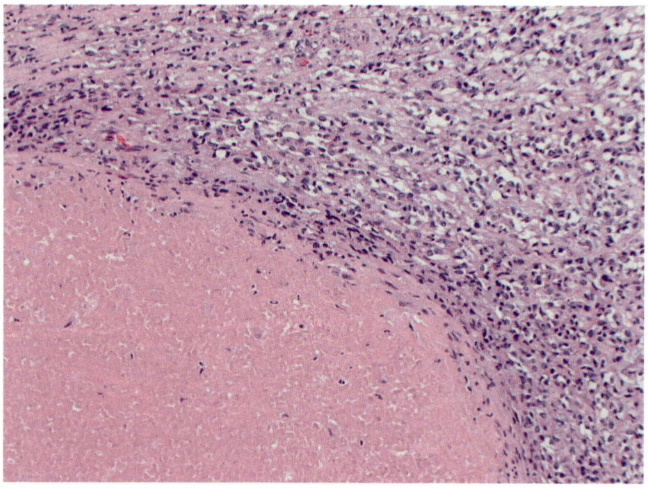

Fig. 7.30 Epithelioid cells with tumor cell necrosis (40×)

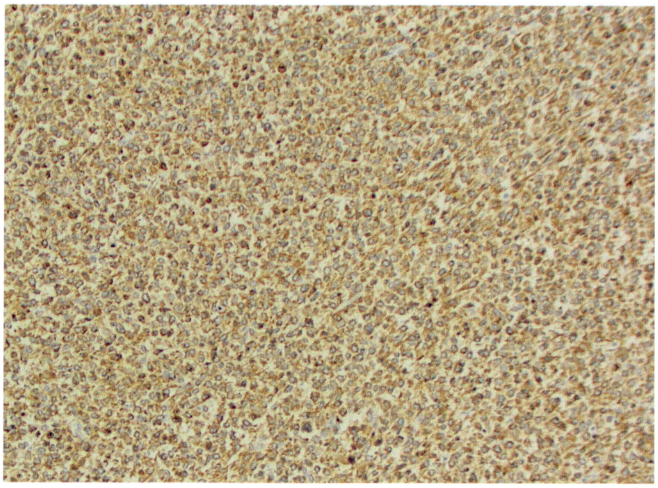

Fig. 7.31 Desmin is diffusely positive in the neoplastic cells (40×)

  - The neoplastic cells are radially arranged around blood vessels.
  - Positive for melanocytic and smooth muscle markers.
  - See Part II, Sect. 7.10.
- Uterine tumor resembling ovarian sex cord-stromal tumor (UTROSCT)
  - A well-circumscribed nodular lesion with variable cell morphologies.
  - See Part II, Sect. 8.1.
- Undifferentiated uterine sarcoma
  - Heterogenous group of tumors with no identifiable line of differentiation (negative for smooth muscle markers).
  - Sheets of uniform or pleomorphic epithelioid and spindle cells with high mitotic activity.
  - Adequate sampling is required to rule out other diagnostic entities such as carcinosarcoma, adenosarcoma, and high-grade ESS.

7.8.1.4 Clinical Significance

- Patients with ELMS have a shorter disease-specific survival than the matched cohort from patients with non-epithelioid LMS [33].

7.9 Cellular Leiomyoma

7.9.1 Received as a Second Opinion for Endometrial Stromal Nodule or Low-Grade ESS

7.9.1.1 Key Diagnostic Features

- In gross examination, the cut surface is tan to yellow and in soft consistency [34].
- The tumor has irregular margins with surrounding myometrium or cleft-like spaces (Fig. 7.32). The neoplastic

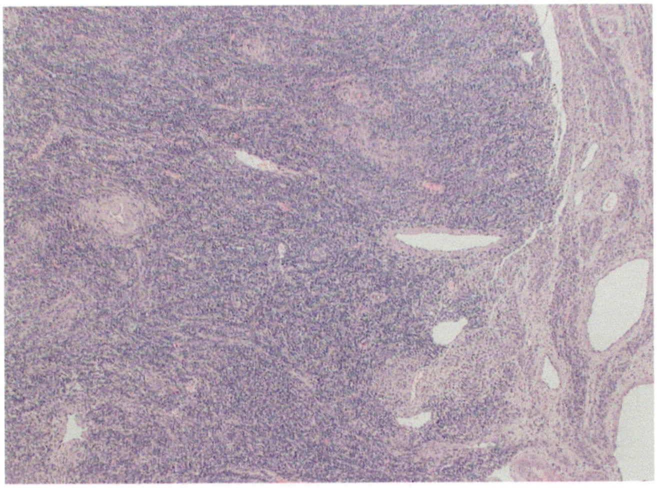

Fig. 7.32 Highly cellular sheets of small blue cells are separated from the myometrium with a cleft-like space (right upper corner) (40×)

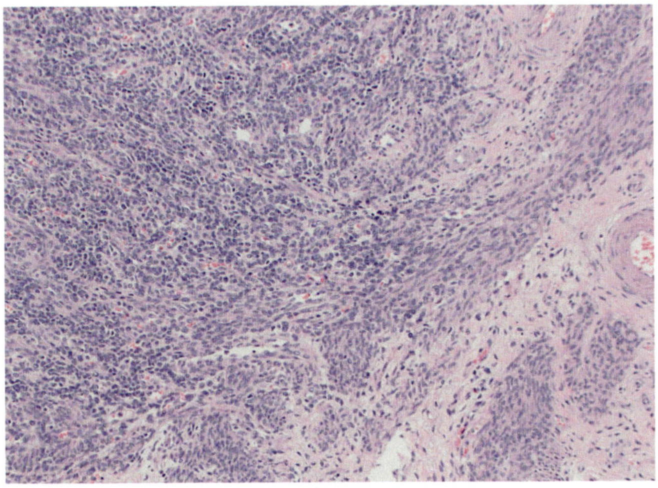

Fig. 7.33 The neoplastic cells merge with the surrounding myometrium (100×)

cells might extend into the adjacent myometrium (Fig. 7.33).

- The cellularity is dense with scattered, thick-walled vessels (Fig. 7.34). In some samples, there might be small vessel proliferation and cuffing of cells around vessels. It might resemble the whorls around arterioles of endometrial stromal tumors.
- Cellular leiomyomas might contain highly cellular areas alternating with normocellular areas.

7.9.1.2 Ancillary Studies

- Immunoreactive with desmin, SMA, and h-caldesmon. CD10 can be positive for up to 50% of cellular leiomyomas [35].

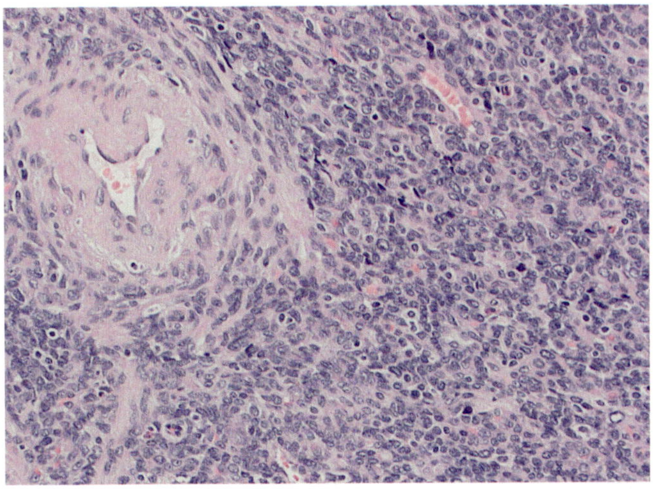

Fig. 7.34 The neoplastic cells are uniform without cytological atypia. Hyalinized, thick-walled blood vessels are scattered throughout the lesion (100×)

7.9.1.3 Differential Diagnosis

- Low-grade endometrial stromal sarcoma (LESS)
  - Fascicular growth pattern, thick-walled blood vessels, merging of neoplastic cells with surrounding myometrium, cleft-like spaces at the periphery, and diffuse immunoreactivity with smooth muscle markers are features that favor cellular leiomyoma over LGESS [36].
- Endometrial stroma nodules (ESN)
  - ESN might have margin irregularities but not overt invasion into the myometrium. Finger-like projections or satellite islands <3 mm and <3 in number are allowed for the diagnosis of ESN [32].

7.9.1.4 Clinical Significance

- Misdiagnosing as an ESN has no clinical consequences, but the survival of patients with LGESS depends on the disease stage. Clinical follow-up is necessary for patients with LGESS [37].

7.10 Perivascular Epithelioid Cell Neoplasm (PEComa)

7.10.1 A 37-Year-Old Woman with Uterine Fibroid

7.10.1.1 Key Diagnostic Features

- Well-circumscribed or invasive borders.
- Nested or diffuse pattern of proliferation of either spindle cells (Fig. 7.35), more frequently epithelioid cells (Fig. 7.36).

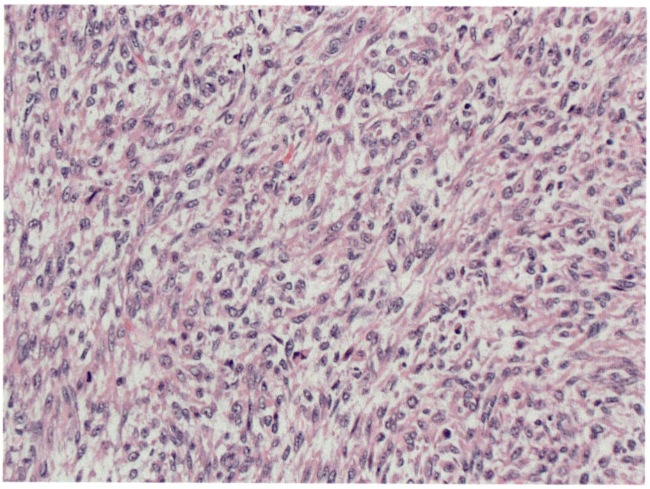

Fig. 7.35 Spindle cell component of the PEComa. The cells have foamy cytoplasm. Nuclear atypia is mild to moderate degree (100×)

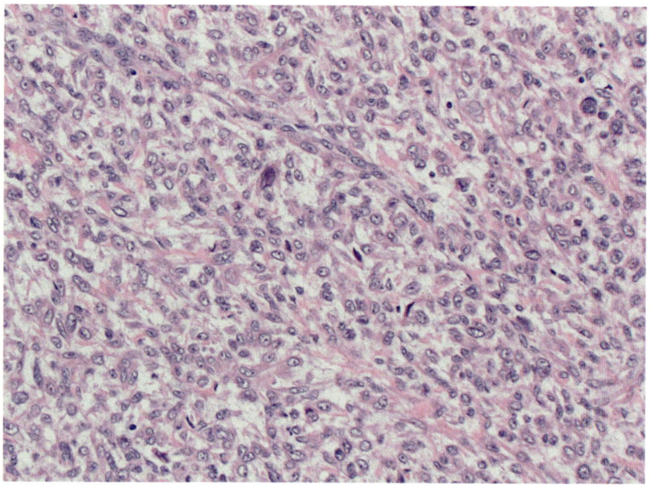

Fig. 7.36 Epithelioid cells in nested and diffuse patterns (200×)

- The majority of neoplastic cells have well-defined borders with clear to eosinophilic granular cytoplasm.
- Nuclear atypia and mitotic activity are variable.
- Macronucleoli, multinucleated giant cells, intranuclear pseudoinclusions, spider-like giant cells (Fig. 7.37), rhabdoid cells, and melanin pigment can be present [38].
- There might be extensive sclerosing in PEComa (sclerosing type) [39].
- Vessels are thin and ectatic (Fig. 7.38). A perivascular/radial distribution of tumor cells is present in less than 25% oftumors [40].

7.10.1.2 Ancillary Studies

- Positive immunostains: HMB45 (99%) (Fig. 7.39), Melan-A, Cathepsin-K, desmin, SMA, h-caldesmon, melanoma-associated antigen (PNL2) [41].

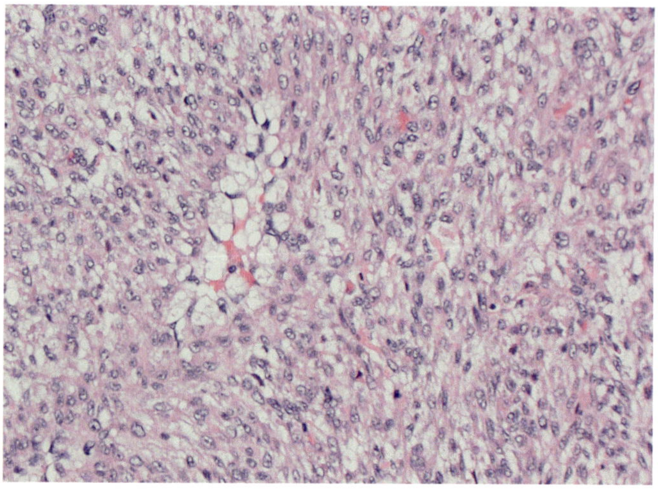

Fig. 7.37 Cells resembling spider cells of adult rhabdomyoma (200×)

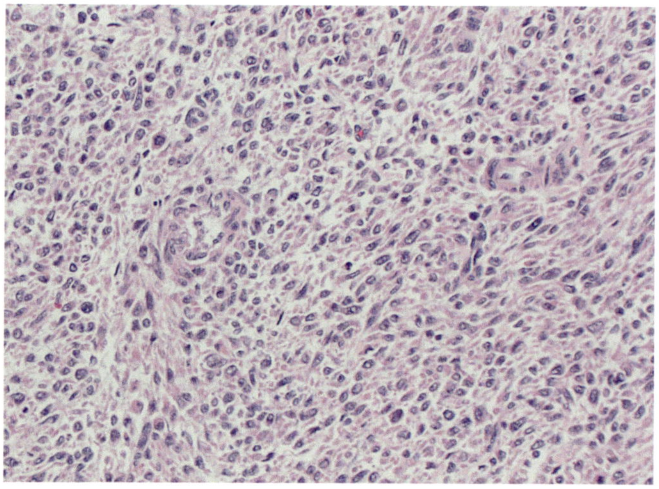

Fig. 7.38 The vasculature is thin-walled in this field (200×)

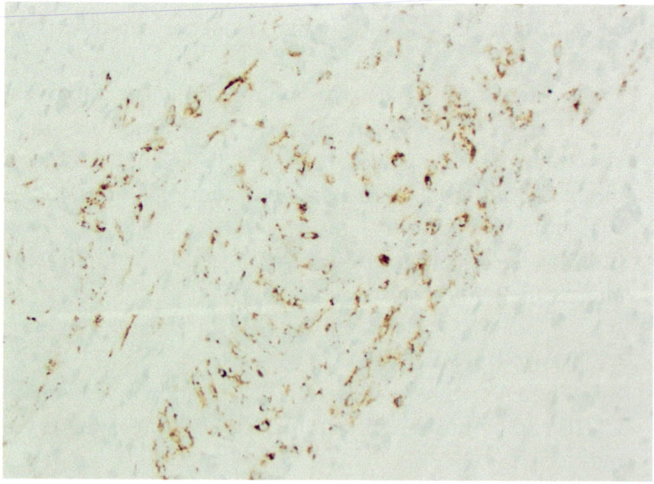

Fig. 7.39 HMB45 is focally positive (200×)

- Extent of staining with melanocytic markers is variable (focal to diffuse).
- *TFE3* rearrangement and *TSC* 1 and 2 mutations are detected in PEComa samples [42, 43]. *TSC* mutations and *TFE3* fusions are mutually exclusive.

7.10.1.3 Differential Diagnosis

- Epithelioid smooth muscle tumors
  - Thick-walled vessels.
  - Perinuclear vacuoles, diffuse eosinophilic cytoplasm (not granular) [44].
  - See Part II, Sect. 7.8.
- Alveolar soft part sarcoma
  - Arranged in nests and sheets and comprised of large polygonal cells with abundant clear, eosinophilic, or granular cytoplasm.
  - Negative for melanocytic and smooth muscle markers.
  - TFE3 and Cathepsin-K are positive.

7.10.1.4 Clinical Significance

- The presence of two of the following morphological features indicates a malignant clinical behavior: (1) Tumor size >5 cm. (2) Infiltrative borders. (3) High nuclear grade. (4) Mitotic count >1 per 50 mm square. (5) Necrosis. (6) Vascular invasion [32].

7.11 Solitary Fibrous Tumor (SFT)

7.11.1 A 39-Year-Old Woman with Fibroids

7.11.1.1 Key Diagnostic Features

- Usually well-circumscribed lesions of the myometrium with hyper- and hypocellular areas of spindle cell proliferation (Fig. 7.40).
- Dilated branching (staghorn/hemangiopericytoma-like) vasculature (Fig. 7.41).
- Patternless proliferation of spindle cells (Fig. 7.42).
- Unusual morphological features include a fatty component, diffuse stromal hyalinization, myxoid stroma, and giant-cell angiofibroma-like features [45].

7.11.1.2 Ancillary Studies

- *NAB2-STAT6* gene fusion is present in most SFTs [46, 47]. STAT6 is a sensitive and specific marker of SFT by immunohistochemistry [48].
- CD34 is expressed in 90% of SFT [49].

7.11.1.3 Differential Diagnosis

- Cellular leiomyoma
  - Spindle/ovoid cells with scant cytoplasm with fascicular pattern.

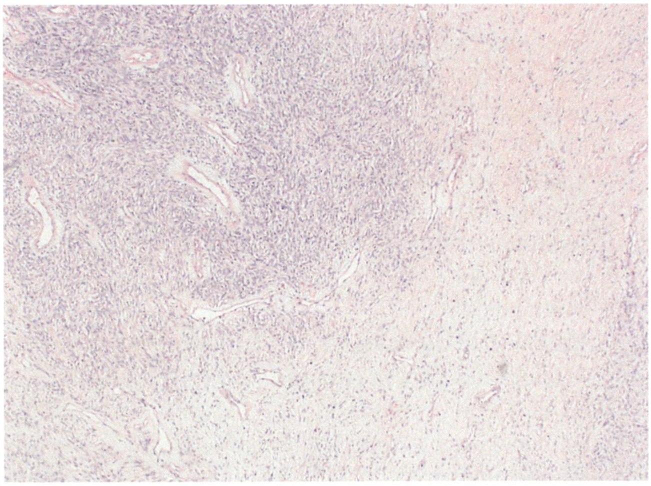

Fig. 7.40 Hypercellular and hypocellular areas of spindle cell proliferation within the myometrium (40×)

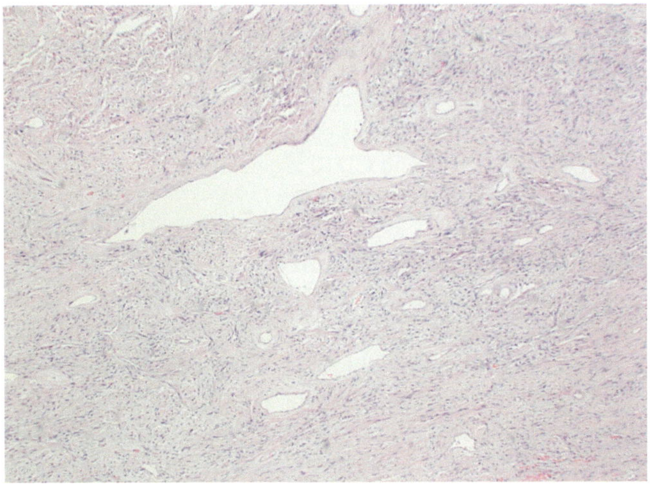

Fig. 7.41 Prominent staghorn-type vasculature in this field (40×)

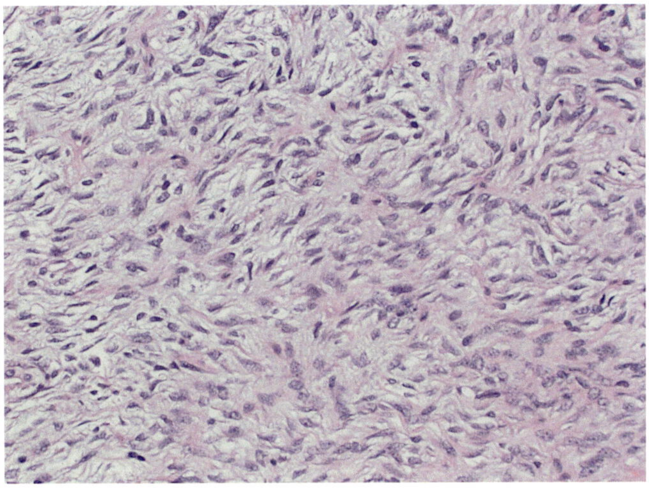

Fig. 7.42 Patternless growth of spindle cells without any cytological atypia or mitotic activity (200×)

- The presence of thick-walled blood vessels and cleft-like spaces supports the diagnosis.
- Positive for smooth muscle markers. STAT6 is not expressed.
- See Part II, Sect. 7.9.

- Low-grade endometrial stromal sarcoma
  - Ovoid cells with scant cytoplasm, resembling proliferative-type endometrial stromal cells, arranged in diffuse sheets with varying degrees of hyalinization.
  - Thin-walled capillaries.
  - A finger-like pattern of permeative myoinvasion.
  - STAT 6 is not expressed.
- Inflammatory myofibroblastic tumor
  - Spindle and epithelioid myofibroblastic cells admixed with lymphoplasmacytic infiltrates in a fascicular pattern or myxoid stroma.
  - The lesion borders can be infiltrative or well-circumscribed.
  - Cytological atypia is mild to moderate.
  - Rearrangements involving the *ALK* (anaplastic lymphoma kinase) gene at 2p23 result in positive ALK staining by immunohistochemistry [50].
  - Desmin, SMA, and CD10 are positive.
  - STAT 6 might be positive.

7.11.1.4 Clinical Significance

- A stratification model for risk assessment of clinical behavior based on age, tumor size, mitotic activity, and tumor necrosis is available [51]. The long-term follow-up is limited for gynecologic cases. In rare case reports, uterine SFT with low mitotic counts presents with lung metastasis [52]. SFT in the gynecological tract might be better considered as a tumor with uncertain malignant potential.

7.12 Myxoid Leiomyosarcoma (MLMS)

7.12.1 A 63-Year-Old Woman with a Pelvic Mass

7.12.1.1 Key Diagnostic Features

- In gross examination, the lesion is gelatinous, mucoid, or myxoid.
- Cellularity can be variable (low-to-high cellularity) or uniformly hypercellular (Fig. 7.43). The hypocellular areas have myxoid/mucinous pools. Nuclei are cigar-shaped, and cytoplasm is eosinophilic.
- If one of the following criteria is fulfilled, the smooth muscle lesion is myxoid LMS per current WHO diagnostic criteria: infiltrative borders (Fig. 7.44), moderate to severe cytological atypia (Fig. 7.45), tumor cell necrosis, or more than 1 mitosis per 10 high-power fields (Fig. 7.46).

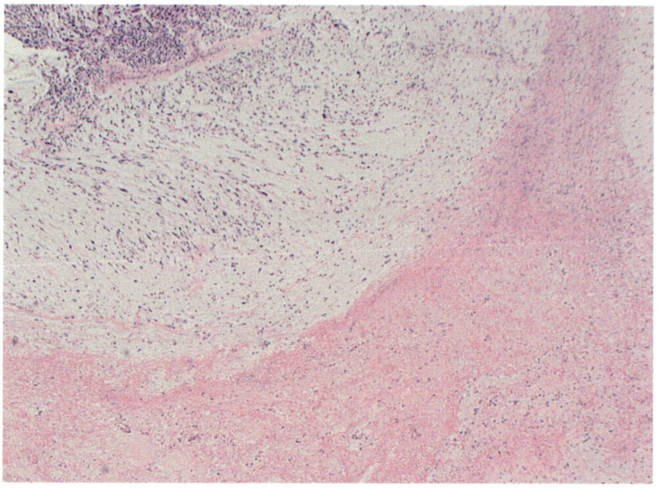

Fig. 7.43 Smooth muscle tumor with myxoid stroma and necrosis (40×)

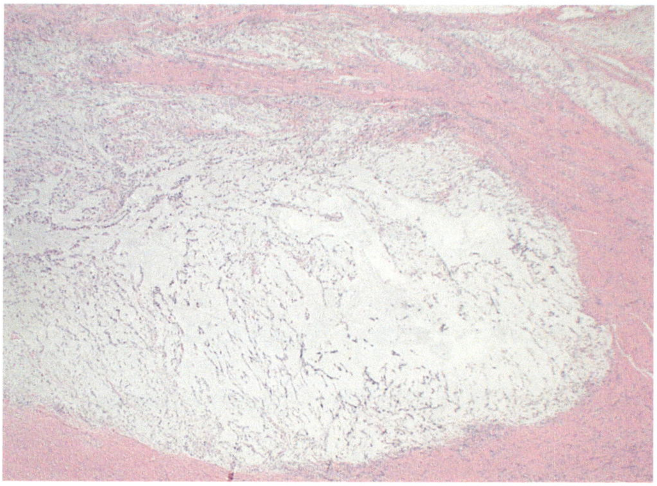

Fig. 7.44 The lesion has irregular/infiltrative borders with the myometrium (40×)

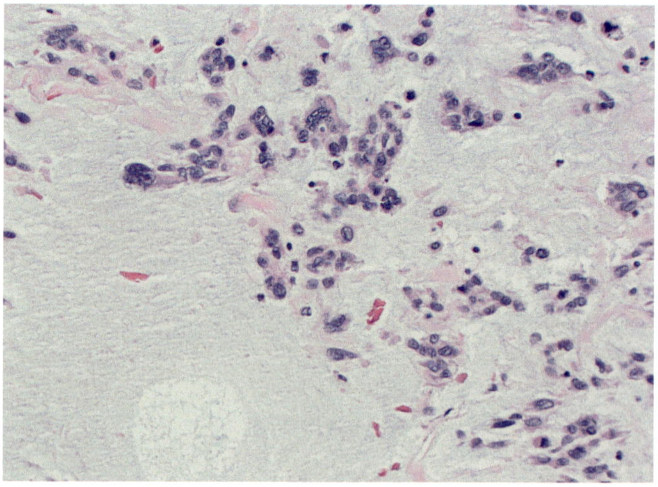

Fig. 7.45 The cytological atypia is moderate to severe (200×)

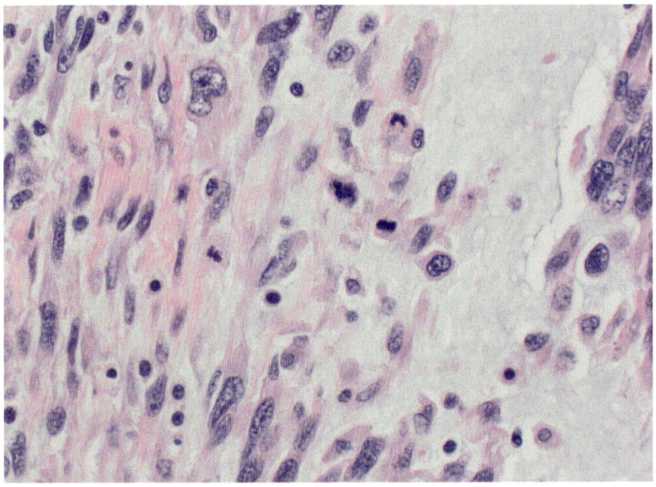

Fig. 7.46 The mitotic figures within the myxoid areas (200×)

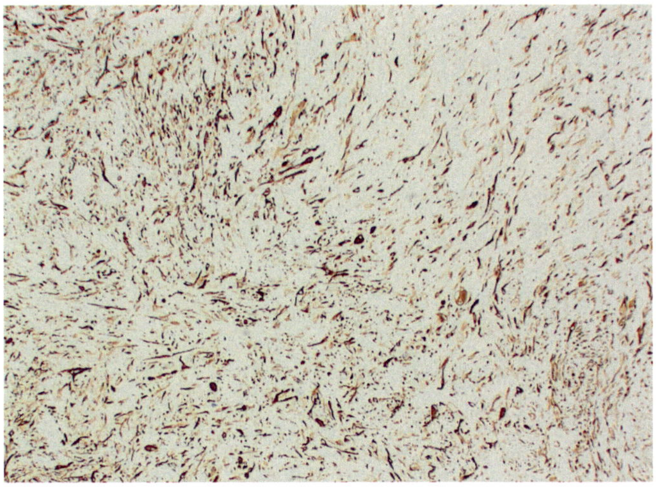

Fig. 7.47 Immunostain for desmin is diffusely positive (100×)

7.12.1.2 Ancillary Studies

- At least one smooth muscle marker is expressed in large series [53] (Fig. 7.47).
- *PLAG1* fusion is detected in around 25% of myxoid LMS cases [54].
- Alcian blue highlights the myxoid background (Fig. 7.48).

7.12.1.3 Differential Diagnosis

- Leiomyoma with myxoid or hydropic change
  - Myometrial or lymphovascular invasion, cytological atypia, mitotic figures, and tumor cell necrosis are the morphological features of myxoid LMS. An extensive sampling might be required to identify characteristic morphological features in some lesions.
  - See Part II, Sect. 7.1.
- High-grade endometrial stromal sarcoma (HGESS) with *BCOR* genetic abnormalities

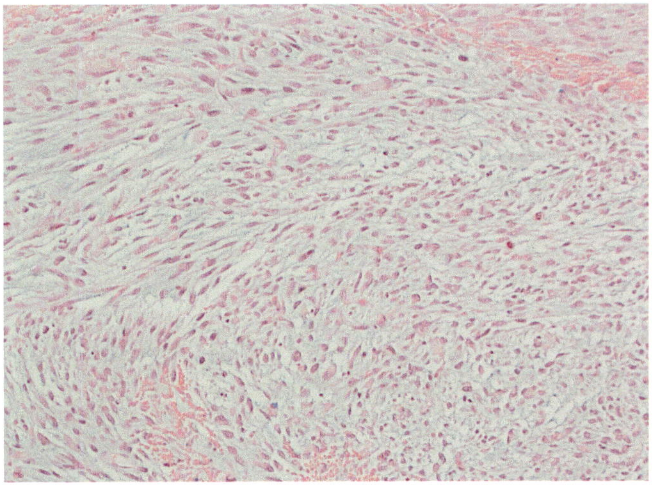

Fig. 7.48 Alcian blue highlights the myxoid background (100×)

  - In general, endometrial or nodal involvement favors HGESS over myxoid LMS.
  - X-linked BCL-6 co-repressor *(BCOR)* plays a role in suppressing gene transcription and maintaining tissue homeostasis and gene silencing through epigenetic mechanisms [55].
  - *ZC3H7B–BCOR* fusion-positive HGESS is bulky polypoid masses that involve the endomyometrium and exhibit tongue-like and expansile myometrial invasion. Haphazard fascicles of spindle cells are associated with variable amounts of myxoid matrix. Collagen plaques and arteriolar vasculature without perivascular whorling are frequently present. The cells have intermediate-sized ovoid to spindled and occasionally rounded nuclei with even chromatin and inconspicuous. The cytoplasm is usually scant to moderate and eosinophilic [56, 57].
  - CD10, Cyclin D1, BCOR (50%), SMA (<50%), and h-caldesmon are expressed by immunohistochemistry. Desmin is negative in HGESS with *ZC3H7B-BCOR* fusion [58].
  - HGESS with *BCOR* internal tandem duplication (ITD) often consists of three components: high-grade spindle cells resembling those in *ZC3H7B-BCOR* tumors, high-grade round cells, and low-grade spindle cells. There is an overlap between morphologies of *ZC3H7B-BCOR* tumors and those harboring *BCOR* ITD.
  - Cyclin D1, CD10, and BCOR are positive, and desmin is focally positive in HGESS with *BCOR* ITD [59].
- *YWHAE–NUTM2* fusion-positive HGESS
  - A pure myxoid or fibromyxoid ESS. Most examples have a distinctive high-grade round cell and low-grade fibromyxoid components.
  - The round cell component harbors *YWHAE–NUTM2* gene fusion.

- CD10, ER, and PR: positive in low-grade component. Cyclin D1 and BCOR are variable positive.
- LGESS with myxoid change
  - Admixture of conventional and variant morphology.
  - CD10 is diffusely positive.
- Myxoid inflammatory myofibroblastic tumor (IMT)
  - Morphological patterns include myxoid, compact/fascicular, and hyalinized types.
  - ALK expression and confirmation of *ALK1* rearrangement are diagnostic for IMT.

7.12.1.4 Clinical Significance

- The prognosis is worse compared to that of spindle-cell (conventional) LMS. A mitotic rate of ≥5 mitoses per 10 high-power fields is a risk factor for death from the disease [53].

7.13 Mullerian Adenosarcoma (MA) with Sarcomatous Overgrowth

7.13.1 A 72-Year-Old Woman with Postmenopausal Bleeding

7.13.1.1 Key Diagnostic Features

- MA is a biphasic tumor with an admixture of benign glandular epithelium and low-grade sarcoma, usually of endometrial stromal type. A leaf-like appearance resembling phyllodes tumor of the breast, at least focally, is characteristic of MA (Fig. 7.49).
- MA can arise in the endometrium, endocervix, or extrauterine locations [60] or from adenomyosis [61].
- The glandular component can demonstrate squamous or mucinous metaplasia [62].
- The stroma typically concentrates around the glands, forming periglandular cuffs (Fig. 7.50). Bulging of periglandular stroma into the gland lumen (Fig. 7.51) is common. Mitotic figures are easily identified around periglandular stroma (Fig. 7.52).
- Sarcomatous overgrowth is usually high-grade and defined as the presence of pure sarcoma without a glandular component in an area occupying at least 25% of the lesion (Fig. 7.53).
- Morphologic features of sarcomatous overgrowth include severe cytologic atypia, brisk mitotic activity, and necrosis. Rhabdomyoblastic differentiation (Fig. 7.54) is the most common high-grade sarcoma type observed in MA with sarcomatous overgrowth.
- The morphological features associated with an increased risk of recurrence in MA are the presence of myometrial invasion and sarcomatous overgrowth [62].

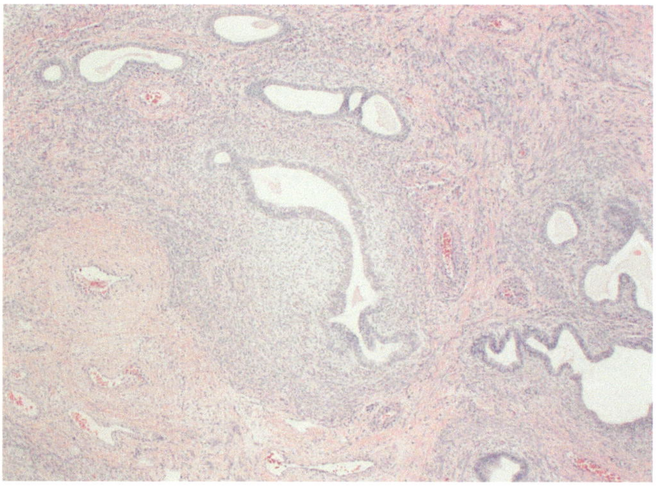

Fig. 7.50 Dense periglandular stromal condensation and compression into glandular lumen (100×)

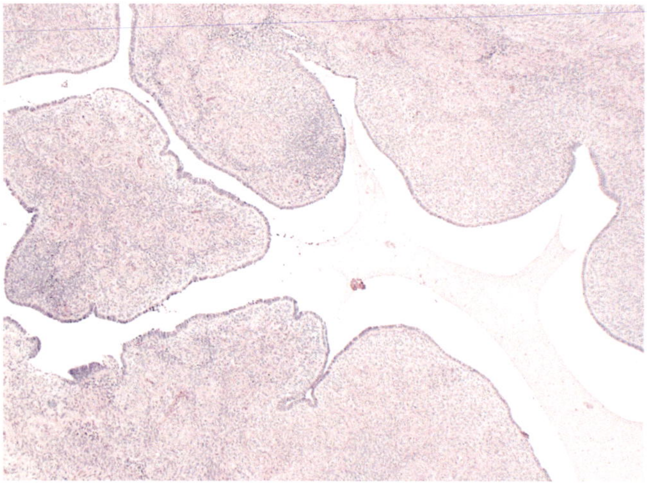

Fig. 7.49 MA has phyllodes-like (leaf-like) architecture with papillary fronds (40×)

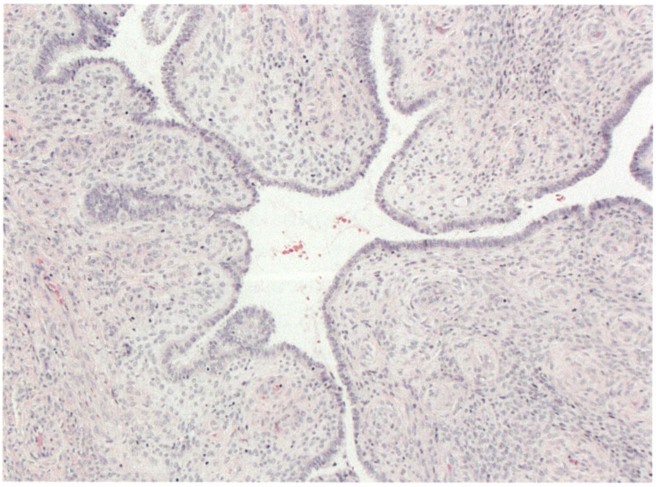

Fig. 7.51 Bulging of periglandular stroma into gland lumen (100×)

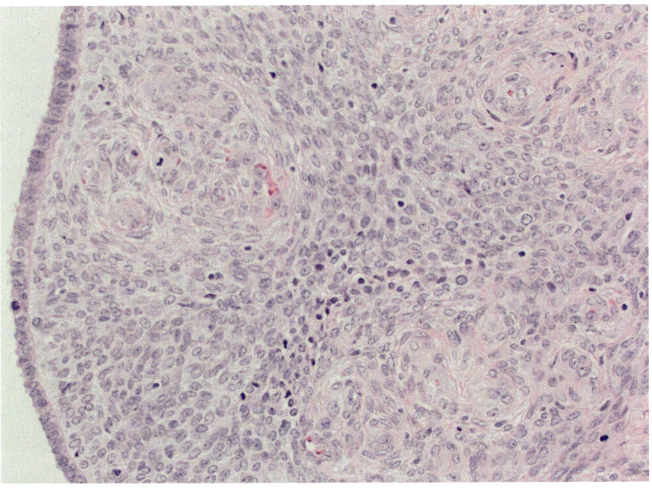

Fig. 7.52 Mitotic figures are easily identified around periglandular stroma (200×)

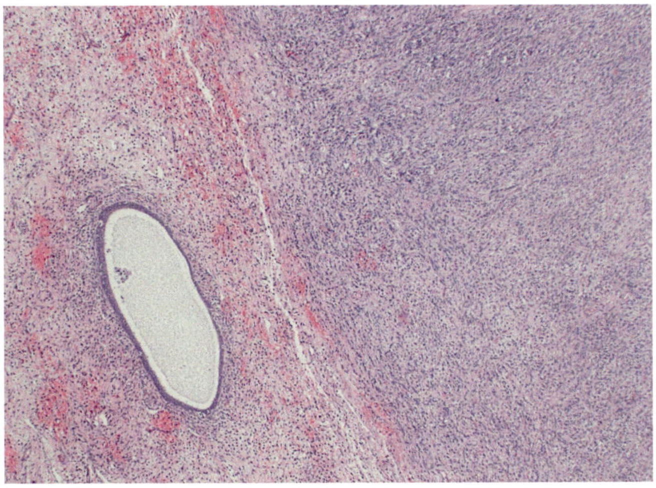

Fig. 7.53 The MA with low-grade sarcoma on the left and the sarcomatous overgrowth with high-grade sarcomatous elements on the right side of the figure (40×)

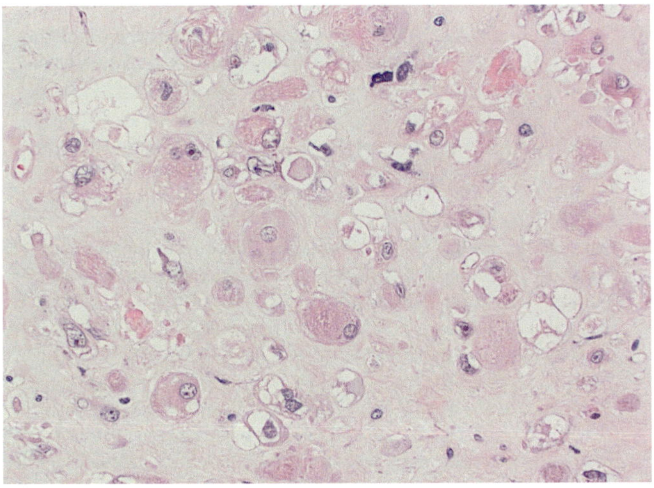

Fig. 7.54 High-grade heterologous rhabdomyosarcoma component in the MA with sarcomatous overgrowth (400×)

7.13.1.2 Ancillary Studies

- The cell proliferation markers are expressed more strongly in MA with sarcomatous overgrowth than in typical MA. On the other hand, the marker expression of cell differentiation (CD10 and PR) is higher in MA than in MA with sarcomatous overgrowth [63].
- ER, PR, WT1, and CD10 are positive in MA without sarcomatous overgrowth. The expressions of all markers are lost in MA with sarcomatous overgrowth. SMA, desmin, and CD34 can have variable positivity in the stromal component of MA [64].

7.13.1.3 Differential Diagnosis of MA with Sarcomatous Overgrowth

- Carcinosarcoma
  - Both epithelial and mesenchymal elements are high-grade tumors.
  - Carcinomatous and sarcomatous components are spatially distinct.
- Mixed endometrioid adenocarcinoma and Müllerian adenosarcoma
  - Adenocarcinoma can arise in close spatial association with MA [65].
  - The endometrioid carcinoma component is clonally related to the MA.
- Embryonal rhabdomyosarcoma (ERMS)
  - The most useful morphological feature is the lack of leaf-like architecture in ERMS. The glands preserve their normal architecture.
  - The immunostaining profile overlaps with the MA.
  - Almost all gynecologic ERMS and 20% of MA harbor *DICER1* mutations [66].
  - See Part III, Sect. 9.10.
- Undifferentiated uterine sarcoma
  - There is no glandular component of the lesion.
  - Inadequate sampling might lead to this diagnosis if the sections do not contain conventional MA component in an MA with sarcomatous overgrowth.

7.13.1.4 Clinical Significance

- The 2-year progression-free and overall survival drop from 100% in MA to 20% in MA with sarcomatous overgrowth [67].

References

1. Clement PB, Young RH, Scully RE. Diffuse, perinodular, and other patterns of hydropic degeneration within and adjacent to uterine leiomyomas. Problems in differential diagnosis. Am J Surg Pathol. 1992;16(1):26–32.
2. Prayson RA, Goldblum JR, Hart WR. Epithelioid smooth-muscle tumors of the uterus: a clinicopathologic study of 18 patients. Am J Surg Pathol. 1997;21(4):383–91.
3. Kaminski PF, Tavassoli FA. Plexiform tumorlet: a clinical and pathologic study of 15 cases with ultrastructural observations. Int J Gynecol Pathol. 1984;3(2):124–34.

4. Lou YF, Shi XP, Song ZZ. Intravenous leiomyomatosis of the uterus with extension to the right heart. Cardiovasc Ultrasound. 2011;9:25.
5. Clement PB, Young RH, Scully RE. Intravenous leiomyomatosis of the uterus. A clinicopathological analysis of 16 cases with unusual histologic features. Am J Surg Pathol. 1988;12(12):932–45.
6. Ordulu Z, Nucci MR, Dal Cin P, Hollowell ML, Otis CN, Hornick JL, et al. Intravenous leiomyomatosis: an unusual intermediate between benign and malignant uterine smooth muscle tumors. Mod Pathol. 2016;29(5):500–10.
7. Lu B, Liu Q, Tang L, Ma Y, Shi H. Intravenous leiomyomatosis: molecular analysis of 17 cases. Pathology. 2020;52(2):213–7.
8. Deng Y, Song B. Three case reports of intravenous leiomyomatosis with intracardiac extensions. Thorac Cardiovasc Surg Rep. 2020;9(1):e40–e3.
9. Tavassoli FA, Norris HJ. Peritoneal leiomyomatosis (leiomyomatosis peritonealis disseminata): a clinicopathologic study of 20 cases with ultrastructural observations. Int J Gynecol Pathol. 1982;1(1):59–74.
10. Yu BR, Lee SY, Cho DH. Leiomyomatosis peritonealis disseminata with endometriosis. BMJ Case Rep. 2021;14(7).
11. Ma KF, Chow LT. Sex cord-like pattern leiomyomatosis peritonealis disseminata: a hitherto undescribed feature. Histopathology. 1992;21(4):389–91.
12. Chen X, Liu H, Shi H, Fan Q, Sun D, Lang J. Leiomyomatosis peritonealis disseminata following laparoscopic surgery with uncontained morcellation: 13 cases from one institution. Front Surg. 2021;8:788749.
13. Patton KT, Cheng L, Papavero V, Blum MG, Yeldandi AV, Adley BP, et al. Benign metastasizing leiomyoma: clonality, telomere length and clinicopathologic analysis. Mod Pathol. 2006;19(1):130–40.
14. Posligua L, Silva EG, Deavers MT, Merino MJ, Malpica A. Low-grade smooth muscle tumors of the primary and the secondary mullerian system: a proposed concept of multicentricity. Int J Gynecol Pathol. 2012;31(6):547–55.
15. Li J, Dai S. Leiomyomatosis peritonealis disseminata: a clinical analysis of 13 cases and literature review. Int J Surg Pathol. 2020;28(2):163–8.
16. Sharma P, Chaturvedi KU, Gupta R, Nigam S. Leiomyomatosis peritonealis disseminata with malignant change in a post-menopausal woman. Gynecol Oncol. 2004;95(3):742–5.
17. Roth LM, Reed RJ, Sternberg WH. Cotyledonoid dissecting leiomyoma of the uterus. The Sternberg tumor. Am J Surg Pathol. 1996;20(12):1455–61.
18. Roth LM, Reed RJ. Dissecting leiomyomas of the uterus other than cotyledonoid dissecting leiomyomas: a report of eight cases. Am J Surg Pathol. 1999;23(9):1032–9.
19. Smith CC, Gold MA, Wile G, Fadare O. Cotyledonoid dissecting leiomyoma of the uterus: a review of clinical, pathological, and radiological features. Int J Surg Pathol. 2012;20(4):330–41.
20. Roth LM, Kirker JA, Insull M, Whittaker J. Recurrent cotyledonoid dissecting leiomyoma of the uterus. Int J Gynecol Pathol. 2013;32(2):215–20.
21. Bennett JA, Weigelt B, Chiang S, Selenica P, Chen YB, Bialik A, et al. Leiomyoma with bizarre nuclei: a morphological, immunohistochemical and molecular analysis of 31 cases. Mod Pathol. 2017;30(10):1476–88.
22. Joseph NM, Solomon DA, Frizzell N, Rabban JT, Zaloudek C, Garg K. Morphology and immunohistochemistry for 2SC and FH aid in detection of fumarate hydratase gene aberrations in uterine leiomyomas from Young patients. Am J Surg Pathol. 2015;39(11):1529–39.
23. Chan E, Rabban JT, Mak J, Zaloudek C, Garg K. Detailed morphologic and immunohistochemical characterization of myomectomy and hysterectomy specimens from women with hereditary leiomyomatosis and renal cell carcinoma syndrome (HLRCC). Am J Surg Pathol. 2019;43(9):1170–9.
24. Oliva E. Practical issues in uterine pathology from banal to bewildering: the remarkable spectrum of smooth muscle neoplasia. Mod Pathol. 2016;29(Suppl 1):S104–20.
25. Croce S, Young RH, Oliva E. Uterine leiomyomas with bizarre nuclei: a clinicopathologic study of 59 cases. Am J Surg Pathol. 2014;38(10):1330–9.
26. Chen L, Yang B. Immunohistochemical analysis of p16, p53, and Ki-67 expression in uterine smooth muscle tumors. Int J Gynecol Pathol. 2008;27(3):326–32.
27. Mills AM, Ly A, Balzer BL, Hendrickson MR, Kempson RL, McKenney JK, et al. Cell cycle regulatory markers in uterine atypical leiomyoma and leiomyosarcoma: immunohistochemical study of 68 cases with clinical follow-up. Am J Surg Pathol. 2013;37(5):634–42.
28. Veras E, Malpica A, Deavers MT, Silva EG. Mitosis-specific marker phospho-histone H3 in the assessment of mitotic index in uterine smooth muscle tumors: a pilot study. Int J Gynecol Pathol. 2009;28(4):316–21.
29. Jones MA, Young RH, Scully RE. Endometrial adenocarcinoma with a component of giant cell carcinoma. Int J Gynecol Pathol. 1991;10(3):260–70.
30. Liegl-Atzwanger B, Heitzer E, Flicker K, Müller S, Ulz P, Saglam O, et al. Exploring chromosomal abnormalities and genetic changes in uterine smooth muscle tumors. Mod Pathol. 2016;29(10):1262–77.
31. Fischer JV, Mejia-Bautista M, Vadasz B, Yin P, Bulun S, Tanner EJ, et al. Uterine leiomyosarcoma associated with leiomyoma with bizarre nuclei: histology and genomic analysis of 2 cases. Int J Gynecol Pathol. 2022;41(6):552–65.
32. WHO Classification of Tumours Editorial Board. Female genital tumours, vol. 4. 5th ed. Lyon: International Agency for Research on Cancer; 2020. WHO Classification of Tumours Series.
33. Chapel DB, Nucci MR, Quade BJ, Parra-Herran C. Epithelioid leiomyosarcoma of the uterus: modern outcome-based appraisal of diagnostic criteria in a large institutional series. Am J Surg Pathol. 2022;46(4):464–75.
34. Oliva E. Cellular mesenchymal tumors of the uterus: a review emphasizing recent observations. Int J Gynecol Pathol. 2014;33(4):374–84.
35. Oliva E, Young RH, Amin MB, Clement PB. An immunohistochemical analysis of endometrial stromal and smooth muscle tumors of the uterus: a study of 54 cases emphasizing the importance of using a panel because of overlap in immunoreactivity for individual antibodies. Am J Surg Pathol. 2002;26(4):403–12.
36. Oliva E, Young RH, Clement PB, Bhan AK, Scully RE. Cellular benign mesenchymal tumors of the uterus. A comparative morphologic and immunohistochemical analysis of 33 highly cellular leiomyomas and six endometrial stromal nodules, two frequently confused tumors. Am J Surg Pathol. 1995;19(7):757–68.
37. Smith ES, Jansen C, Miller KM, Chiang S, Alektiar KM, Hensley ML, et al. Primary characteristics and outcomes of newly diagnosed low-grade endometrial stromal sarcoma. Int J Gynecol Cancer. 2022;32(7):882–90.
38. Bennett JA, Braga AC, Pinto A, Van de Vijver K, Cornejo K, Pesci A, et al. Uterine PEComas: a morphologic, immunohistochemical, and molecular analysis of 32 tumors. Am J Surg Pathol. 2018;42(10):1370–83.
39. Hornick JL, Fletcher CD. Sclerosing PEComa: clinicopathologic analysis of a distinctive variant with a predilection for the retroperitoneum. Am J Surg Pathol. 2008;32(4):493–501.
40. Bennett JA, Oliva E. Perivascular epithelioid cell tumors (PEComa) of the gynecologic tract. Genes Chromosomes Cancer. 2021;60(3):168–79.
41. Valencia-Guerrero A, Pinto A, Anderson WJ, Trevisan G, Nucci MR, Hirsch MS. PNL2: a useful adjunct biomarker to HMB45 in the diagnosis of uterine perivascular epithelioid cell tumor (PEComa). Int J Gynecol Pathol. 2020;39(6):529–36.

42. Schoolmeester JK, Dao LN, Sukov WR, Wang L, Park KJ, Murali R, et al. TFE3 translocation-associated perivascular epithelioid cell neoplasm (PEComa) of the gynecologic tract: morphology, immunophenotype, differential diagnosis. Am J Surg Pathol. 2015;39(3):394–404.
43. Agaram NP, Sung YS, Zhang L, Chen CL, Chen HW, Singer S, et al. Dichotomy of genetic abnormalities in PEComas with therapeutic implications. Am J Surg Pathol. 2015;39(6):813–25.
44. Folpe AL, Kwiatkowski DJ. Perivascular epithelioid cell neoplasms: pathology and pathogenesis. Hum Pathol. 2010;41(1):1–15.
45. Yang EJ, Howitt BE, Fletcher CDM, Nucci MR. Solitary fibrous tumour of the female genital tract: a clinicopathological analysis of 25 cases. Histopathology. 2018;72(5):749–59.
46. Robinson DR, Wu YM, Kalyana-Sundaram S, Cao X, Lonigro RJ, Sung YS, et al. Identification of recurrent NAB2-STAT6 gene fusions in solitary fibrous tumor by integrative sequencing. Nat Genet. 2013;45(2):180–5.
47. Chmielecki J, Crago AM, Rosenberg M, O'Connor R, Walker SR, Ambrogio L, et al. Whole-exome sequencing identifies a recurrent NAB2-STAT6 fusion in solitary fibrous tumors. Nat Genet. 2013;45(2):131–2.
48. Doyle LA, Vivero M, Fletcher CD, Mertens F, Hornick JL. Nuclear expression of STAT6 distinguishes solitary fibrous tumor from histologic mimics. Mod Pathol. 2014;27(3):390–5.
49. Dermawan JK, Rubin BP, Kilpatrick SE, Gjorgova Gjeorgjievski S, Fritchie KJ, Goldblum JR, et al. CD34-negative solitary fibrous tumor: a clinicopathologic study of 25 cases and comparison with their CD34-positive counterparts. Am J Surg Pathol. 2021;45(12):1616–25.
50. Parra-Herran C, Quick CM, Howitt BE, Dal Cin P, Quade BJ, Nucci MR. Inflammatory myofibroblastic tumor of the uterus: clinical and pathologic review of 10 cases including a subset with aggressive clinical course. Am J Surg Pathol. 2015;39(2):157–68.
51. Demicco EG, Wagner MJ, Maki RG, Gupta V, Iofin I, Lazar AJ, et al. Risk assessment in solitary fibrous tumors: validation and refinement of a risk stratification model. Mod Pathol. 2017;30(10):1433–42.
52. Strickland KC, Nucci MR, Esselen KM, Muto MG, Chopra S, George S, et al. Solitary fibrous tumor of the uterus presenting with lung metastases: a case report. Int J Gynecol Pathol. 2016;35(1):25–9.
53. Parra-Herran C, Schoolmeester JK, Yuan L, Dal Cin P, Fletcher CD, Quade BJ, et al. Myxoid leiomyosarcoma of the uterus: a clinicopathologic analysis of 30 cases and review of the literature with reappraisal of its distinction from other uterine myxoid mesenchymal neoplasms. Am J Surg Pathol. 2016;40(3):285–301.
54. Arias-Stella JA 3rd, Benayed R, Oliva E, Young RH, Hoang LN, Lee CH, et al. Novel PLAG1 gene rearrangement distinguishes a subset of uterine myxoid leiomyosarcoma from other uterine myxoid mesenchymal tumors. Am J Surg Pathol. 2019;43(3):382–8.
55. Fan Z, Yamaza T, Lee JS, Yu J, Wang S, Fan G, et al. BCOR regulates mesenchymal stem cell function by epigenetic mechanisms. Nat Cell Biol. 2009;11(8):1002–9.
56. Hoang LN, Aneja A, Conlon N, Delair DF, Middha S, Benayed R, et al. Novel high-grade endometrial stromal sarcoma: a morphologic mimicker of myxoid leiomyosarcoma. Am J Surg Pathol. 2017;41(1):12–24.
57. Lewis N, Soslow RA, Delair DF, Park KJ, Murali R, Hollmann TJ, et al. ZC3H7B-BCOR high-grade endometrial stromal sarcomas: a report of 17 cases of a newly defined entity. Mod Pathol. 2018;31(4):674–84.
58. Chiang S, Lee CH, Stewart CJR, Oliva E, Hoang LN, Ali RH, et al. BCOR is a robust diagnostic immunohistochemical marker of genetically diverse high-grade endometrial stromal sarcoma, including tumors exhibiting variant morphology. Mod Pathol. 2017;30(9):1251–61.
59. Mariño-Enriquez A, Lauria A, Przybyl J, Ng TL, Kowalewska M, Debiec-Rychter M, et al. BCOR internal tandem duplication in high-grade uterine sarcomas. Am J Surg Pathol. 2018;42(3):335–41.
60. Gallardo A, Prat J. Mullerian adenosarcoma: a clinicopathologic and immunohistochemical study of 55 cases challenging the existence of adenofibroma. Am J Surg Pathol. 2009;33(2):278–88.
61. Talia KL, Naaman Y, McCluggage WG. Uterine adenosarcoma originating in adenomyosis: report of an extremely rare phenomenon and review of published literature. Int J Gynecol Pathol. 2021;40(4):342–8.
62. Clement PB, Scully RE. Mullerian adenosarcoma of the uterus: a clinicopathologic analysis of 100 cases with a review of the literature. Hum Pathol. 1990;21(4):363–81.
63. Mbatani N, Olawaiye AB, Prat J. Uterine sarcomas. Int J Gynaecol Obstet. 2018;143(Suppl 2):51–8.
64. Soslow RA, Ali A, Oliva E. Mullerian adenosarcomas: an immunophenotypic analysis of 35 cases. Am J Surg Pathol. 2008;32(7):1013–21.
65. El Hallani S, Arora R, Lin DI, Måsbäc A, Mateoiu C, McCluggage WG, et al. Mixed endometrioid adenocarcinoma and Müllerian adenosarcoma of the uterus and ovary: clinicopathologic characterization with emphasis on its distinction from carcinosarcoma. Am J Surg Pathol. 2021;45(3):374–83.
66. Apellaniz-Ruiz M, McCluggage WG, Foulkes WD. DICER1-associated embryonal rhabdomyosarcoma and adenosarcoma of the gynecologic tract: pathology, molecular genetics, and indications for molecular testing. Genes Chromosomes Cancer. 2021;60(3):217–33.
67. Tanner EJ, Toussaint T, Leitao MM Jr, Hensley ML, Soslow RA, Gardner GJ, et al. Management of uterine adenosarcomas with and without sarcomatous overgrowth. Gynecol Oncol. 2013;129(1):140–4.

8 Miscellaneous Uterine Lesions

8.1 Uterine Tumor Resembling Ovarian Sex Cord Tumors (UTROSCT)

8.1.1 A 50-Year-Old Woman with Vaginal Bleeding

8.1.1.1 Key Diagnostic Features

- Usually, well-circumscribed nodular lesions with morphological patterns resembling ovarian sex cord tumors (Fig. 8.1).
- Multiple growth patterns, including sheets, cords, nests, trabeculae (Fig. 8.2), and tubules without any endometrial stromal component [1].
- A smooth muscle component might be present within the lesion or at the periphery by entrapment of the surrounding myometrium (Fig. 8.3). Follicle-like spaces might alternate with the diffuse sheet of cells (Fig. 8.4).

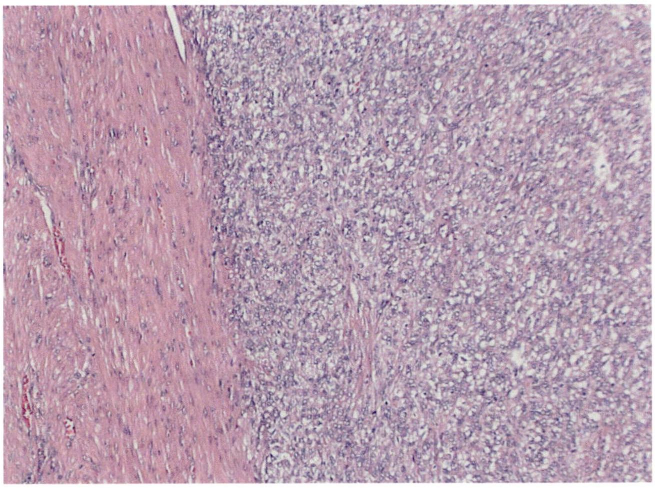

Fig. 8.1 Nodular lesion with well-circumscribed borders (40×)

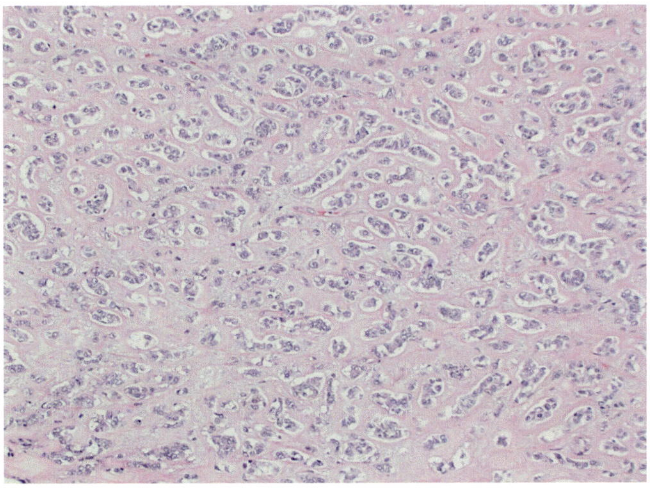

Fig. 8.2 The neoplastic cells form cords, nests, and trabeculae (100×)

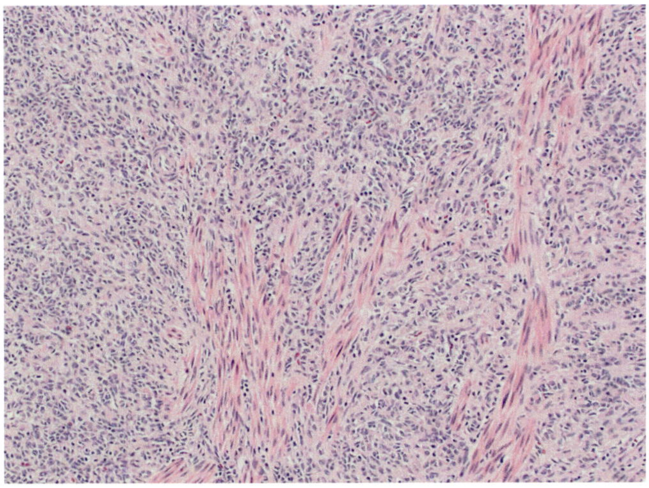

Fig. 8.3 A smooth muscle component within the lesion is present in this field (200×)

O. Saglam, *Challenging Cases in Gynecologic Surgical Pathology*, https://doi.org/10.1007/978-3-031-51656-6_8

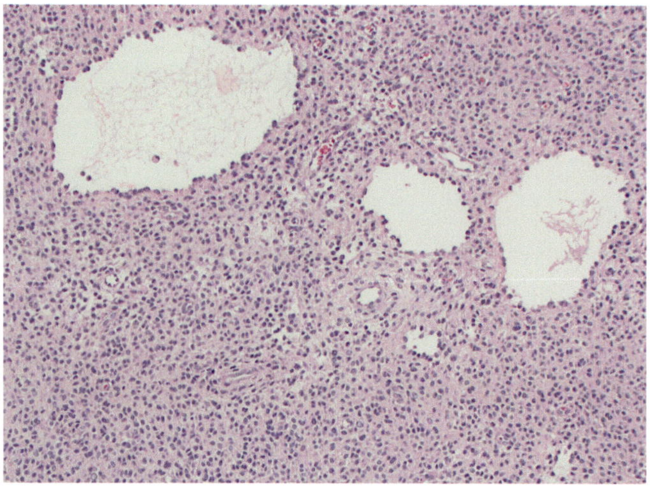

Fig. 8.4 Follicle-like spaces alternate with diffuse sheets of neoplastic cells (200×)

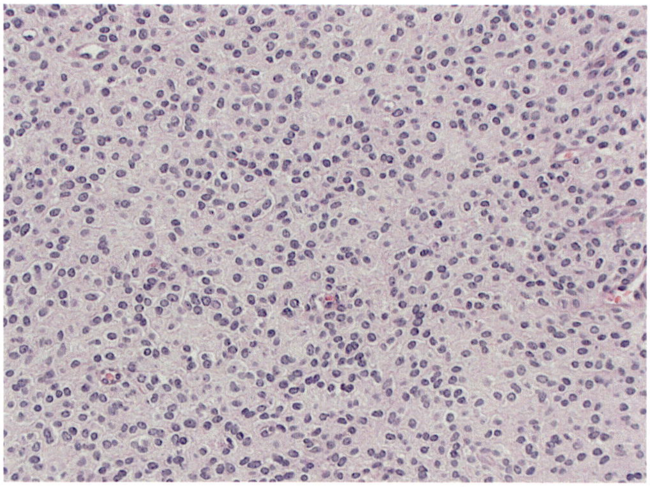

Fig. 8.5 Epithelioid cells with mild nuclear atypia and eosinophilic cytoplasm (200×)

- Cytological features are variable from scant to abundant pale, eosinophilic (Fig. 8.5), or foamy appearance. Nuclei are usually mildly atypical and might be pushed eccentrically and gain rhabdoid cell morphology (Fig. 8.6).

8.1.1.2 Ancillary Studies

- Multiple lineage positivity with varying percentages, including sex cord markers (inhibin, calretinin, SF11, Melan A), epithelial markers (cytokeratin-usually focal), smooth muscle markers (desmin, h-caldesmon, actin), CD10, ER, and PR [2]. A panel approach is necessary in the application of ancillary studies.

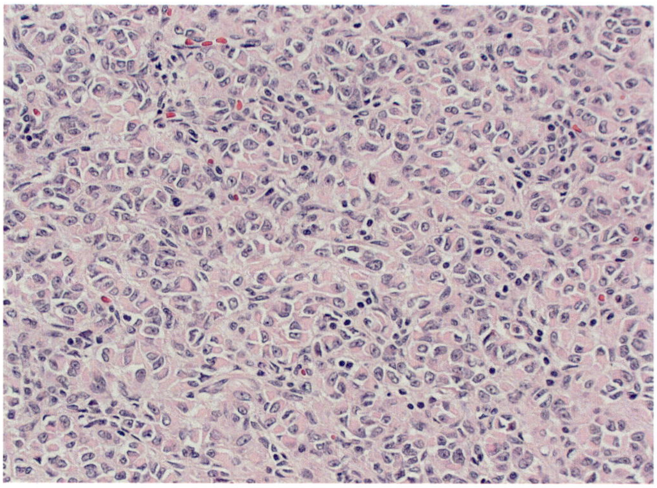

Fig. 8.6 The rhabdoid cell morphology is associated with adverse disease outcomes (200×)

8.1.1.3 Differential Diagnosis

- Epithelioid leiomyoma
  - Round, polygonal, and epithelioid cells with cytoplasmic clearing.
  - Lack of sex cord marker expression in epithelioid leiomyoma.
  - See Part II, Sect. 7.9.
- Low-grade endometrial stromal sarcoma with sex cord elements
  - Sex cord component is minor (less than 10%).
  - Typical tongue-like myometrial invasion pattern.
  - Tumor cells whorl around the delicate vessels.
- Endometrioid carcinoma with sex cord-like features
  - Small, hollow tubules, anastomosing cords or trabeculae.
  - Merging of sertoliform elements with typical endometrioid carcinoma or squamous epithelium at some foci.
  - Cytokeratin and EMA are diffusely positive, and sex cord markers are negative.

8.1.1.4 Clinical Significance

- UTROSCT usually has a benign clinical course. In rare cases, it might recur locally or even metastasize. There is limited data to predict clinical outcome [1].
- Tumor size (>5 cm), infiltrative borders, increased mitotic activity (≥3 per 10 high power fields), necrosis, moderate cytological atypia, and rhabdoid morphology are among the adverse prognostic features [3].
- *ESR1-NCOA2* fusions are associated with aggressive clinical behavior [4].

References

1. Moore M, McCluggage WG. Uterine tumour resembling ovarian sex cord tumour: first report of a large series with follow-up. Histopathology. 2017;71(5):751–9.
2. Croce S, de Kock L, Boshari T, Hostein I, Velasco V, Foulkes WD, et al. Uterine tumor resembling ovarian sex cord tumor (UTROSCT) commonly exhibits positivity with sex cord markers FOXL2 and SF-1 but lacks FOXL2 and DICER1 mutations. Int J Gynecol Pathol. 2016;35(4):301–8.
3. Boyraz B, Watkins JC, Young RH, Oliva E. Uterine tumors resembling ovarian sex cord tumors: a clinicopathologic study of 75 cases emphasizing features predicting adverse outcome and differential diagnosis. Am J Surg Pathol. 2023;47(2):234–47.
4. Bennett JA, Lastra RR, Barroeta JE, Parilla M, Galbo F, Wanjari P, et al. Uterine tumor resembling ovarian sex cord stromal tumor (UTROSCT): a series of 3 cases with extensive rhabdoid differentiation, malignant behavior, and ESR1-NCOA2 fusions. Am J Surg Pathol. 2020;44(11):1563–72.

Part III

Uterine Cervix Pathology Cases

9 Uncommon Tumors and Mimickers of Cancer

9.1 Mesonephric Hyperplasia (MH)

9.1.1 A 45-Year-Old Woman with a History of Endocervical Adenocarcinoma In Situ, the Entire Cervical Tissue Submitted for Microscopic Examination

9.1.1.1 Key Diagnostic Features

- Small embryonic remnants of mesonephric ducts can persist in broad ligaments, the lateral wall of the cervix, and the vagina.
- Mesonephric remnants can present in four categories: (1) lobular mesonephric hyperplasia, (2) diffuse mesonephric hyperplasia, (3) mesonephric ductal hyperplasia, and (4) mesonephric carcinoma [1]. The division of benign proliferations is arbitrary.
- Mesonephric hyperplasia is defined as a proliferation of mesonephric tubules measuring >6 mm in a single dimension (Fig. 9.1).

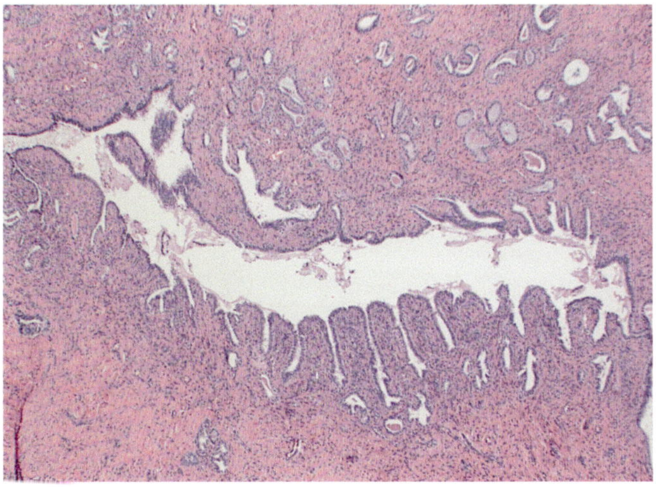

Fig. 9.1 Mesonephric hyperplasia with centrally located duct and surrounding tubules (40×)

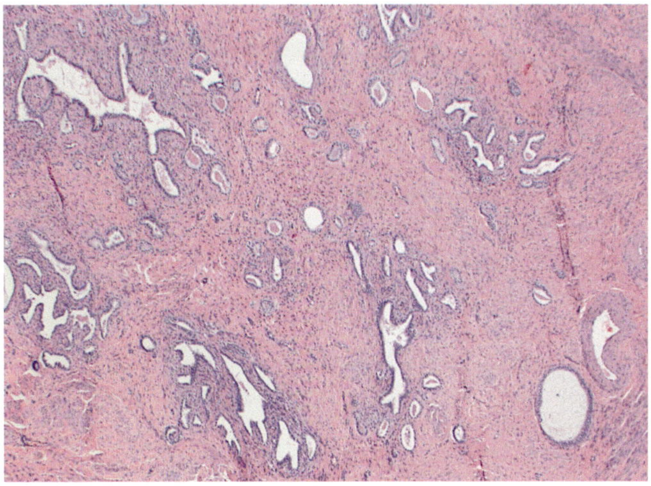

Fig. 9.2 In lobular hyperplasia, there is a clustering of tubules. The tubules preserve well-circumscribed lobular architecture (100×)

- In the lobular type, there is a clustered growth pattern (Fig. 9.2). The small, orderly proliferation of mesonephric tubules is arranged in a lobular architecture with or without a central duct. Densely eosinophilic intraluminal secretions are at least focally present. The tubules are lined by single cuboidal epithelium (Fig. 9.3).
- In diffuse MH, the tubules lack a clustered appearance but are still separated by the stroma. There is no cytological atypia or mitotic activity.
- Ductal-type MH is distinguished from lobular or diffuse MH by the presence of a myoepithelial cell layer and micropapillary tufting [2]. There might be luminal cilia focally, but mucin is absent. Ductal hyperplasia lacks densely eosinophilic secretions unless there are associated small tubules.

9.1.1.2 Ancillary Studies

- Intraluminal secretions are positive with Periodic Acid-Schiff.

O. Saglam, *Challenging Cases in Gynecologic Surgical Pathology*, https://doi.org/10.1007/978-3-031-51656-6_9

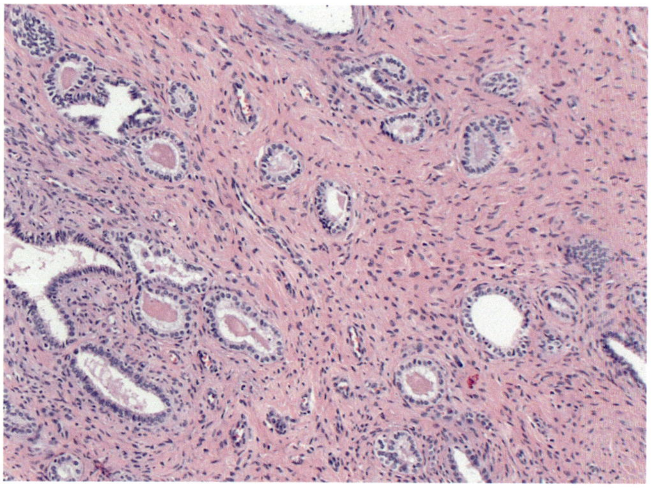

Fig. 9.3 Dense eosinophilic luminal secretions point out possible mesonephric lineage. The cytological features are bland without mitotic activity in benign proliferations (200×)

- CD10 has apical/luminal staining of mesonephric remnants/hyperplasia and carcinoma.
- GATA3, calretinin, and PAX8 stain mesonephric-type epithelium [3].

9.1.1.3 Differential Diagnosis

- Diffuse mesonephric hyperplasia versus mesonephric carcinoma
  - Mesonephric carcinoma presents as a mass lesion. The tubules are closely packed without any intervening stroma. The presence of cytological atypia and mitosis supports carcinoma diagnosis.
  - Mesonephric carcinoma might have a background diffuse mesonephric hyperplasia.
  - In contrast to mesonephric carcinoma, mesonephric hyperplasia lacks *KRAS/NRAS* mutations [4].
- Endometrioid adenocarcinoma involving cervix
  - The presence of mucinous and squamous differentiation is helpful in addition to the lack of mesonephric marker expression.

9.1.1.4 Clinical Significance

- Presence of diffuse MH should trigger additional samples to rule out microscopic foci of mesonephric carcinoma.

9.2 Endocervicosis

9.2.1 A 29-Year-Old Woman with Pelvic Pain

9.2.1.1 Key Diagnostic Features

- Benign Mullerian glandular proliferation of mucinous type involving the outer wall of the uterine cervix (Fig. 9.4), paracervical fibroadipose tissue (Fig. 9.5), and urinary bladder [5, 6].
- The size of glands and glandular arrangement is variable (Fig. 9.6). The complex architecture like gland fusion or cribriform appearances is not a morphological feature.
- The glands are lined by a single layer of cuboidal or epithelial cells with pale mucinous cytoplasm. Focally, other features of Mullerian-type epithelium and stroma, such as ciliated cells or endometrial stroma, can be present.
- No cytological atypia or mitotic figures.
- Extravasated mucin might be associated with a stromal reaction.

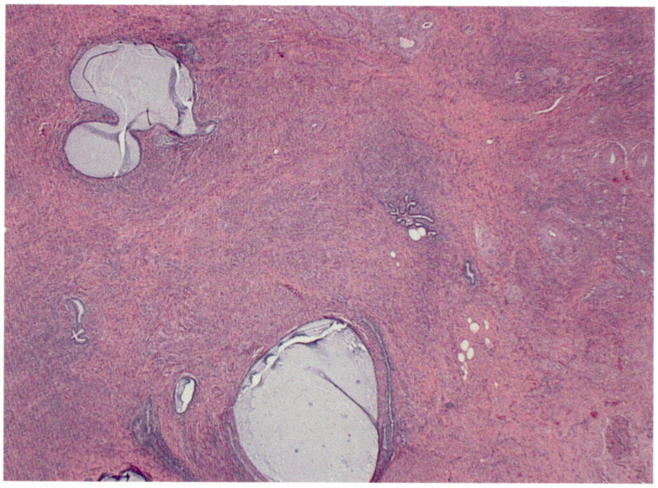

Fig. 9.4 Endocervical-type glands within the deep endocervical stroma have irregular size and shape. There is an uninvolved zone of cervical stroma between surface epithelium (not in the picture) and endocervicosis (40×)

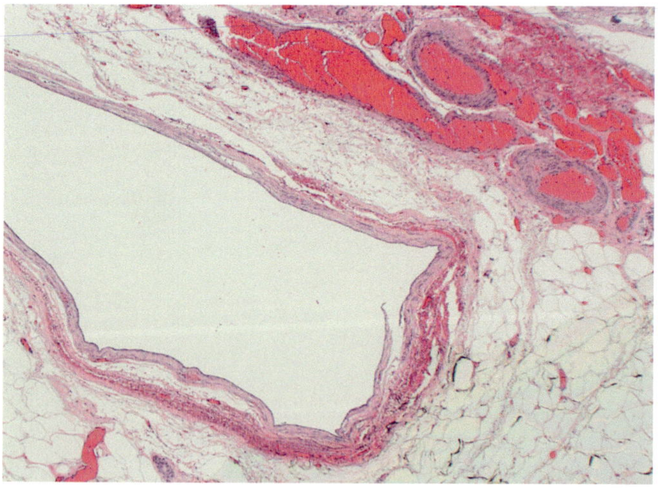

Fig. 9.5 The glandular epithelium is extending into the parametrial adipose tissue (100×)

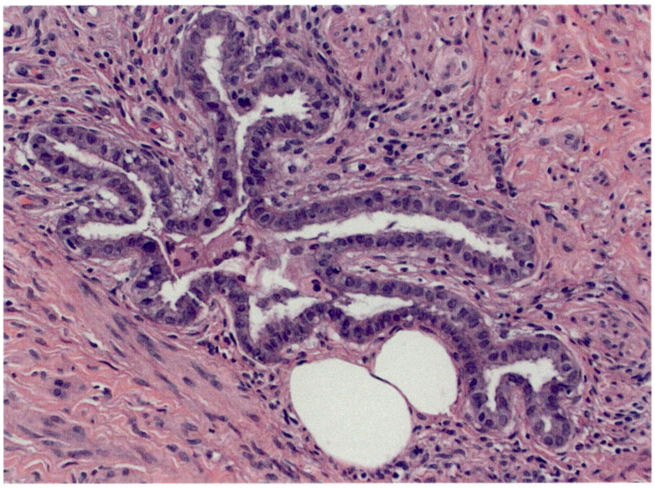

Fig. 9.6 The gland is irregular and surrounded by fibrotic stroma and inflammatory cells. The lining epithelium has cilia and no cytological atypia (100×)

9.2.1.2 Ancillary Studies

- None.

9.2.1.3 Differential Diagnosis

- Well-differentiated gastrointestinal-type adenocarcinoma (adenoma malignum)
  - Cystically dilated or irregular glands lined by gastric/pyloric-type epithelium with abundant clear to pinkish cytoplasm infiltrate the cervical wall with minimal stromal reaction.
  - See Part III, Sect. 9.4.
- Metastatic mucinous adenocarcinoma
  - Infiltrating pattern with stromal reaction and at least focal cytologic atypia.
  - Lymphovascular invasion supports metastatic carcinoma.

9.2.1.4 Clinical Significance

- Endocervicosis might involve axillary or intramammary lymph nodes [7, 8]. Mucinous adenocarcinoma can arise in the background of endocervicosis [9]. Endocervicosis is a diagnostic pitfall for both benign and malignant proliferations.

9.3 HPV-Associated Invasive Endocervical Adenocarcinoma (EAC) with Silva Pattern A

9.3.1 A 39-Year-Old Woman with Atypical Glandular Cells in PAP Smear

9.3.1.1 Key Diagnostic Features

- Silva morphological patterns of invasion apply only to HPV-associated invasive endocervical adenocarcinomas and stratify invasion patterns into three groups [10].
- Pattern A shows well-demarcated glands with rounded contours, frequently forming groups with no destructive stromal invasion, no single cells or cell detachment, and no lymphovascular invasion (Figs. 9.7, 9.8, and 9.9). Complex intraglandular growth, such as cribriform or papillary architecture, is acceptable without solid growth. The depth of the tumor or in relation to large vessels is not relevant.
- Pattern B shows localized (limited, early) destructive stromal invasion (Fig. 9.10). Individual or small groups of tumor cells are separated from a rounded gland in a focally desmoplastic or inflamed stroma (Fig. 9.11). Pattern C shows diffuse destructive stromal invasion. The growth pattern is confluent or solid (Fig. 9.12).

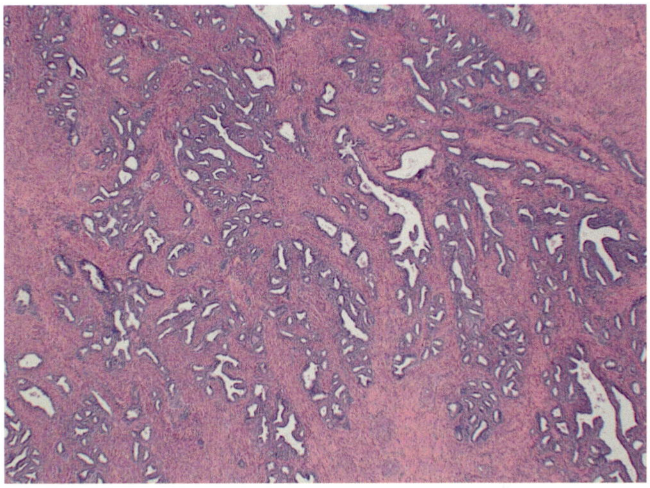

Fig. 9.7 Invasive well-differentiated endocervical adenocarcinoma with Silva pattern A. There is no stromal reaction around the rounded clusters of glandular epithelia (20×)

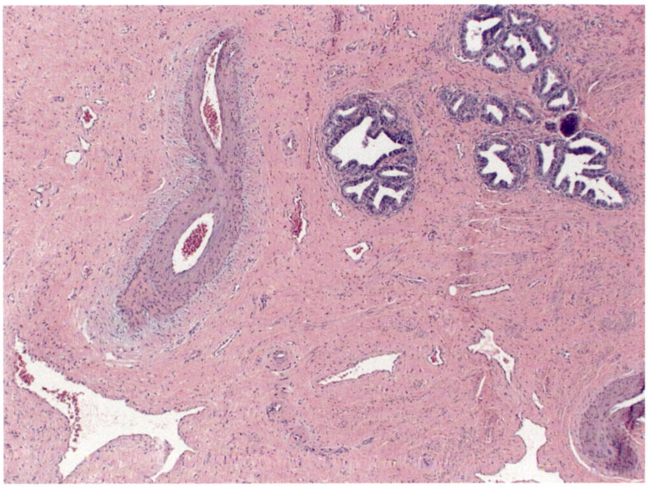

Fig. 9.8 The groups of neoplastic glands are next to deep, large cervical vessels (40×)

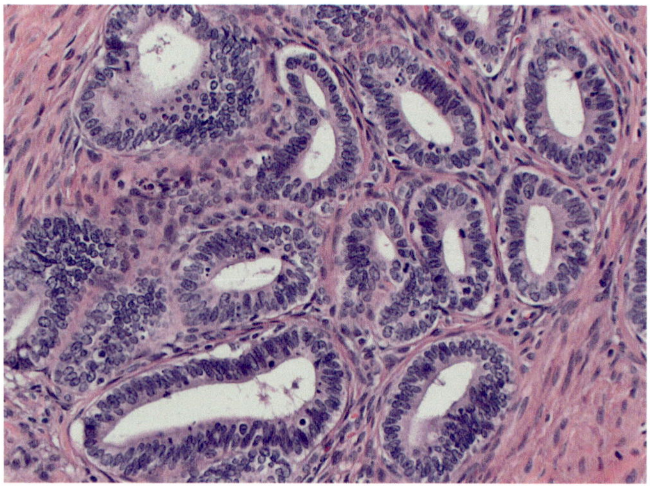

Fig. 9.9 Cytological features of usual-type (HPV-associated) adenocarcinoma resemble those of adenocarcinoma in situ, including nuclear stratification, hyperchromasia, and apical mitosis (100×)

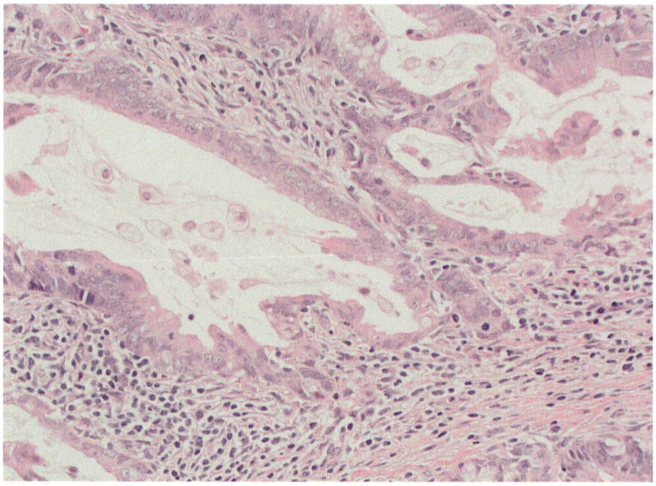

Fig. 9.11 Pattern B: Individual or small groups of cells are budding from neoplastic glands (200×)

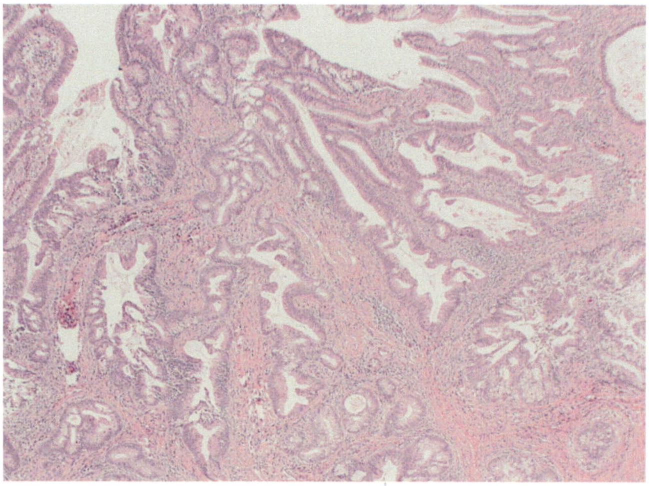

Fig. 9.10 Pattern B: There is a localized stromal desmoplastic reaction (40×)

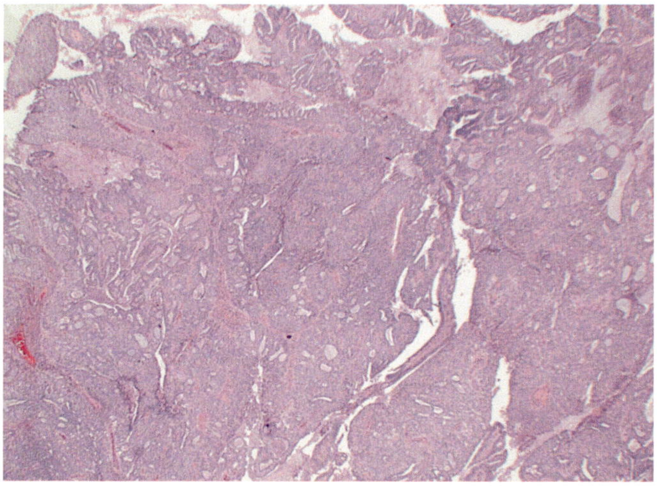

Fig. 9.12 Pattern C: Solid and confluent growth pattern (40×)

9.3.1.2 Ancillary Studies

- Immunostain for p16 (a surrogate marker of human papilloma virus infection) and in situ hybridization studies for high-risk HPV infection are block-positive in around 82–87% of samples [11].

9.3.1.3 Differential Diagnosis

- The worst pattern seen in a given tumor is the one to be reported (i.e., tumors with pattern A and focal pattern B, should be classified as pattern B).
- In exophytic tumors, the Silva pattern is evaluated at the tumor base within the cervical wall and not within the exophytic portion of the neoplasm.
- Exophytic lesions are challenging because their gross size by itself might determine the stage according to the current FIGO system [12].
- The confluent growth is described as gland or papillary structures with little intervening stroma or mucin lakes with tumor cells within the cervical stroma filling 4× field (5 mm) [13].

9.3.1.4 Clinical Significance

- The Silva pattern-based classification of HPV-associated invasive adenocarcinomas predicts the risk of lymph node metastasis and recurrences. Samples with pattern A are all stage I disease with negative lymph nodes and no recurrences, pattern B tumors rarely have metastatic lymph nodes, and only 23.8% of cases with pattern C have lymph node metastases in an international study that led the pattern classification [14].

9.4 Gastric-Type Endocervical Adenocarcinoma (HPV-Independent Adenocarcinoma) (GAS)

9.4.1 A 55-Year-Old Woman with Watery Vaginal Discharge

9.4.1.1 Key Diagnostic Features

- A spectrum of differentiation from well-differentiated form (minimal deviation adenocarcinoma/adenoma malignum) to overtly malignant tumors [15].
- The mucinous-type lining epithelium is similar to gastric/pyloric-type epithelium with abundant clear to pinkish cytoplasm due to neutral mucin (Figs. 9.13 and 9.14) in contrast to dark purple acidic mucin of the normal endocervical glands. Cystically dilated glands are scattered in the cervical stroma (Fig. 9.15) in well-differentiated tumors.

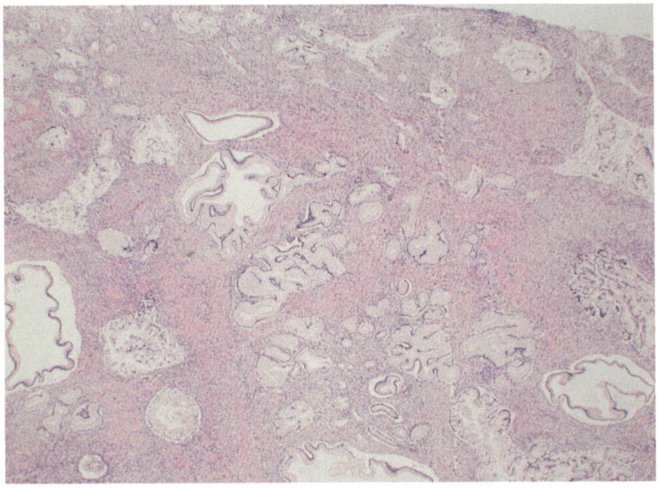

Fig. 9.13 Irregularly shaped mucinous-type glandular epithelium invading cervical stroma (20×)

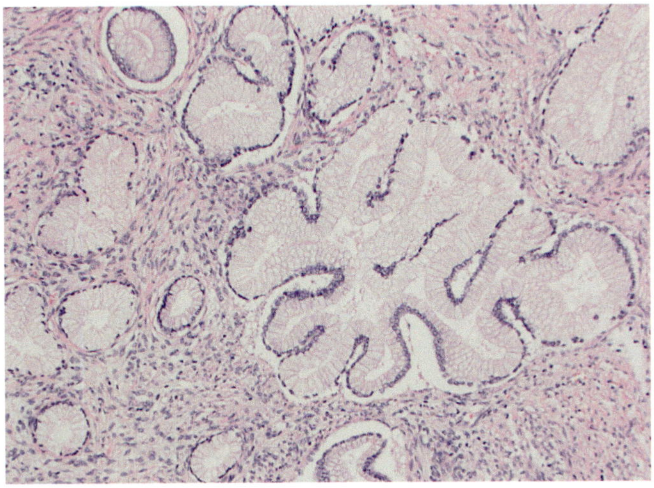

Fig. 9.14 Claw-like glands lined by mucinous epithelium with abundant pink cytoplasm, well-defined cell borders (pyloric type epithelium), and basally located uniform nuclei (100×)

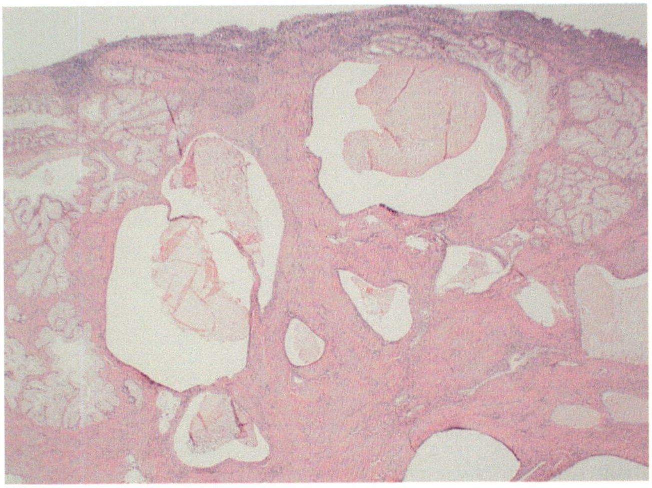

Fig. 9.15 Cystically dilated glands are scattered among mucinous/pyloric-type glandular epithelium (40×)

- There might be minimal to mild stromal reaction. The cytological atypia is usually minimal and localized in well-differentiated cancers. The nuclei are basally located and uniform (Fig. 9.16).
- Lobular endocervical glandular hyperplasia (LEGH)/pyloric gland metaplasia is a benign form of gastric metaplasia [16, 17] and can be found next to the lesion.
- Gastric-type adenocarcinoma in situ or atypical lobular endocervical glandular hyperplasia is the potential precursor of the GAS [15, 18].

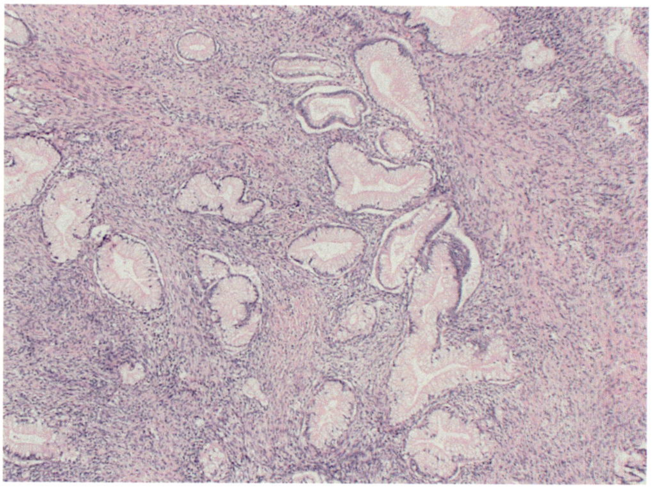

Fig. 9.16 There is minimal stromal desmoplastic reaction (40×)

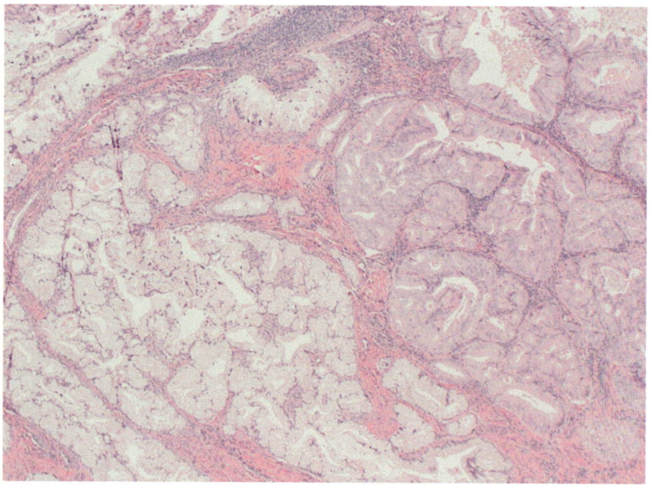

Fig. 9.17 Gastric-type adenocarcinoma (left) and usual-type endocervical adenocarcinoma (right) can be present together in rare lesions (100×)

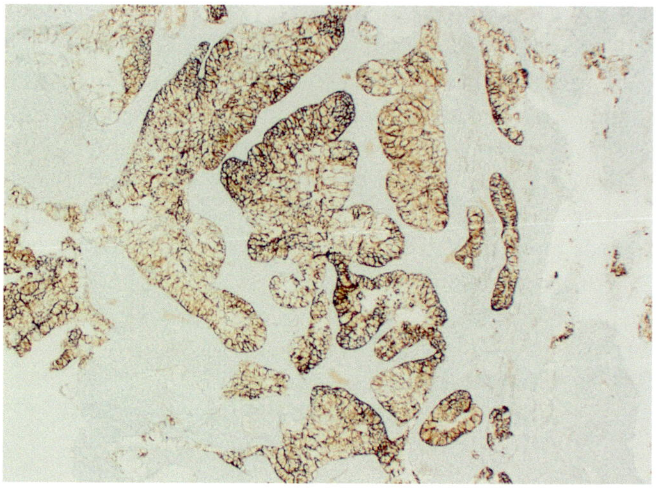

Fig. 9.18 Immunostain for MUC6 is positive in gastric-type adenocarcinoma (100×)

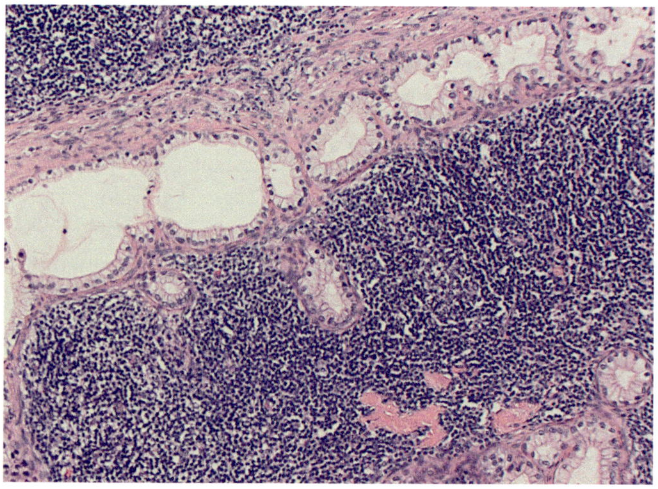

Fig. 9.19 Gastric-type adenocarcinoma involving pelvic lymph nodes (100×)

- An admixture of GAS and HPV-associated adenocarcinoma can be seen together (Fig. 9.17).

9.4.1.2 Ancillary Studies

- HK1083 [19], MUC6 (poor specificity) (Fig. 9.18) [17]: positive; PAX8, CK7, CK20, CEA: varying positivity
- P53 immunostain: mutant pattern (20–57%) [18, 20, 21]
- P16 and HPV molecular testing: negative [18]

9.4.1.3 Differential Diagnosis

- Metastatic mucinous adenocarcinoma to cervix
  - Clinical and imaging correlation is required. The morphology can be similar or identical.
- Atypical lobular endocervical glandular hyperplasia
  - A lesion with the architecture of LEGH together with four of the following atypical features: (1) nuclear enlargement, (2) irregular nuclear contour, (3) distinct nucleoli, (4) coarse chromatin texture, (5) loss of polarity, (6) occasional mitotic figures, (7) apoptotic bodies and nuclear debris in the lumen, and (8) infoldings of epithelium or distinct papillary projections with delicate fibrovascular stroma [22]. It might be challenging to distinguish atypical LEGH from GAS unless there is a mass lesion.

9.4.1.4 Clinical Significance

- GAS is an aggressive type of cervical adenocarcinoma. Patients with GAS have worse disease-free and overall survival than patients with HPV-associated adenocarcinoma [23, 24]. In a large case series, half of the patients with GAS (20 out of 40) have lymph node metastasis [24] (Fig. 9.19). GAS might be associated with Peutz-Jeghers syndrome (*STK11* germline mutation) [25].

9.5 Neurotrophic Tyrosine Receptor Kinase *(NTRK)*-Rearranged Spindle Cell Neoplasm

9.5.1 A 31-Year-Old Woman with Cervical Mass Lesion

9.5.1.1 Key Diagnostic Features

- Lesions can be polypoid or confined to cervical stroma with well-circumscribed or infiltrative borders [26] (Figs. 9.20, 9.21, and 9.22).
- The spindle cells proliferate in haphazard fascicles or herringbone patterns, resembling fibrosarcoma. Focal areas of whorled architecture can also be present. The neoplastic cells have intermediate-sized nuclei and small nucleoli [27] (Fig. 9.23).

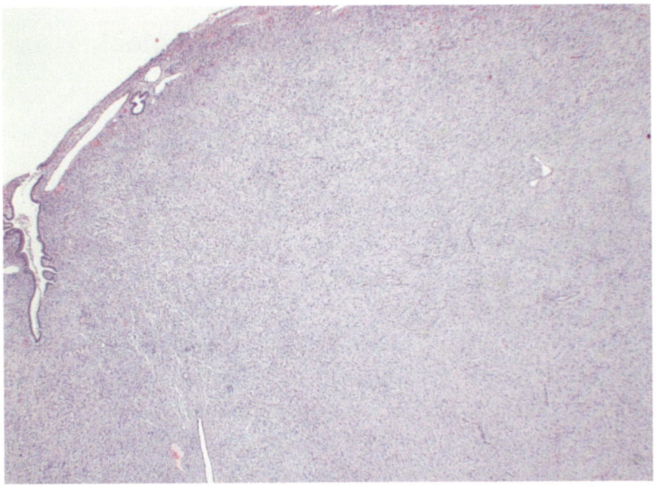

Fig. 9.20 *NTRK*-rearranged spindle cell neoplasm of the cervix with diffuse proliferation pattern (20×)

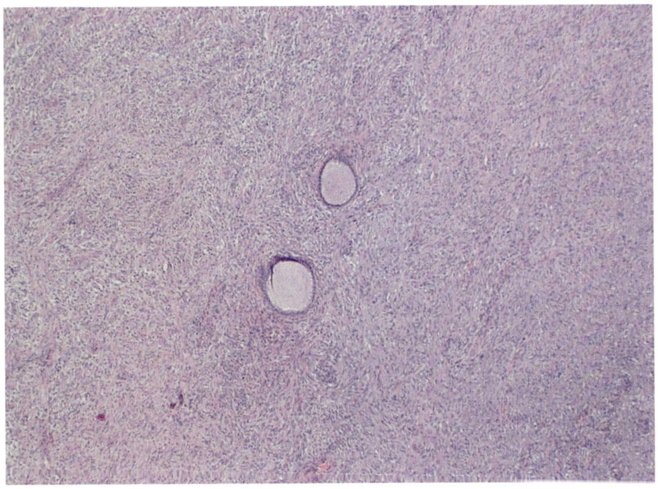

Fig. 9.21 There are entrapped benign endocervical glands among spindle cells (40×)

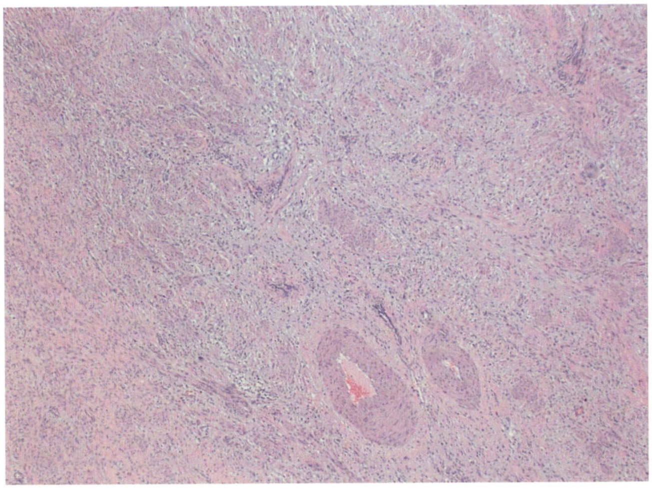

Fig. 9.22 The lesion has infiltrative borders (40×)

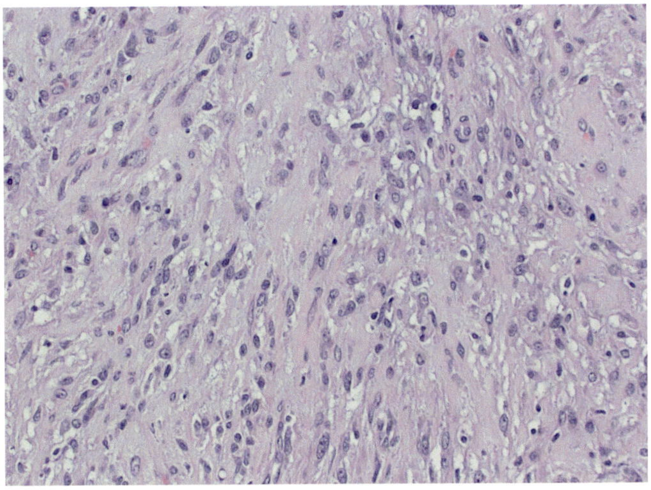

Fig. 9.23 The cytological atypia is mild to moderate (200×)

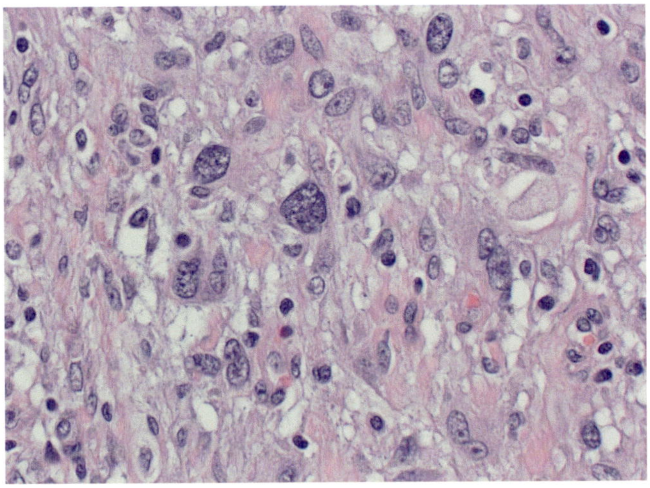

Fig. 9.24 Rare multinucleated atypical cells can be present (400×)

- Hyalinized vessels can be prominent in some cases. Entrapment of benign glands is also a frequent morphological feature (Fig. 9.21).
- Rare pleomorphic cells might be present (Fig. 9.24). Diffuse severe cytological atypia is rare. The mitotic activity might be low to brisk [26, 27].

9.5.1.2 Ancillary Studies

- Pan-Trk (Trk A, Trk B, and Trk C) immunostaining detects *NTRK* fusions, and the expression can be focal (Fig. 9.25) or diffuse. *NTRK* fusion assays have higher specificity [28, 29].
- S100 and CD34 are coexpressed in most cases. CD10, SMA, ER, PR, and cyclin D1 might be focal positive [30].
- Desmin and SOX10: negative

9.5.1.3 Differential Diagnosis

- Solitary fibrous tumor (SFT)
  - Staghorn vasculature might be a morphological feature in *NTRK*-rearranged spindle cell neoplasm [30], but the majority has vague branching vessels. The degree of cytologic atypia, cellularity, and elongated fascicular pattern in cervical *NTRK*-rearranged spindle cell neoplasm is rarely seen in SFT.
  - SFT is CD34 positive but S100 negative. STAT 6 is a specific marker of SFT.
  - See Part II, Sect. 7.11 (SFT of the uterus).
- Leiomyosarcoma (LMS)
  - The cells in leiomyosarcoma have abundant eosinophilic cytoplasm and are arranged in more uniform fascicles. Smooth muscle markers (desmin, smooth muscle actin, and h-caldesmon) are positive in LMS.
- Low-grade endometrial stromal sarcoma (ESS)
  - The neoplastic cells resemble proliferative-type endometrial stromal cells with prominent plexiform vascular pattern. The majority of ESS expresses hormone receptors and CD10 and are negative for S100 and CD34.
- Malignant peripheral nerve sheath tumor
  - Might have fibrosarcoma-like fascicular growth.
  - SOX10 and S100 are patchy positive.
  - Loss of nuclear expression of H3K27Me3.
- Monophasic synovial sarcoma (SS)
  - SS may show areas of alternating cellular density.
  - SS can express S100 and also cytokeratin and EMA.

9.5.1.4 Clinical Significance

- Patients with tumors harboring *NTRK* fusions have shown high response rates to tropomyosin receptor kinase inhibitors [31].

9.6 Epithelioid Trophoblastic Tumor (ETT)

9.6.1 A 34-Year-Old Woman with Vaginal Bleeding

9.6.1.1 Key Diagnostic Features

- The anatomical location is cervix/lower uterine segment (50%), uterine corpus (35%), and extrauterine sites [32].
- Well-circumscribed, nodular lesion with an expansile growth pattern [33] (Fig. 9.26).
- Broad zones of necrosis are often present (Fig. 9.27).
- The neoplastic cells have granular, eosinophilic, or clear cytoplasm with a distinct cell membrane and round nuclei with at least moderate cytological atypia.
- The neoplastic cells can colonize under the mucosal surface and might look like high-grade squamous intraepithelial lesions under low-power examination (Fig. 9.28).

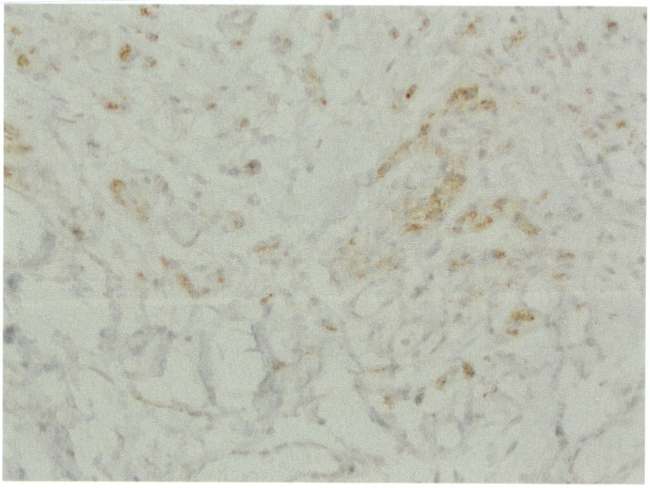

Fig. 9.25 Immunostain for pan-Trk is focal cytoplasmic positive (40×)

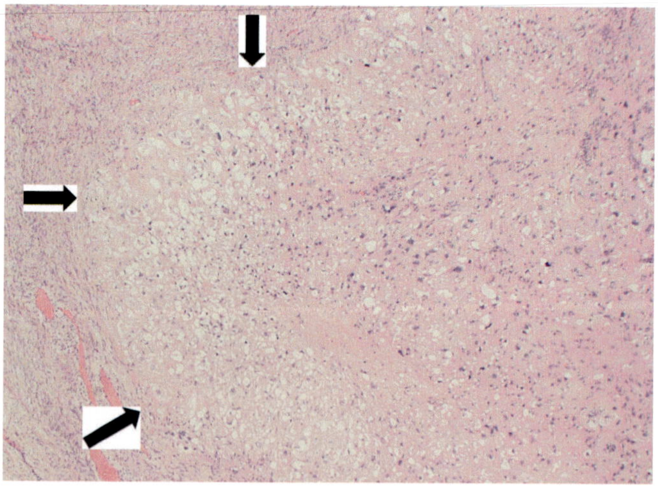

Fig. 9.26 ETT has an expansile growth pattern and well-circumscribed borders. Arrows are at the stromal interface (40×)

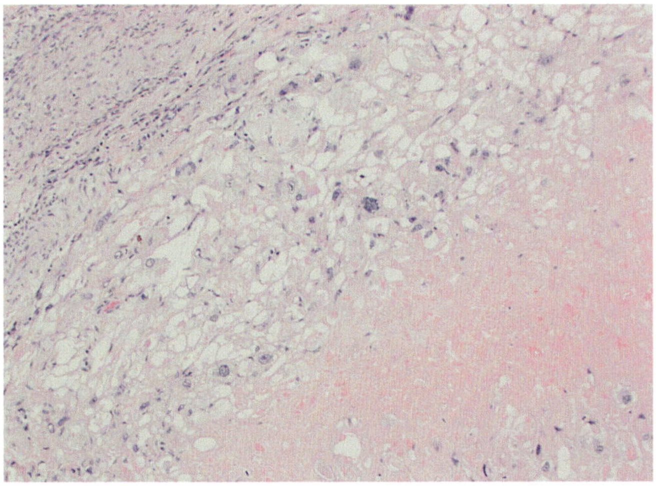

Fig. 9.27 The right lower third is a necrotic zone. At the center of the picture, a proliferation of intermediate-type trophoblasts with moderate nuclear atypia and cytoplasmic clearing is noticeable. The cell borders are distinct (100×)

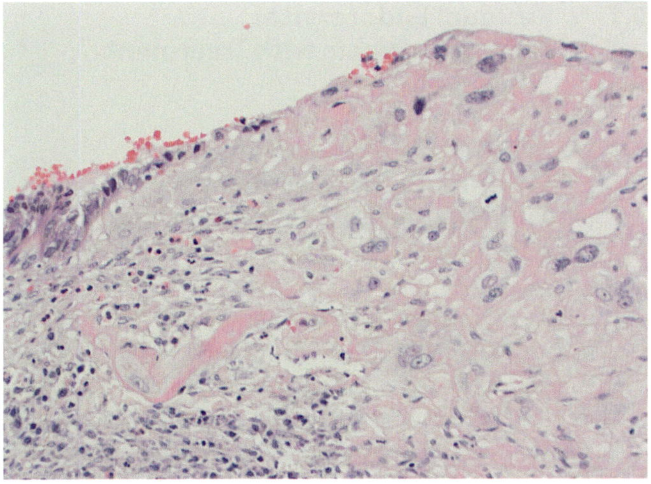

Fig. 9.29 Hyalinized extracellular material seen among the neoplastic cells, which might be interpreted as keratin at lower power examination (200×)

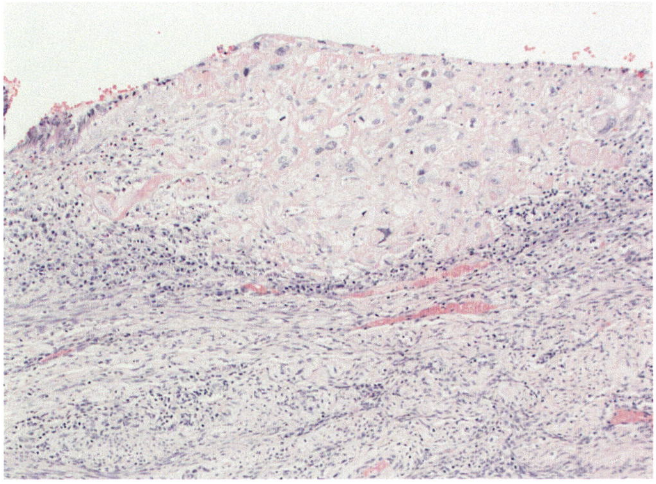

Fig. 9.28 The neoplastic cells are colonized under the native endocervical lining epithelium (100×)

- Eosinophilic hyaline-like material might be present among the tumor nests, mimicking keratin formation (Fig. 9.29).

9.6.1.2 Ancillary Studies

- Mild to moderate elevation of serum hCG (less than 2500 mIU/mL) is detectable in 80% of the cases [34].
- Inhibin-alpha, GATA-3 (80% of cases) [35], P63 [36], and cyclin E are diffusely positive, and human placental lactogen (hPL) is scattered positive in ETT.

9.6.1.3 Differential Diagnosis

- Squamous cell carcinoma (SCC) (anatomical site: cervix and lower uterine segment)
  - The presence of keratin formation, intercellular bridges, and background squamous intraepithelial neoplasia is compatible with SCC diagnosis.
  - Diffuse P16 staining [37], positive CK5/6, and positive HPV molecular testing support SCC diagnosis.
- Placental site nodule (PSN) (endocervical curetting specimens)
  - A benign counterpart of ETT.
  - Well-circumscribed, oval nodules or plaques of less than 5 mm in size.
  - Cyclin E staining score is higher in ETT than in PSN [37].
  - Ki-67 proliferative index is less than 8% in PSN [38].
- Atypical placental site nodule (APSN) (curetting specimen)
  - The larger size of the nodule (between 5 and 10 mm), increased cellularity, marked nuclear atypia, increased mitotic activity, and Ki-67 proliferation index between 8 and 10%.
  - Malignant gestational trophoblastic disease (GTD) is associated with 14% of APSN [39]. Clinical and imaging work-up is required to rule out GTD.
- Epithelioid leiomyosarcoma
  - Smooth muscle markers (desmin, SMA, caldesmon) are positive.
  - See Part II, Sect. 7.8.

9.6.1.4 Clinical Significance

- ETT is not sensitive to chemotherapy. Hysterectomy is the primary mode of treatment in most cases, and surgery also plays an essential role in metastatic diseases, including resection of solitary lung lesions [40].

9.7 Residual Endocervical Adenocarcinoma with Treatment Effect

9.7.1 A 47-Year-Old Woman Received Chemoradiation Treatment for Endocervical Adenocarcinoma a Year Ago

9.7.1.1 Key Diagnostic Features

- After radiation therapy, normal endocervical glandular epithelium becomes sparse and widely spaced [41]. The lining epithelium consists of large cells with a slight increase in N/C ratio, well-defined intercellular borders, and eosinophilic or finely vacuolated cytoplasm. Nuclei frequently show loss of polarity with prominent eosinophilic nucleoli and evenly dispersed chromatin.
- Sequential changes of the neoplastic cells after radiation therapy are the following: Cytoplasmic changes appear first, followed by nuclear changes such as enlargement of nuclei, multinucleation, chromatin clumping, pyknosis, karyorrhexis and loss of nuclei, and wrinkling (Fig. 9.30). To distinguish bizarre benign forms from persistent cancer cells might be difficult [42].
- The stroma around the neoplastic cells is thickened, swollen, or desmoplastic (Figs. 9.31 and 9.32). Other changes in the stroma are calcifications, cholesterol clefts, foamy macrophages, and thickened blood vessels [43].
- Complex architecture, such as cribriform appearance, is not a therapy-related change.
- In nonresponsive cases, neoplastic cells do not show particular morphological changes, with nuclei and cytoplasm looking essentially the same as in the pretreatment biopsies. The histological grading of the tumor remains the same in comparison to the pretreatment biopsy.

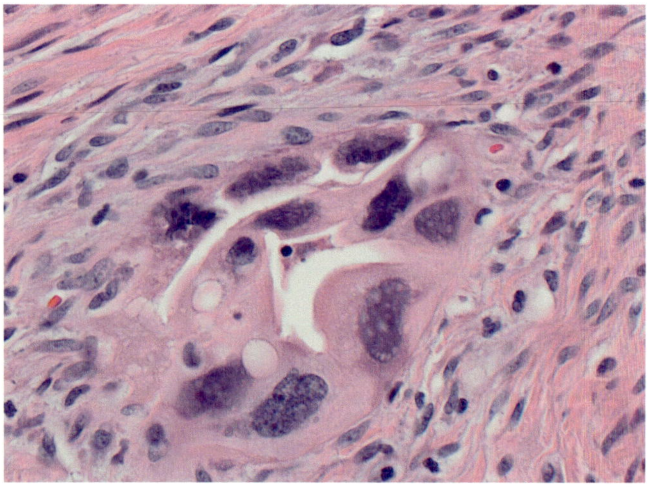

Fig. 9.30 Uterine cervical section after chemoradiation therapy for endocervical adenocarcinoma. Cytological changes include cytoplasmic vacuolation, multinucleation, one or two prominent nucleoli, and loss of chromatin details (200×)

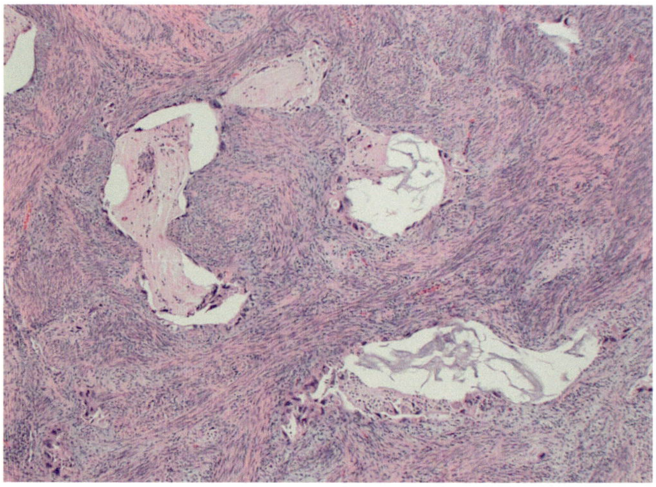

Fig. 9.31 Residual adenocarcinoma is composed of dilated irregular glands lined by cells with attenuated or hyperchromatic nuclei (40×)

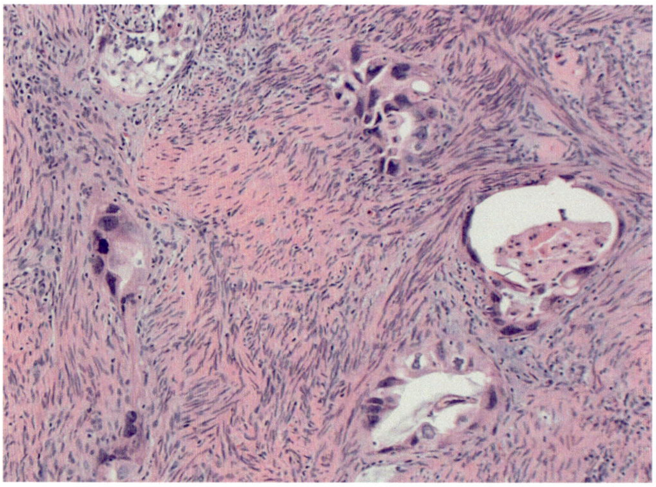

Fig. 9.32 The surrounding stroma is thickened and desmoplastic (100×)

9.7.1.2 Ancillary Studies

- Overexpression of p53 by immunohistochemistry is associated with low response to chemotherapy [44].

9.7.1.3 Differential Diagnosis

- There are overlapping cytological changes of benign glandular epithelium and residual adenocarcinoma of the endocervix. The presence of complex gland formation and single cells in isolation or groups are the morphological features of residual adenocarcinoma (Fig. 9.33).

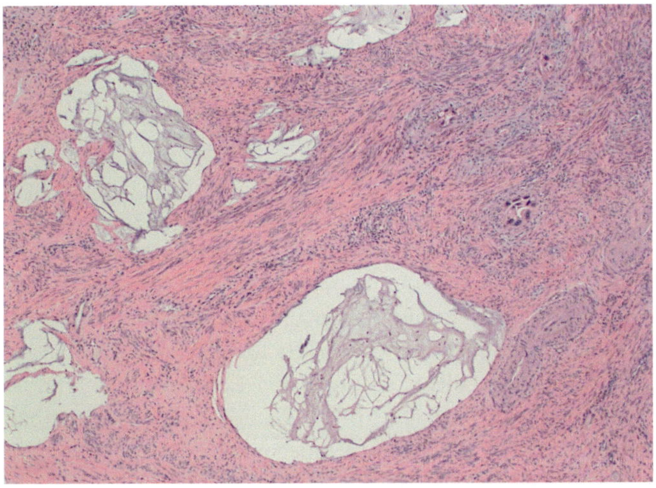

Fig. 9.33 The mucinous pools replace neoplastic glandular epithelium. On the right side of the image, the small glands and single cells represent residual carcinoma (40×)

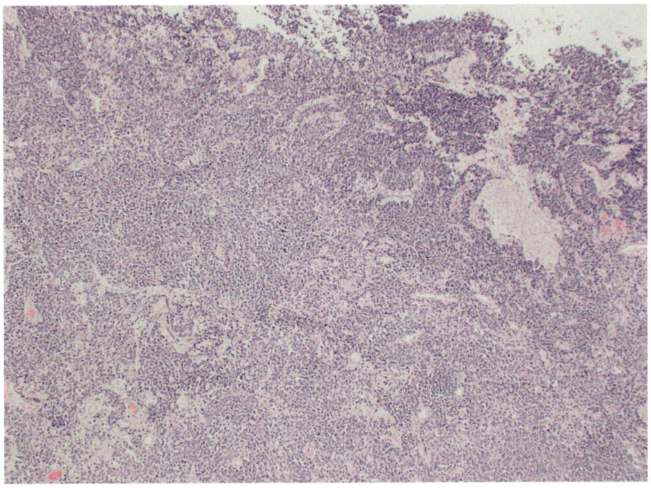

Fig. 9.34 Small cell neuroendocrine carcinoma of the cervix with a solid pattern (40×)

9.7.1.4 Clinical Significance

- Pelvic exenteration might be a treatment of choice for recurrent cervical cancer after concurrent chemoradiation therapy [45].

9.8 Small Cell Neuroendocrine Carcinoma of the Cervix (SCNEC)

9.8.1 A 48-Year-Old Woman with Postcoital Bleeding

9.8.1.1 Key Diagnostic Features

- Small blue cells with high N/C ratios arranged in solid (Fig. 9.34), nested, or trabecular architecture.
- The nuclei are hyperchromatic with inconspicuous nucleoli (Fig. 9.35). Apoptotic bodies and mitotic figures are numerous.
- Nuclei might appear focally slightly spindled (Fig. 9.36).
- In mixed NEC and adenocarcinoma samples, a transition zone from adenocarcinoma to NEC can be identified (Figs. 9.37 and 9.38).

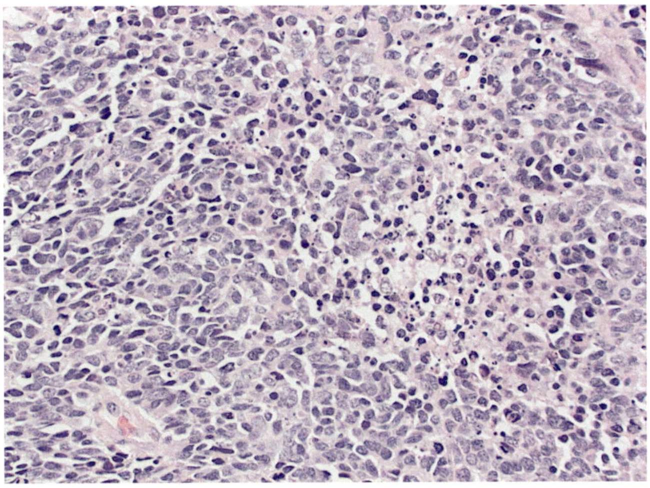

Fig. 9.35 Nuclei have a salt and pepper chromatin appearance. Scattered foci of apoptotic bodies are also present (200×)

9.8.1.2 Ancillary Studies

- Synaptophysin, chromogranin, CD56, SATB2 [46], TTF1 and CDX2 [47], and INSM1 [48] are variable positive.
- Diffuse block p16 staining pattern.
- High-risk HPV (16 and 8) is detected in 72% of the NEC of the cervix [48].
- Keratins and neuroendocrine markers might be negative in the NEC of the cervix [49].

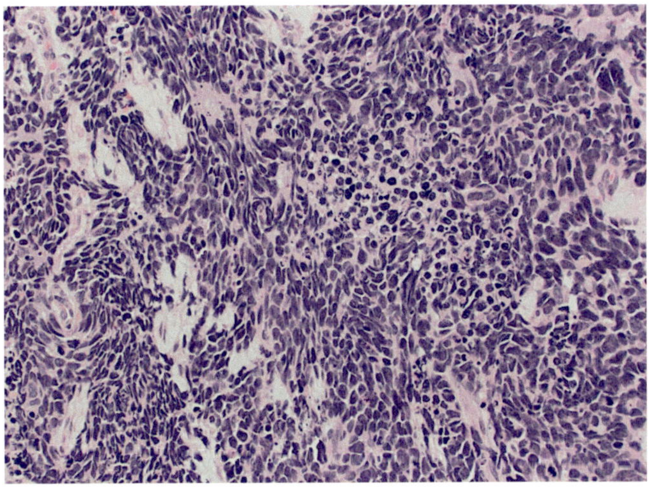

Fig. 9.36 High nuclear-cytoplasmic ratios and focally spindled nuclei (200×)

9.8.1.3 Differential Diagnosis

- Metastatic NEC from other anatomical sites

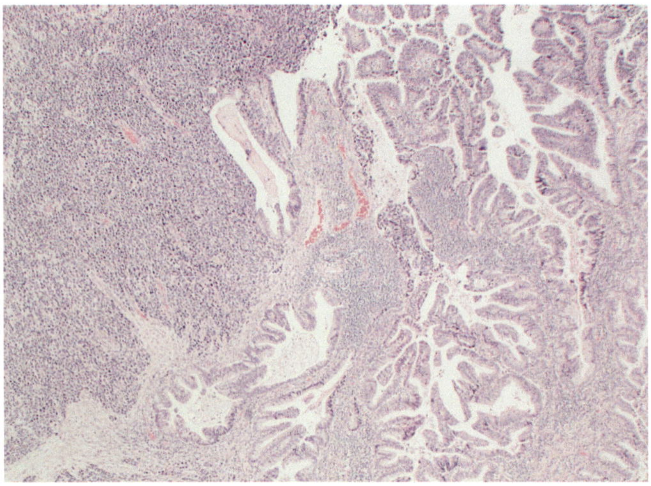

Fig. 9.37 Sharp demarcation between usual-type endocervical adenocarcinoma and SCNEC (40×)

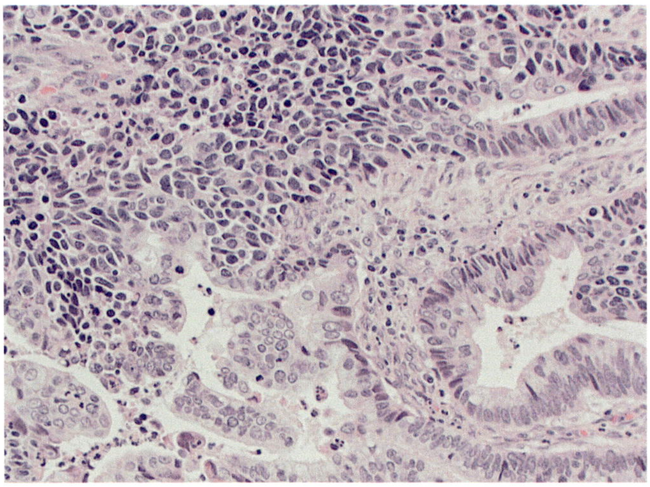

Fig. 9.38 The area of transition between adenocarcinoma and SCNEC (200×)

  - Clinical and imaging correlation is required. The morphology and immunostaining profiles are similar in primary and metastatic NEC
- Poorly differentiated squamous cell carcinoma (PSCC)
  - Identification of differentiated component supports the diagnosis.
  - P63 might be expressed in the NEC of the cervix [50].
  - A panel of high molecular weight keratins and neuroendocrine markers is required instead of a single antibody.

9.8.1.4 Clinical Significance

- Patients with SCNEC of the cervix have high mortality rates because of early lymphatic spread and high incidence of nodal or distant metastasis [51].

9.9 Stratified Mucin-Producing Intraepithelial Lesion (SMILE)

9.9.1 A 28-Year-Old Woman with Atypical Glandular Cells in PAP Smear

9.9.1.1 Key Diagnostic Features

- Rare high-grade cervical precancerous lesion, variant of cervical adenocarcinoma in situ [52]
- The lesion is composed of stratified epithelium with mucin throughout all cell layers and peripherally located basal/reserve cells [53] (Fig. 9.39). Large confluent mucin droplets can produce diffuse vacuoles or honeycombed patterns. The spectrum includes neoplastic epithelia with fewer cell layers resembling gland-like structures. In addition to cytological atypia, apical mitoses and apoptotic bodies are supportive of diagnosis.
- SMILE is associated with conventional CIN2–3, endocervical adenocarcinoma in situ, invasive adenocarcinoma, adenosquamous carcinoma, papillary squamous neoplasms, and invasive stratified mucin-producing carcinoma [53–55].

9.9.1.2 Ancillary Studies

- CK14 and p63 expressions are lost (lack of squamous differentiation).
- P16 is diffusely (on-block) positive (Fig. 9.40) [56].
- Ki67 proliferation index is high (over 30%) [57].

9.9.1.3 Differential Diagnosis

- Squamous metaplasia involving endocervical glands

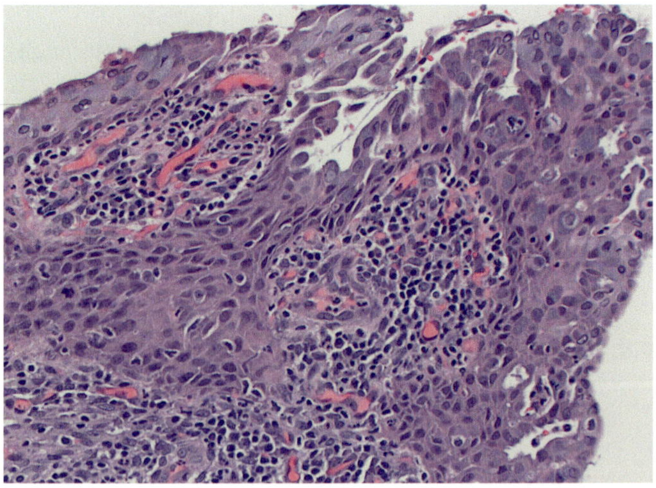

Fig. 9.39 SMILE (right side of the picture) is located at the surface next to the dysplastic squamous epithelium (left side of the picture). The stratified epithelium has mucin-producing cells throughout all layers and gland-like structures. The basal/reserve cells are located peripherally. Nuclei are enlarged and hyperchromatic (100×)

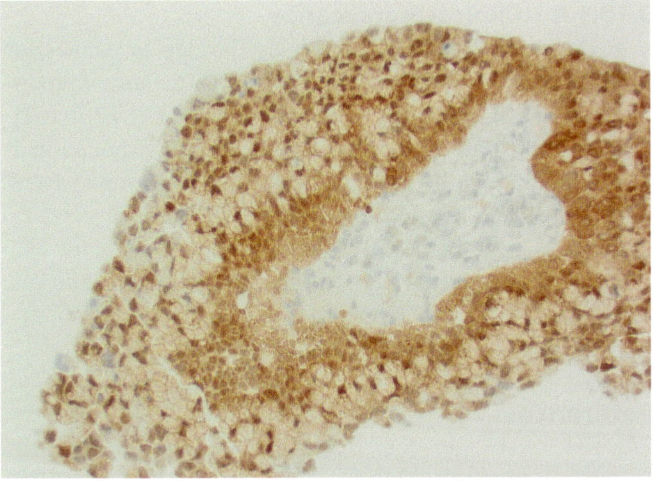

Fig. 9.40 P16 is on-block positive in SMILE (100×)

- SMILE has abnormal cells typically throughout the epithelium with relatively little reduction in nuclear density in the surface epithelial cells.
- Multinucleated cells with uniform nuclei and opaque chromatin might be present in metaplastic squamous epithelium.
- Mucin production in metaplasia concentrates in the middle and upper epithelial layers. In contrast, all layers have mucin-producing cells in SMILE.
- The proliferative index by Ki67 is high (diffuse) in SMILE. P16 is either negative or patchy positive in squamous metaplasia.

- Squamous intraepithelial lesion (SIL)
  - The mucinous cells are predominantly confined to the surface layers in SIL.
  - One morphological feature that can distinguish SMILE from conventional SIL is the conspicuous spacing of nuclei in the lower to middle epithelial layers due to the presence of cytoplasmic mucin [53].
  - P16 and KI67 are not helpful in differential diagnosis, but mucicarmine is diffusely positive in SMILE.
- Benign SMILE [58]
  - Epithelial stratification, intracytoplasmic mucin in all layers of epithelium, paler cytoplasm than adjacent endocervical epithelium, low nuclear to cytoplasmic ratio, rare sometimes apical mitoses, and absence of apoptotic bodies.
  - P16 is negative in benign lesions.

9.9.1.4 Clinical Significance

- The pathology report should clarify that the management of SMILE is similar to that of endocervical adenocarcinoma in situ.

9.10 Embryonal Rhabdomyosarcoma (ERMS), Botryoid Type

9.10.1 A 46-Year-Old Woman with Cervical Polyp

9.10.1.1 Key Diagnostic Features

- Polypoid lesions usually covered by squamous epithelium.
- Hypercellular stroma composed of small primitive blue cells condenses around benign glandular epithelium or beneath the surface epithelium (cambium layer) (Figs. 9.41, 9.42, and 9.43).

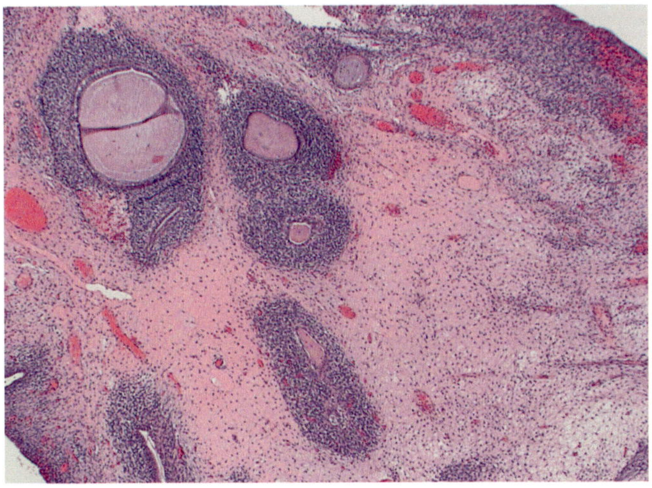

Fig. 9.41 ERMS botryoid type exhibits a hypercellular cambium layer around the benign cervical glands. The lesion has polypoid architecture (40×)

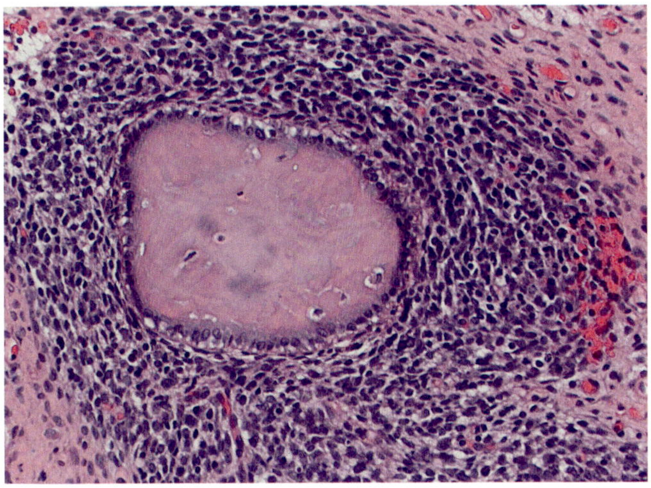

Fig. 9.42 The hypercellular stroma is composed of small blue cells with high nuclear-cytoplasmic ratios (200×)

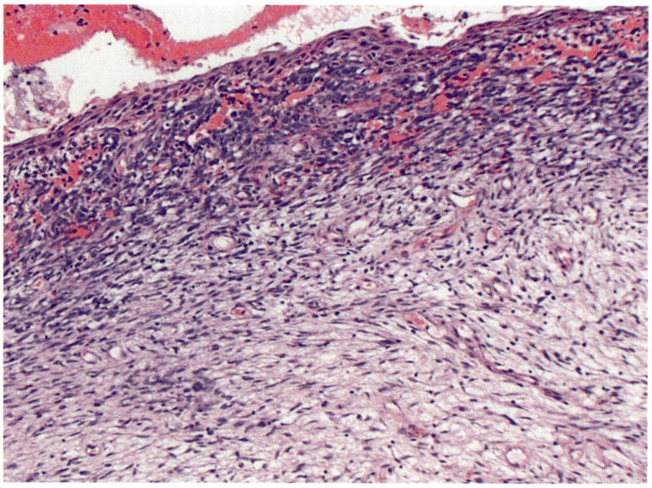

Fig. 9.43 The attenuated squamous epithelium and less cellular edematous areas under the cambium layer (hypercelluar zone) (100×)

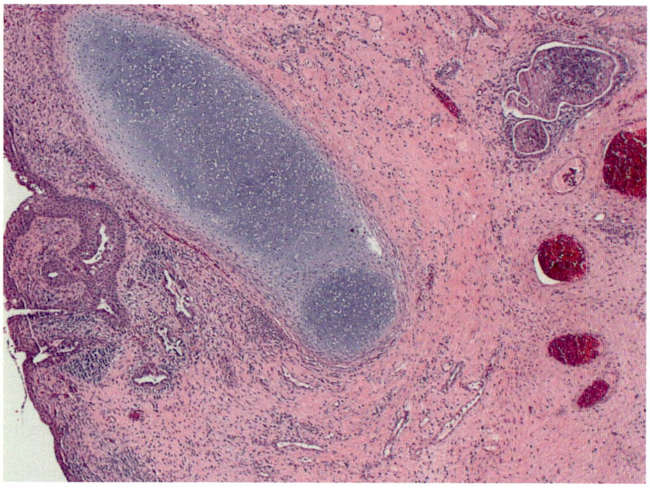

Fig. 9.44 The chondroid tissue is benign fetal type (40×)

- The stroma alternates in cellularity with hypercellular and hypocellular edematous areas [59].
- The mitotic activity is brisk in the hypercellular stroma.
- There might be fetal-type cartilage (Fig. 9.44) (45% of tumors) within the stroma [60]. In recent studies, presence of cartilaginous nodules is associated with *DICER1* gene alterations [61].

9.10.1.2 Ancillary Studies

- MYOD1, myogenin, desmin, myoglobin: positive and SMA: negative

9.10.1.3 Differential Diagnosis

- Mullerian adenosarcoma
  - The glandular epithelium has typical leaf-like (phyllodes-like) architecture in Mullerian adenosarcoma.
  - See Part II, Sect. 7.13.

9.10.1.4 Clinical Significance

- ERMS of the uterine cervix may develop in connection with the pleuropulmonary blastoma familial tumor predisposition syndrome (germline mutations in *DICER1*) [62].
- Harboring pathogenic variants of *DICER1* mutation is reportedly high in adult patients with ERMS (up to 100% of samples: five cervices and four uterine corpora) (median age: 36) [63]. In another study, patients with DICER1 syndrome are younger than nonsyndromic patients (16 versus 24 years) [64].

References

1. Ferry JA, Scully RE. Mesonephric remnants, hyperplasia, and neoplasia in the uterine cervix. A study of 49 cases. Am J Surg Pathol. 1990;14(12):1100–11.
2. Roy SF, Wong J, Latour M, Reichetzer B, Rahimi K. Ductal-type mesonephric duct/remnant hyperplasia: distinguished from lobular or diffuse mesonephric hyperplasia by the presence of a myoepithelial cell layer and micropapillary tufting. Pathology. 2022;54(3):378–81.
3. Howitt BE, Nucci MR. Mesonephric proliferations of the female genital tract. Pathology. 2018;50(2):141–50.
4. Mirkovic J, Schoolmeester JK, Campbell F, Miron A, Nucci MR, Howitt BE. Cervical mesonephric hyperplasia lacks KRAS/NRAS mutations. Histopathology. 2017;71(6):1003–5.
5. Clement PB, Young RH. Endocervicosis of the urinary bladder. A report of six cases of a benign Müllerian lesion that may mimic adenocarcinoma. Am J Surg Pathol. 1992;16(6):533–42.
6. Young RH, Clement PB. Endocervicosis involving the uterine cervix: a report of four cases of a benign process that may be confused with deeply invasive endocervical adenocarcinoma. Int J Gynecol Pathol. 2000;19(4):322–8.
7. Mukonoweshuro P, McCluggage WG. Endocervicosis involving axillary lymph nodes: first case report. Int J Gynecol Pathol. 2014;33(6):620–3.
8. Jebakumar D, Asirvatham JR. Endocervicosis in an intramammary lymph node. Int J Surg Pathol. 2022;30(7):784–8.
9. Nakaguro M, Tsuzuki T, Shimada S, Taki T, Tsuchiyama M, Kitamura A, et al. Adenocarcinoma arising in urinary bladder endocervicosis. Pathol Int. 2016;66(2):108–13.
10. Roma AA, Diaz De Vivar A, Park KJ, Alvarado-Cabrero I, Rasty G, Chanona-Vilchis JG, et al. Invasive endocervical adenocarcinoma: a new pattern-based classification system with important clinical significance. Am J Surg Pathol. 2015;39(5):667–72.
11. Stolnicu S, Hoang L, Soslow RA. Recent advances in invasive adenocarcinoma of the cervix. Virchows Arch. 2019;475(5):537–49.
12. Corrigendum to "Revised FIGO staging for carcinoma of the cervix uteri" [Int J Gynecol Obstet. 145(2019):129–35]. Int J Gynaecol Obstet. 2019;147(2):279–80.
13. Alvarado-Cabrero I, Parra-Herran C, Stolnicu S, Roma A, Oliva E, Malpica A. The silva pattern-based classification for HPV-associated invasive endocervical adenocarcinoma and the distinction between in situ and invasive adenocarcinoma: relevant issues and recommendations from the International Society of Gynecological Pathologists. Int J Gynecol Pathol. 2021;40(Suppl 1):S48–s65.
14. Roma AA, Mistretta TA, Diaz De Vivar A, Park KJ, Alvarado-Cabrero I, Rasty G, et al. New pattern-based personalized risk stratification system for endocervical adenocarcinoma with important clinical implications and surgical outcome. Gynecol Oncol. 2016;141(1):36–42.

15. Mikami Y. Gastric-type mucinous carcinoma of the cervix and its precursors—historical overview. Histopathology. 2020;76(1):102–11.
16. Nucci MR, Clement PB, Young RH. Lobular endocervical glandular hyperplasia, not otherwise specified: a clinicopathologic analysis of thirteen cases of a distinctive pseudoneoplastic lesion and comparison with fourteen cases of adenoma malignum. Am J Surg Pathol. 1999;23(8):886–91.
17. Mikami Y, Hata S, Fujiwara K, Imajo Y, Kohno I, Manabe T. Florid endocervical glandular hyperplasia with intestinal and pyloric gland metaplasia: worrisome benign mimic of "adenoma malignum". Gynecol Oncol. 1999;74(3):504–11.
18. Talia KL, Stewart CJR, Howitt BE, Nucci MR, McCluggage WG. HPV-negative gastric type adenocarcinoma in situ of the cervix: a spectrum of rare lesions exhibiting gastric and intestinal differentiation. Am J Surg Pathol. 2017;41(8):1023–33.
19. Ishii K, Hosaka N, Toki T, Momose M, Hidaka E, Tsuchiya S, et al. A new view of the so-called adenoma malignum of the uterine cervix. Virchows Arch. 1998;432(4):315–22.
20. Wong RW, Ralte A, Grondin K, Talia KL, McCluggage WG. Endometrial gastric (gastrointestinal)-type mucinous lesions: report of a series illustrating the spectrum of benign and malignant lesions. Am J Surg Pathol. 2020;44(3):406–19.
21. Lu S, Shen D, Zhao Y, Kang N, Wang X. Primary endocervical gastric-type adenocarcinoma: a clinicopathologic and immunohistochemical analysis of 23 cases. Diagn Pathol. 2019;14(1):72.
22. Mikami Y, Kiyokawa T, Hata S, Fujiwara K, Moriya T, Sasano H, et al. Gastrointestinal immunophenotype in adenocarcinomas of the uterine cervix and related glandular lesions: a possible link between lobular endocervical glandular hyperplasia/pyloric gland metaplasia and 'adenoma malignum'. Mod Pathol. 2004;17(8):962–72.
23. Kojima A, Mikami Y, Sudo T, Yamaguchi S, Kusanagi Y, Ito M, et al. Gastric morphology and immunophenotype predict poor outcome in mucinous adenocarcinoma of the uterine cervix. Am J Surg Pathol. 2007;31(5):664–72.
24. Karamurzin YS, Kiyokawa T, Parkash V, Jotwani AR, Patel P, Pike MC, et al. Gastric-type endocervical adenocarcinoma: an aggressive tumor with unusual metastatic patterns and poor prognosis. Am J Surg Pathol. 2015;39(11):1449–57.
25. Garg S, Nagaria TS, Clarke B, Freedman O, Khan Z, Schwock J, et al. Molecular characterization of gastric-type endocervical adenocarcinoma using next-generation sequencing. Mod Pathol. 2019;32(12):1823–33.
26. Chiang S, Cotzia P, Hyman DM, Drilon A, Tap WD, Zhang L, et al. NTRK fusions define a novel uterine sarcoma subtype with features of fibrosarcoma. Am J Surg Pathol. 2018;42(6):791–8.
27. Mills AM, Karamchandani JR, Vogel H, Longacre TA. Endocervical fibroblastic malignant peripheral nerve sheath tumor (neurofibrosarcoma): report of a novel entity possibly related to endocervical CD34 fibrocytes. Am J Surg Pathol. 2011;35(3):404–12.
28. Hechtman JF, Benayed R, Hyman DM, Drilon A, Zehir A, Frosina D, et al. Pan-Trk immunohistochemistry is an efficient and reliable screen for the detection of NTRK fusions. Am J Surg Pathol. 2017;41(11):1547–51.
29. Gatalica Z, Xiu J, Swensen J, Vranic S. Molecular characterization of cancers with NTRK gene fusions. Mod Pathol. 2019;32(1):147–53.
30. Nilforoushan N, Wethington SL, Nonogaki H, Gross J, Vang R, Xing D. NTRK-fusion sarcoma of the uterine cervix: report of 2 cases with comparative clinicopathologic features. Int J Gynecol Pathol. 2022;41(6):642–8.
31. Khotskaya YB, Holla VR, Farago AF, Mills Shaw KR, Meric-Bernstam F, Hong DS. Targeting TRK family proteins in cancer. Pharmacol Ther. 2017;173:58–66.
32. Shih IM, Kurman RJ. Epithelioid trophoblastic tumor: a neoplasm distinct from choriocarcinoma and placental site trophoblastic tumor simulating carcinoma. Am J Surg Pathol. 1998;22(11):1393–403.
33. Kurman RJ, Shih Ie M. Discovery of a cell: reflections on the checkered history of intermediate trophoblast and update on its nature and pathologic manifestations. Int J Gynecol Pathol. 2014;33(4):339–47.
34. Palmer JE, Macdonald M, Wells M, Hancock BW, Tidy JA. Epithelioid trophoblastic tumor: a review of the literature. J Reprod Med. 2008;53(7):465–75.
35. Banet N, Gown AM, Shih Ie M, Kay Li Q, Roden RB, Nucci MR, et al. GATA-3 expression in trophoblastic tissues: an immunohistochemical study of 445 cases, including diagnostic utility. Am J Surg Pathol. 2015;39(1):101–8.
36. McCarthy WA, Paquette C, Gundogan F, Lawrence WD. Comparison of p63 and p40 immunohistochemical stains to distinguish epithelioid trophoblastic tumor from other trophoblastic lesions. Int J Gynecol Pathol. 2018;37(4):401–4.
37. Mao TL, Seidman JD, Kurman RJ, Shih Ie M. Cyclin E and p16 immunoreactivity in epithelioid trophoblastic tumor—an aid in differential diagnosis. Am J Surg Pathol. 2006;30(9):1105–10.
38. Shih Ie M. Trophogram, an immunohistochemistry-based algorithmic approach, in the differential diagnosis of trophoblastic tumors and tumorlike lesions. Ann Diagn Pathol. 2007;11(3):228–34.
39. Kaur B, Short D, Fisher RA, Savage PM, Seckl MJ, Sebire NJ. Atypical placental site nodule (APSN) and association with malignant gestational trophoblastic disease; a clinicopathologic study of 21 cases. Int J Gynecol Pathol. 2015;34(2):152–8.
40. Ngan HYS, Seckl MJ, Berkowitz RS, Xiang Y, Golfier F, Sekharan PK, et al. Diagnosis and management of gestational trophoblastic disease: 2021 update. Int J Gynaecol Obstet. 2021;155 Suppl 1(Suppl 1):86–93.
41. Lesack D, Wahab I, Gilks CB. Radiation-induced atypia of endocervical epithelium: a histological, immunohistochemical and cytometric study. Int J Gynecol Pathol. 1996;15(3):242–7.
42. Gupta S, Mukherjee K, Gupta YN, Kumar M. Sequential radiation changes in cytology of vaginal smears in carcinoma of cervix uteri during radiotherapy. Int J Gynaecol Obstet. 1987;25(4):303–8.
43. Zannoni GF, Vellone VG, Carbone A. Morphological effects of radiochemotherapy on cervical carcinoma: a morphological study of 50 cases of hysterectomy specimens after neoadjuvant treatment. Int J Gynecol Pathol. 2008;27(2):274–81.
44. Saito T, Takehara M, Tanaka R, Lee R, Horie M, Wataba K, et al. Correlation between responsiveness of neoadjuvant chemotherapy and apoptosis-associated proteins for cervical adenocarcinoma. Gynecol Oncol. 2004;92(1):284–92.
45. Chiantera V, Rossi M, De Iaco P, Koehler C, Marnitz S, Ferrandina G, et al. Survival after curative pelvic exenteration for primary or recurrent cervical cancer: a retrospective multicentric study of 167 patients. Int J Gynecol Cancer. 2014;24(5):916–22.
46. Inzani F, Angelico G, Santoro A, Travaglino A, Insabato L, Raffone A, et al. SATB2 is expressed in neuroendocrine carcinoma of the uterine cervix. Virchows Arch. 2022;480(4):873–7.
47. Inzani F, Santoro A, Angelico G, Feraco A, Spadola S, Arciuolo D, et al. Neuroendocrine carcinoma of the uterine cervix: a clinicopathologic and immunohistochemical study with focus on novel markers (Sst2-Sst5). Cancers (Basel). 2020;12(5):1211.
48. Kuji S, Watanabe R, Sato Y, Iwata T, Hirashima Y, Takekuma M, et al. A new marker, insulinoma-associated protein 1 (INSM1), for high-grade neuroendocrine carcinoma of the uterine cervix: analysis of 37 cases. Gynecol Oncol. 2017;144(2):384–90.
49. Howitt BE, Kelly P, McCluggage WG. Pathology of neuroendocrine tumours of the female genital tract. Curr Oncol Rep. 2017;19(9):59.
50. McCluggage WG, Kennedy K, Busam KJ. An immunohistochemical study of cervical neuroendocrine carcinomas: neoplasms that are commonly TTF1 positive and which may express CK20 and P63. Am J Surg Pathol. 2010;34(4):525–32.

51. Satoh T, Takei Y, Treilleux I, Devouassoux-Shisheboran M, Ledermann J, Viswanathan AN, et al. Gynecologic Cancer InterGroup (GCIG) consensus review for small cell carcinoma of the cervix. Int J Gynecol Cancer. 2014;24(9 Suppl 3):S102–8.
52. WHO Classification of Tumours Editorial Board. Female genital tumours, vol. 4. 5th ed. Lyon: International Agency for Research on Cancer; 2020. WHO Classification of Tumours Series.
53. Park JJ, Sun D, Quade BJ, Flynn C, Sheets EE, Yang A, et al. Stratified mucin-producing intraepithelial lesions of the cervix: adenosquamous or columnar cell neoplasia? Am J Surg Pathol. 2000;24(10):1414–9.
54. Onishi J, Sato Y, Sawaguchi A, Yamashita A, Maekawa K, Sameshima H, et al. Stratified mucin-producing intraepithelial lesion with invasive carcinoma: 12 cases with immunohistochemical and ultrastructural findings. Hum Pathol. 2016;55:174–81.
55. Lastra RR, Park KJ, Schoolmeester JK. Invasive stratified mucin-producing carcinoma and stratified mucin-producing intraepithelial lesion (SMILE): 15 cases presenting a spectrum of cervical neoplasia with description of a distinctive variant of invasive adenocarcinoma. Am J Surg Pathol. 2016;40(2):262–9.
56. Boyle DP, McCluggage WG. Stratified mucin-producing intraepithelial lesion (SMILE): report of a case series with associated pathological findings. Histopathology. 2015;66(5):658–63.
57. Stolnicu S, Talia KL, McCluggage WG. The evolving spectrum of precursor lesions of cervical adenocarcinomas. Adv Anat Pathol. 2020;27(5):278–93.
58. Arslanian E, Singh K, Hansen K, Quddus MR. Benign stratified intraepithelial mucinous proliferation of the uterine cervix: significance of a previously unreported potential mimic of SMILE. Ann Diagn Pathol. 2022;60:152025.
59. Li RF, Gupta M, McCluggage WG, Ronnett BM. Embryonal rhabdomyosarcoma (botryoid type) of the uterine corpus and cervix in adult women: report of a case series and review of the literature. Am J Surg Pathol. 2013;37(3):344–55.
60. Daya DA, Scully RE. Sarcoma botryoides of the uterine cervix in young women: a clinicopathological study of 13 cases. Gynecol Oncol. 1988;29(3):290–304.
61. de Kock L, Yoon JY, Apellaniz-Ruiz M, Pelletier D, McCluggage WG, Stewart CJR, et al. Significantly greater prevalence of DICER1 alterations in uterine embryonal rhabdomyosarcoma compared to adenosarcoma. Mod Pathol. 2020;33(6):1207–19.
62. Dehner LP, Jarzembowski JA, Hill DA. Embryonal rhabdomyosarcoma of the uterine cervix: a report of 14 cases and a discussion of its unusual clinicopathological associations. Mod Pathol. 2012;25(4):602–14.
63. Kommoss FKF, Stichel D, Mora J, Esteller M, Jones DTW, Pfister SM, et al. Clinicopathologic and molecular analysis of embryonal rhabdomyosarcoma of the genitourinary tract: evidence for a distinct DICER1-associated subgroup. Mod Pathol. 2021;34(8):1558–69.
64. Devins KM, Young RH, Ghioni M, Burandt E, Bennett JA, Oliva E. Embryonal rhabdomyosarcoma of the uterine cervix: a clinicopathologic study of 94 cases emphasizing issues in differential diagnosis staging, and prognostic factors. Am J Surg Pathol. 2022;46(11):1477–89.

Part IV

Vulvar Pathology Cases

10 Uncommon Tumors and Mimickers of Cancer

10.1 Nodular Hyperplasia (NH) of Bartholin Glands (BG)

10.1.1 A 35-Year-Old Woman with Painless Swelling in the Vulva

10.1.1.1 Key Diagnostic Features

- BG are located in the vulvar vetibule at the posterolateral introitus. The anatomic location is the key to BG's related pathology.
- Differentiation of BG adenoma and NH is an academic exercise.
- BG hyperplasia is a lobulated proliferation of mucinous-type glandular epithelium with the preservation of normal acinar and ductal elements.
- NH is sharply demarcated from the surrounding tissue (Figs. 10.1 and 10.2).
- Bartholin gland adenoma consists of closely packed haphazard proliferation of mucinous acini and tubules containing eosinophilic intraluminal secretions [1]. Residual normal ductal epithelium and acini can be present focally at the periphery of the lesion.

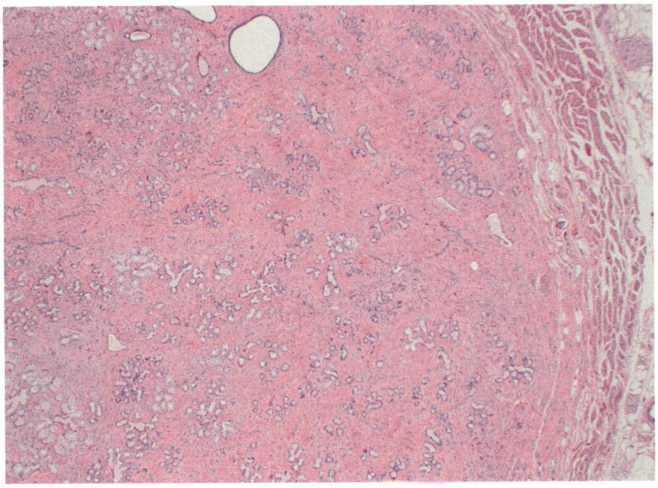

Fig. 10.1 NH of BG is sharply demarcated from the surrounding muscle tissue (20×)

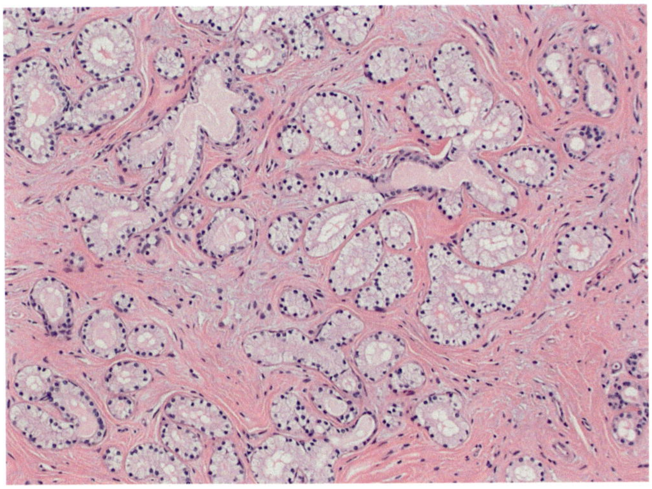

Fig. 10.2 The acinar/lobular architecture is preserved, bland mucinous epithelium lines acini (100×)

10.1.1.2 Ancillary Studies

- Cytokeratin (CAM5.2, AE1/AE3, HMWK), EMA, and polyclonal CEA are positive, and monoclonal CEA is negative in BG adenoma and NH [2].

10.1.1.3 Differential Diagnosis

- BG adenomyoma
  - Well-circumscribed lesion.
  - Compared to NH, a relatively scant acinar component grows in a haphazard pattern within a fibromuscular stroma.
  - Stromal elements are positive for desmin and SMA [1].
- NH with extensive mucin extravasation versus aggressive angiomyxoma (AA) [3]

O. Saglam, *Challenging Cases in Gynecologic Surgical Pathology*, https://doi.org/10.1007/978-3-031-51656-6_10

  - The entrapped stromal cells and vessels with an infiltrative mucinous border might be a diagnostic concern for AA.
  - Mucin stains (PAS and mucicarmine) can confirm sialomucin of BG.
  - See Part IV, Sect. 10.11.
- Bartholin gland carcinoma
  - The anatomic location of the lesion should be around the BG.
  - The presence of a transition area between normal BG and tumor rules out other possible primary cancers.
  - The histological subtypes are squamous carcinoma (most common), adenocarcinoma, adenosquamous carcinoma, transitional cell carcinoma, neuroendocrine carcinoma, and salivary-type carcinomas [4–8].
  - All squamous carcinomas of the BG express p16 diffusely [9].

10.1.1.4 Clinical Significance

- NH and adenoma of BG are benign lesions.

10.2 Hidradenoma Papilliferum (Papillary Hidradenoma) (HP)

10.2.1 A 42-Year-Old Woman with a Solid, Firm Mass Lesion in the Vulva

10.2.1.1 Key Diagnostic Features

- Nodular, usually well-circumscribed lesions composed of complex branching and interconnecting tubules and papillae (Fig. 10.3).
- The most common anatomical location is the interlabial sulcus of the vulva [10].
- The lesion might extend into the overlying epidermis (Fig. 10.4). The lining epithelium is bilayered: columnar secretory-type cells and underlining myoepithelial cells (Fig. 10.5).
- Cystic changes; ulceration of the overlying epidermis; pseudoepitheliomatous hyperplasia; necrosis; metaplastic changes including oxyphilic, squamous, and mucinous metaplasia; and clear cell change of the luminal epithelial or myoepithelial cells are described [11].
- The mitotic figures in high numbers can be present both in epithelial and myoepithelial cells, but this finding does not predict recurrence or a more aggressive outcome [12].

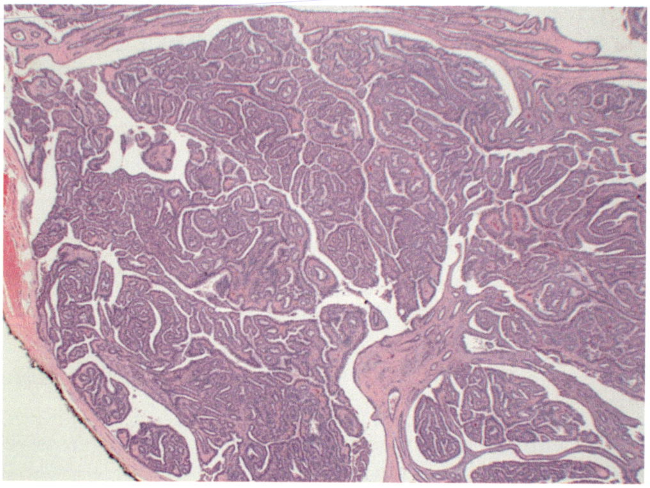

Fig. 10.3 HP is a well-circumscribed nodular lesion with a combination of tubular and papillary architecture (20×)

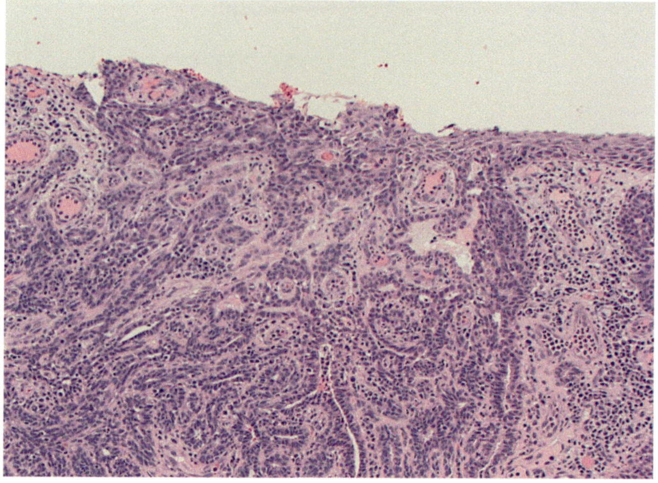

Fig. 10.4 The lesion extends into the surface epithelium with ulcer formation (40×)

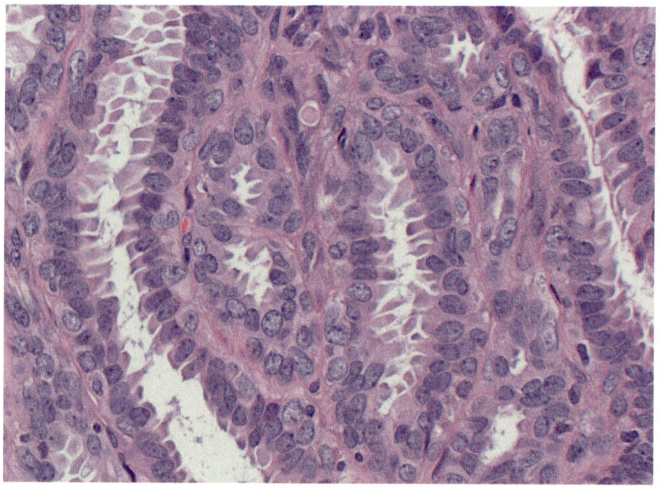

Fig. 10.5 The lining epithelium is bilayered. The columnar epithelium has prominent secretory apical snouting (200×)

10.2.1.2 Ancillary Studies

- Estrogen receptor expression is restricted to epithelial cells, whereas p63 and SMA are exclusively expressed in myoepithelial cells. *PIK3CA* and *AKT1* somatic mutation rates are 29% and 14%, respectively [13].

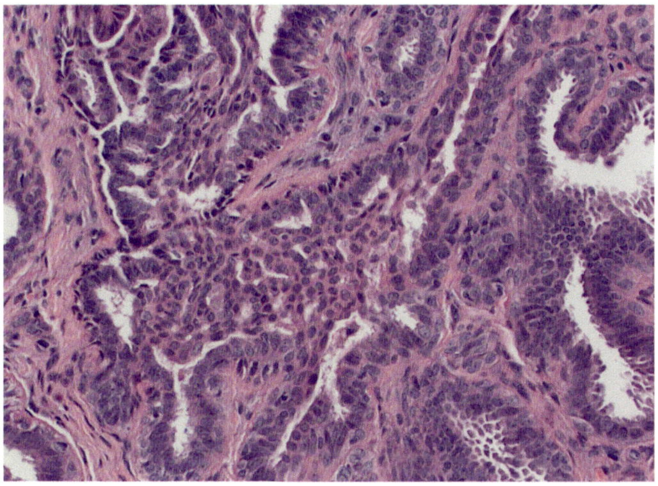

Fig. 10.6 Usual-type epithelial hyperplasia involving HP (200×)

10.2.1.3 Differential Diagnosis

- Changes resembling sclerosing adenosis, usual (Fig. 10.6) and atypical ductal hyperplasia, extramammary Paget's disease of the overlying epidermis, mammary-type intraductal carcinoma, and vulvar apocrine hidradenocarcinoma can arise in HP [11, 14, 15].

10.2.1.4 Clinical Significance

- HP is a benign tumor, but the associated mammary-like epithelial proliferation can be in the spectrum of benign to malignant diseases.

10.3 Molluscum Contagiosum (MC)

10.3.1 A 24-Year-Old Woman Who Is HIV Carrier

10.3.1.1 Key Diagnostic Features

- A pox virus infection, usually transmitted by sexual contact [16].
- An invaginated hyperplastic surface epithelium contains eosinophilic cells with cytoplasmic inclusion bodies (Henderson-Paterson bodies), which distend the keratinocytes [17] (Figs. 10.7, 10.8, and 10.9).
- As the duration of the disease is prolonged, cytoplasmic bodies become more basophilic, and eventually cell lysis occurs [18].

10.3.1.2 Ancillary Studies

N/A.

10.3.1.3 Differential Diagnosis

- Crateriform lesions of the vulva if the viral inclusions are old and scant in the section.

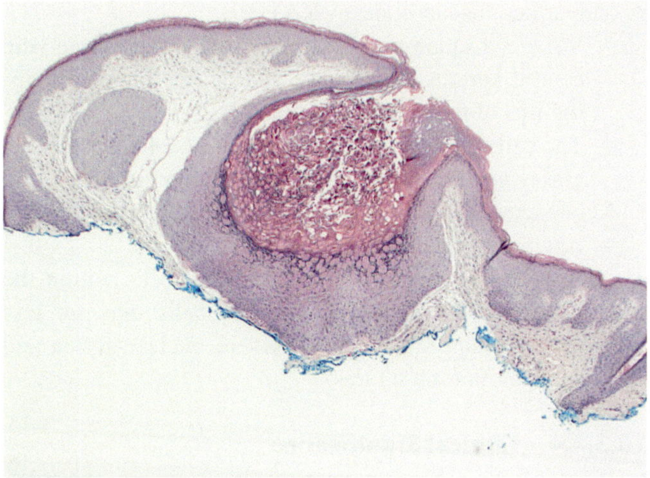

Fig. 10.7 Invaginated hypertrophic epithelium with a central crater filled with virus particles (20×)

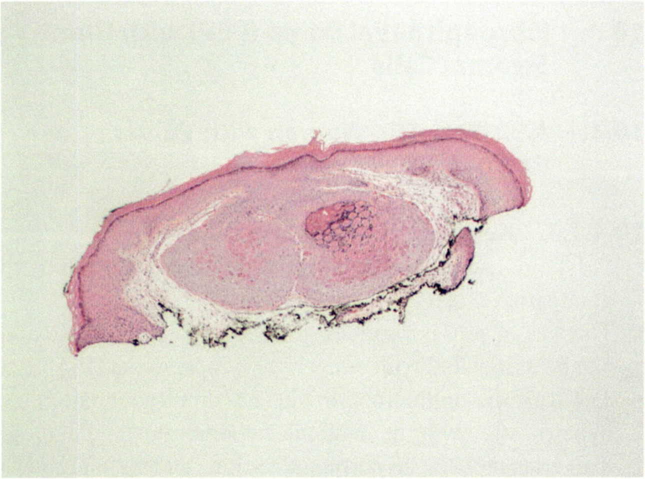

Fig. 10.8 The invaginated squamous epithelium does not extend to the surface in this section (20×)

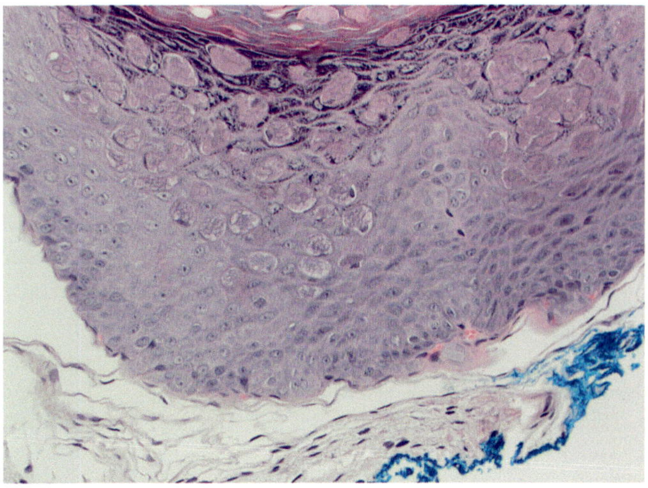

Fig. 10.9 Basophilic cytoplasmic inclusion bodies distend the keratinocytes (200×)

- Vulvar keratoacanthoma (VKA) [19].
  - VKA is a squamous proliferation with a characteristic central keratin-filled crater and buttressing/overhanging lips of the epidermis at the edges.
  - The cells are cytologically bland with an eosinophilic, glassy appearance and have rare mitotic figures.
- Keratoacanthoma-like squamous cell carcinoma [20]
  - Asymmetrical and deeply invasive lesions
  - Irregular distribution of the basaloid cells within the neoplastic lobules of large pink cells that are less glassy in appearance, with severe nuclear atypia and frequent mitotic figures

10.3.1.4 Clinical Significance

- Most lesions regress spontaneously. In others, the treatment of choice is physical destruction by cryotherapy and chemical destruction with cantharidin.

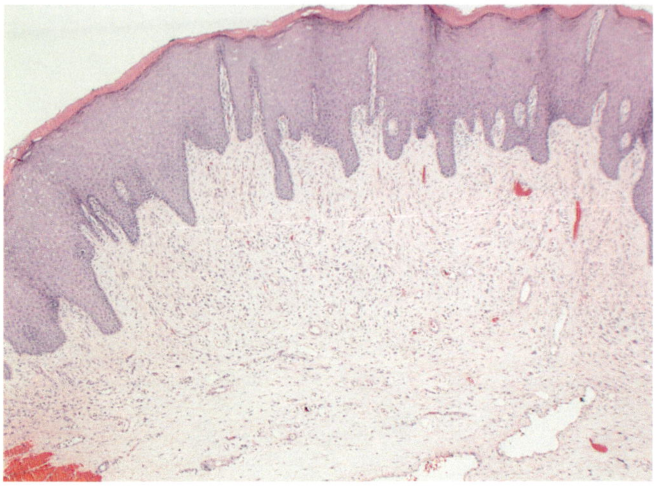

Fig. 10.10 Aggregates of stromal giant cells around the dermo-epidermal junction (40×)

10.4 Fibroepithelial Polyp (FEP) with Giant Stromal Cells

10.4.1 A 32-Year-Old Woman with Vulvar Polyp

10.4.1.1 Key Diagnostic Features

- Polypoid lesion of the vulva, AKA acrochordon with giant stromal cells.
- The size of FEP is variable; giant forms are described and can be associated with congenital lymphedema [21].
- The surface epithelium might be thin (attenuated) or hyperplastic with or without hyperkeratosis. Pagetoid dyskeratosis [22], hyperpigmentation, and hypopigmentation are among the surface epithelial changes. The latter finding is more commonly associated with large pedunculated polyps.
- There are thick-walled blood vessels within the stroma. The stroma might be edematous/myxoid or hypercellular and often contain collagen bundles.
- Giant stromal cells might be a diagnostic concern [23], typically present at the epithelial-stromal interface or adjacent to vessels (Fig. 10.10). The stromal cells can show a significant amount of nuclear pleomorphism, hyperchromasia (Figs. 10.11 and 10.12), and increased mitotic activity (Fig. 10.13) (>10 per 10 high-power fields) with atypical forms, especially during pregnancy [24].

10.4.1.2 Ancillary Studies

- The atypical stromal cells are ER, PR, and desmin positive [25].

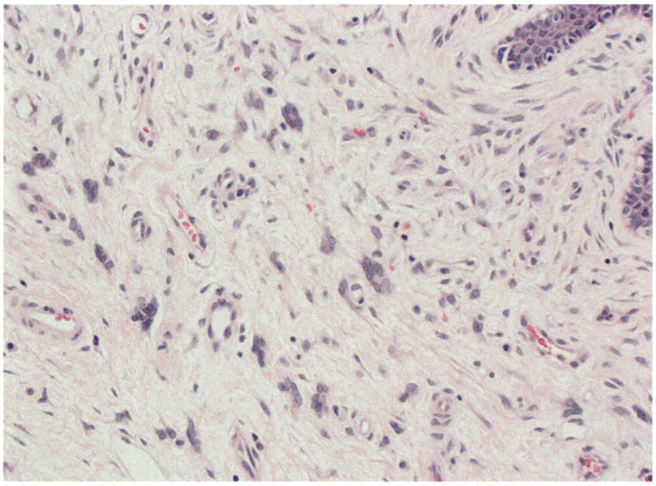

Fig. 10.11 Multinucleated cells around the dermal capillaries in a higher-power field (100×)

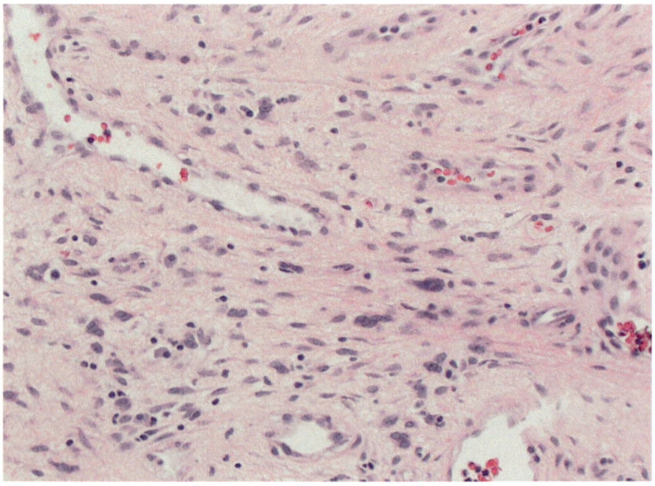

Fig. 10.12 A mixture of stellate and giant cells in the stroma of the polyp (200×)

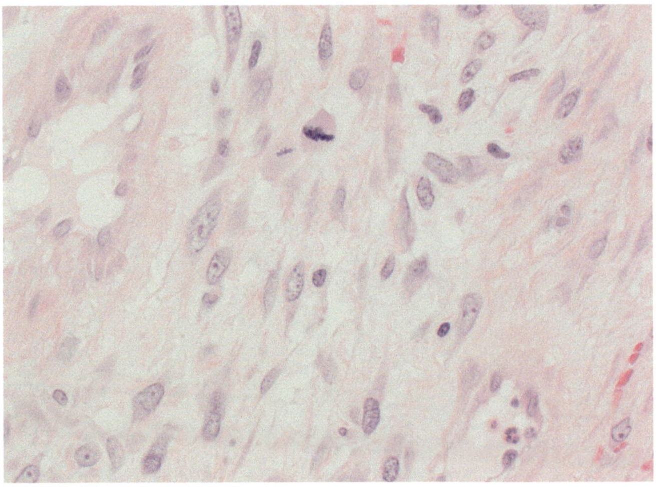

Fig. 10.13 Mitotic figures can be high in number (400×)

10.4.1.3 Differential Diagnosis

- FEP with giant stromal cells versus sarcoma botryoids (SB)
  - FEP with giant stromal cells is a disease in patients of reproductive ages and, more commonly, in pregnant women. SB is usually diagnosed before puberty.
  - The subepithelial hypercellular cambium layer is not present in FEP.
  - Expression of skeletal muscle markers in rhabdomyoblasts supports SB diagnosis.
  - See Part III, Sect. 9.10.
- FEP with myxoid stroma versus superficial angiomyxoma [26]
  - Superficial angiomyxoma is a tumor of cutaneous or subcutaneous sites.
  - Multinodular growth pattern with well-defined borders.
  - Delicate, capillary-sized vessels are typical.
  - A neutrophilic infiltrate and epidermoid cysts (around one-third of cases) may be present.
- FEP with myxoid stroma versus deep (aggressive) angiomyxoma
  - FEP has polypoid architecture and well-circumscribed borders. AA infiltrates deep soft tissue.
  - See Part IV, Sect. 10.11.
- Angiomyofibroblastoma
  - The anatomical location is in the subcutaneous tissue and does not have polypoid architecture.
  - Alternating zones of hyper and hypocellular areas are typical.
  - Prominent vascular component with numerous delicate capillary-sized vessels, with clustering of epithelioid cells around vessels.

10.4.1.4 Clinical Significance

- Complete resection is the treatment of choice, and recurrences are possible after incomplete resection.

10.5 Hibernoma

10.5.1 A 35-Year-Old Woman with a Painless, Soft, and Well-Circumscribed Mass in the Vulva

10.5.1.1 Key Diagnostic Features

- Distinct lobular pattern (Fig. 10.14).
- The cells have granular eosinophilic, multivacuolated cytoplasm, distinct cell membranes, and small central nuclei (Fig. 10.15), intermixed with univacuolar cells resembling lipocytes.
- A myxoid change can be focally present, more common in head and neck cases [27].

10.5.1.2 Ancillary Studies

- Positive immunostains: S100

10.5.1.3 Differential Diagnosis

- Granular cell tumor
  - More uniformly granular cells and lack typical adipocytes.
  - Pseudoepitheliomatous hyperplasia of the overlying squamous epithelium is a frequent finding.
  - In addition to S100, SOX10, CD68, and Inhibin A (small percentage of cases) are positive in granular cell tumors [28].

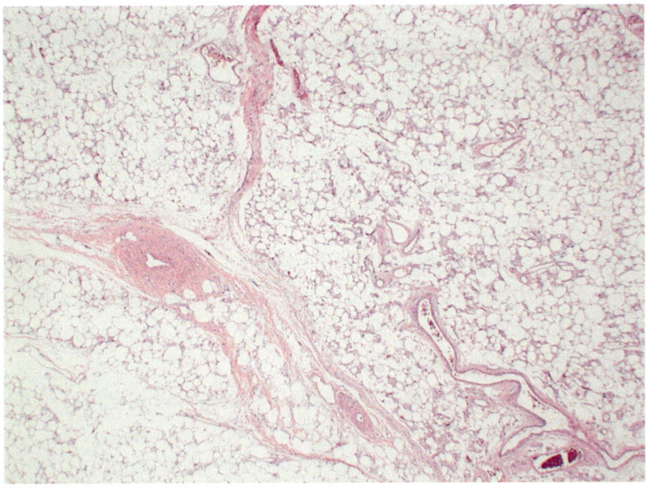

Fig. 10.14 Diffuse sheets of adipocytic proliferation in lobular pattern (20×)

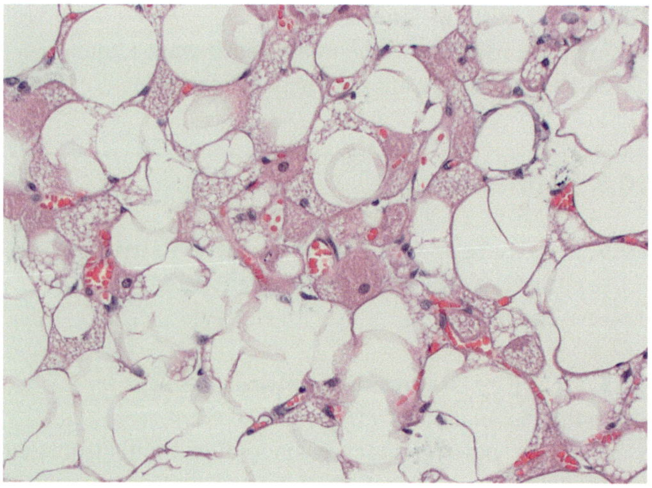

Fig. 10.15 Mixture of cells with granular or multivacuolated cytoplasm and centrally located nuclei and accompanying lipocyte-like cells (200×)

- Lipoblastoma-like tumor of the vulva
  - Exceptionally rare tumor.
  - It is composed of well-delineated large lobules partitioned by fibrous tissue, stromal collagenization, and a prominent arborizing network of thin-walled vessels. The cell types are spindle cells, lipoblasts, and mature adipocytes [29].
  - Lipoblasts are bland and typically small, univacuolated or bivacuolated, and rarely multivacuolated. Spindle cells exhibit indistinct cell borders, scant eosinophilic to inconspicuous cytoplasm, and typically short stubby nuclei.

10.5.1.4 Clinical Significance

- Benign tumor

10.6 Cellular Angiofibroma (CA)

10.6.1 A 65-Year-Old-Woman with a Slow-Growing Vulvar Mass Lesion

10.6.1.1 Key Diagnostic Features

- Well-circumscribed, usually unencapsulated, moderately cellular submucosal lesion composed of bland spindle-shaped cells (Fig. 10.16).
- Vessels might have thick hyalinized walls and hemangiopericytoma-like pattern (Fig. 10.17).
- Localized under submucosal surfaces with an uninvolved tissue between the epithelium and the lesion (Fig. 10.18).
- Adipose tissue, stromal lymphoid aggregates, scattered multinucleated cells, myxoid areas, or focal areas with marked cellular atypia might be a component of the lesion [30].

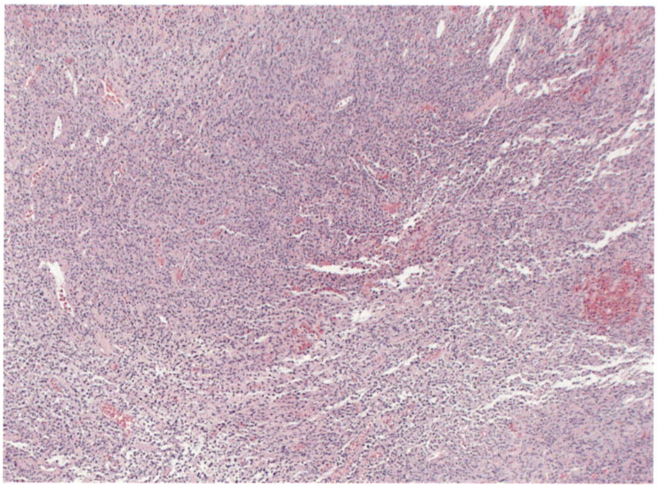

Fig. 10.16 Spindle cell proliferation with hemangiopericytoma-like and hyalinized thin vessels (40×)

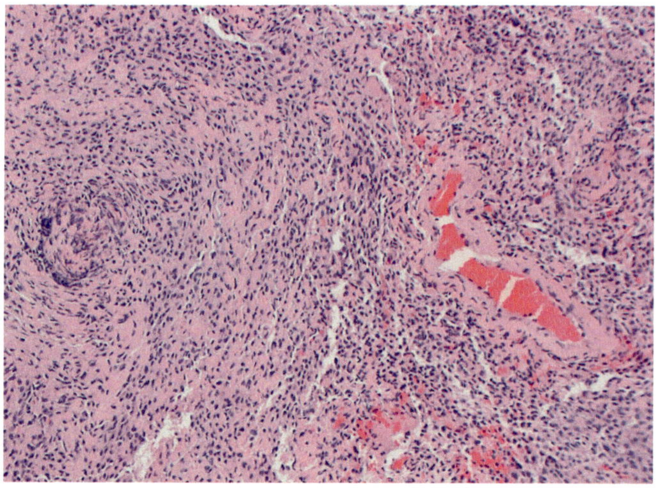

Fig. 10.17 Monotonous spindle cells form short fascicules around hyalinized vessels (100×)

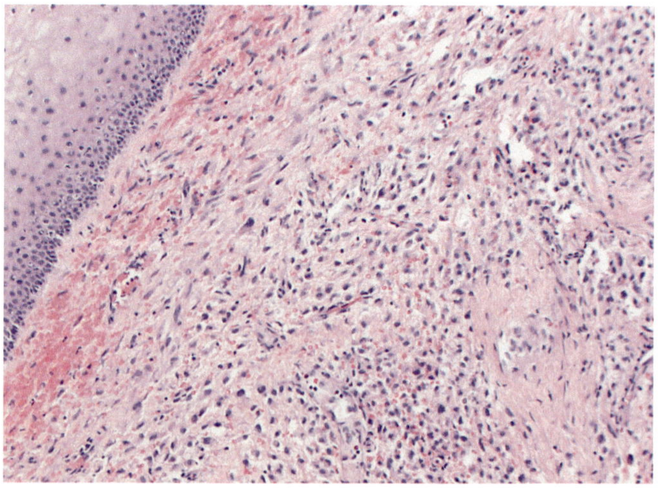

Fig. 10.18 The lesion is under the surface epithelium with a thin rim of uninvolved tissue. There is no true capsule formation (100×)

- Sarcomatous transformation (atypical lipomatous tumor-like component, pleomorphic liposarcoma, and pleomorphic sarcoma) can be admixed without increased risk of metastasis or recurrence (limited follow-up) [31].

10.6.1.2 Ancillary Studies

- Positive immunostains: ER, PR, CD34, S100, vimentin
- Negative immunostains: SMA, desmin, caldesmon
- Monoallelic *RB1/FOXO1* deletion (chromosome 13q12-22) [32, 33]
- Loss of Rb expression by immunohistochemistry

10.6.1.3 Differential Diagnosis

- Fibroepithelial polyp
  - Polypoid, not submucosal.
  - See Part IV, Sect. 10.4.
- Aggressive angiomyxoma
  - Low cellularity of bland, ovoid, and spindle cells embedded in an abundant myxoid stroma.
  - Infiltrative borders.
  - Vimentin, SMA, desmin, ER, PR, and CD34 are positive.
  - See Part IV, Sect. 10.11.
- Angiomyofibroblastoma
  - A well-circumscribed lesion with alternating hypocellular and hypercellular areas.
  - Epithelioid and plasmacytoid cells aggregate around thin-walled blood vessels.
  - Desmin and SMA are positive.

10.6.1.4 Clinical Significance

- Rare local recurrence after adequate excision is described [34].

10.7 Schwannoma with Intralesional Nodularity

10.7.1 A 42-Year-Old Woman with Vulvar Mass

10.7.1.1 Key Diagnostic Features

- Alternating hypercellular (Antoni A) and hypocellular (Antoni B) areas are accentuated with a multinodular appearance. In contrast to plexiform Schwannoma, no fibrous capsule encircles the nodules (Antoni A), and the lesional cells are present between them (Antoni B areas) (Figs. 10.19 and 10.20) [35].
- The nuclei are wavy with tapered ends (Fig. 10.21).
- Verocay bodies (nuclear palisades), inflammatory changes, cystic/pseudoglandular changes, and collagenous spherules can be present.
- Other morphological variants of Schwannoma are also described in the vulva: (1) ancient Schwannoma [36], (2) plexiform Schwannoma [37], and (3) melanotic Schwannoma [38].

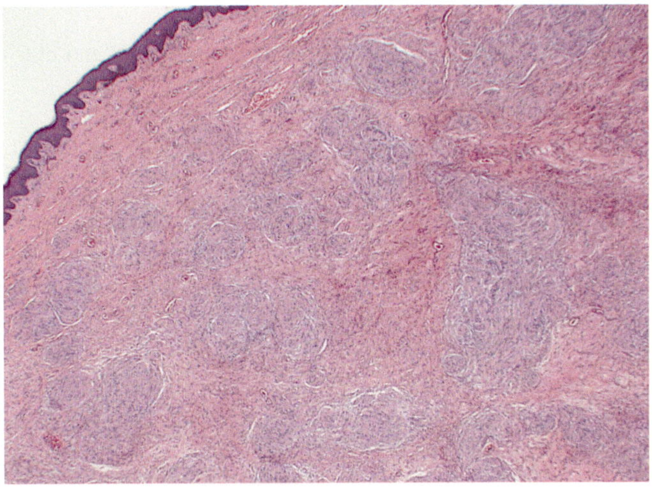

Fig. 10.19 The lesion grows underneath the squamous epithelium. It has well-circumscribed borders (40×)

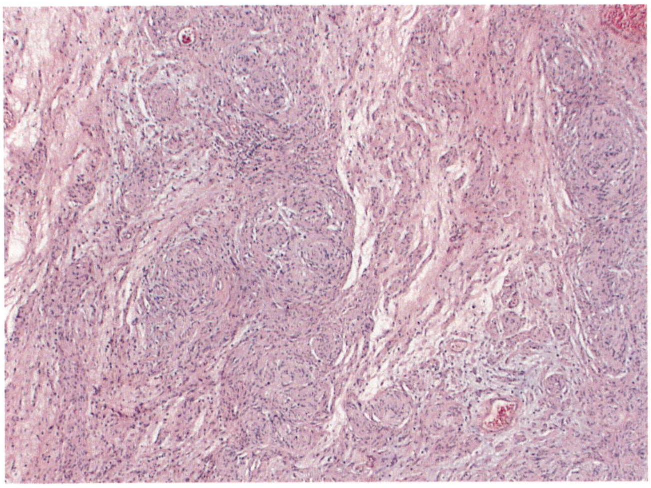

Fig. 10.20 The growth pattern is nodular. There is no fibrous capsule around the nodules. Less cellular areas (Antoni B) have lesional cells (100×)

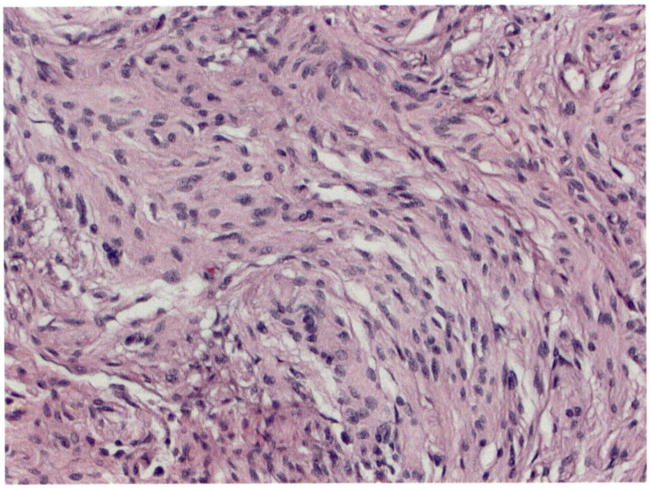

Fig. 10.21 The cells have wavy nuclei with tapered ends (200×)

10.7.1.2 Ancillary Studies

- S100 and SOX10 are diffusely positive; GFAP and cytokeratin might be expressed.

10.7.1.3 Differential Diagnosis

- Plexiform Schwannoma
  - Multinodular growth, composed of well-defined, varying sized-nodules, each separated by fibrous septae.
  - The internodular areas show background stroma without lesional tissue.
- Plexiform neurofibroma
  - Neurofibromas are unencapsulated.
  - There is a tortuous mass of expanded nerve branches in the early stages. Later, the cells spill out of the nerves into soft tissue and become a diffuse lesion composed of small cells with wavy nuclei embedded in a myxoid stroma.
  - S100, SOX10 CD34 (lattice-pattern) EMA, and GLUT1 are positive [39].
- Malignant transformation of Schwannoma (extremely rare)
  - Epithelioid malignant peripheral nerve sheath tumor, rhabdomyosarcoma, and angiosarcoma reportedly might be associated with existing Schwannoma [40].
- Leiomyoma
  - Nuclei have cigar-shaped (blunt) ends. The cytoplasm is eosinophilic with distinct cell membranes.
  - Hyalinized types rarely have a palisading nuclei around hyalinized zones.
  - Smooth muscle markers (SMA, desmin, and caldesmon) are positive in leiomyoma.

10.7.1.4 Clinical Significance

- Schwannoma is associated with the inactivation of the *NF2* gene. The loss of function mutations or deletions in *NF2* cause neurofibromatosis type 2, a multiple tumor-forming disease of the nervous system [41].

10.8 Extramammary Paget Disease (EMPD) with Underlying Adenocarcinoma

10.8.1 A 60-Year-Old Woman with Erythematous and Erosive Lesions in the Vulva

10.8.1.1 Key Diagnostic Features

- Large round cells (Paget cells) within the epidermis and glandular neoplastic epithelium infiltrating underlying stroma (Figs. 10.22 and 10.23).
- The neoplastic cells within the epidermis have round nuclei, prominent nucleoli, and abundant cytoplasm. They can be present in groups around the basement membrane, extend into upper thirds (pagetoid spread), or follow adnexal structures within the dermis (Figs. 10.24 and 10.25).
- The invasive and in situ components can be primary (no internal organ involvement) or can be associated with rectal, bladder, or cervical adenocarcinoma.

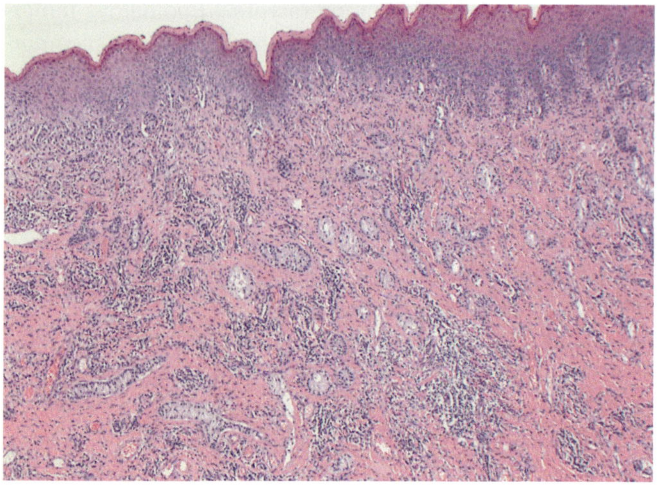

Fig. 10.22 Well-differentiated adenocarcinoma invades dermis and subcutaneous tissue (20×)

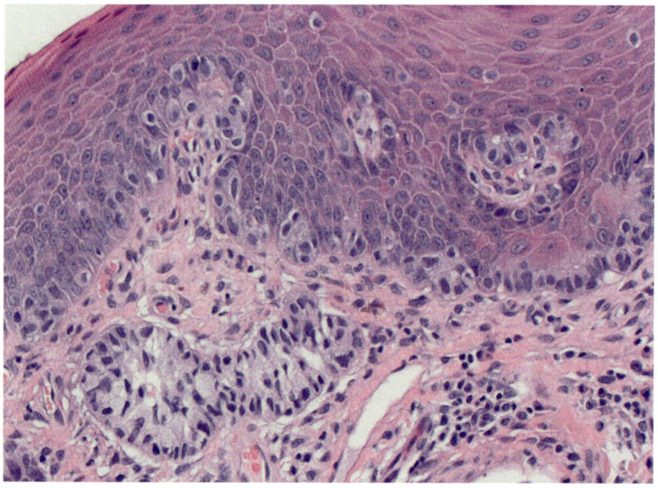

Fig. 10.23 The mucinous-type epithelium lines neoplastic glands (100×). Paget cells within the epithelium and adenocarcinoma have similar cytological features

10.8.1.2 Ancillary Studies

- Her2, CK7, GATA3, EMA, and keratin are positive, and melanoma markers (HM45, Melan A, and S100) are negative.
- CDX2 and CD20 positivity suggests secondary Paget disease with a primary intestinal carcinoma [42, 43].
- Lack of HPV infection does not preclude diffuse p16 positivity in EMPD samples [44].

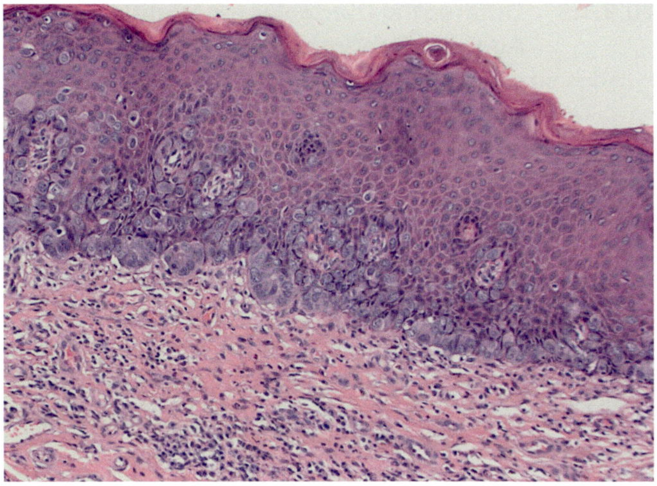

Fig. 10.24 The epithelial disease with aggregates of Paget cells in the lower part of the epithelium. They have large round nuclei and abundant cytoplasm. In contrast to non-invasive disease, the basal layer is not intact (200×)

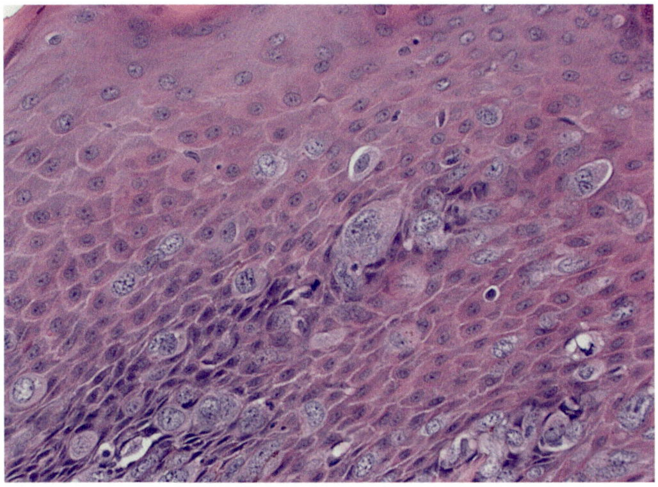

Fig. 10.25 Pagetoid spread involving upper layers of the epidermis (400×)

10.8.1.3 Differential Diagnosis

- Superficial spreading malignant melanoma
  - At the dermoepidermal junction, nests of neoplastic cells are separated by clefts from surrounding keratinocytes.
  - Fine granules in the cytoplasm of the pagetoid cells.
  - HMB45, S100, and Melan A are positive.
- Vulvar intraepithelial neoplasia with Pagetoid cells
  - The epidermis is involved by full-thickness cytological atypia.
  - P16 and P40 (p63) are positive.
- Adnexal involvement in primary EMPD
  - Hair follicles and eccrine ducts are most commonly affected by Paget cells. Patterns of adnexal involvement: (1) spread as single cells, (2) small clusters, (3) gland-like formations, (4) substitution of luminal cells in ducts/coils with preserved peripheral myoepithelial cells resulting in ductal carcinoma in situ-like appearance [45].

10.8.1.4 Clinical Significance

- The association of EMPD with an underlying adenocarcinoma is rare (<5%) and often characterized by more aggressive behavior [46]. The most common carcinoma types are breast analogs (i.e., invasive ductal carcinoma). Rare isolated tumor cells in the dermis are not associated with a worse prognosis [47].

10.9 Basal Cell Carcinoma (BCC) of the Vulva, Nodular/Adenoid Subtype

10.9.1 An 81-Year-Old Woman with Blisters and Itching in the Vulva

10.9.1.1 Key Diagnostic Features

- Well-circumscribed basaloid cells (Fig. 10.26) with peripheral palisading nuclei (Fig. 10.27). Artifactual retraction spaces between the tumor and stroma can be present [48, 49].
- Lobules may be solid or show central cyst formation due to excessive mucin production (pseudo-glandular pattern) (Fig. 10.28). Scattered mitotic figures are common.

10.9.1.2 Ancillary Studies

- Positive immunostains: BerEP4 (Fig. 10.29), p63, 34 beta E12, and P16 [50]

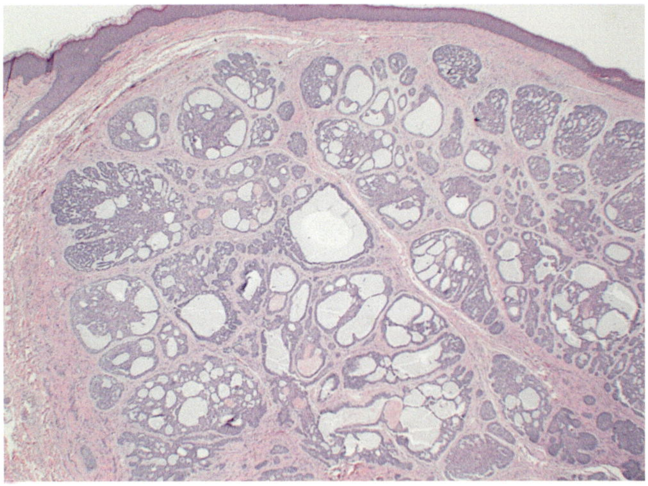

Fig. 10.26 Well-circumscribed and nodular growth of basaloid cells under the surface epithelium (20×)

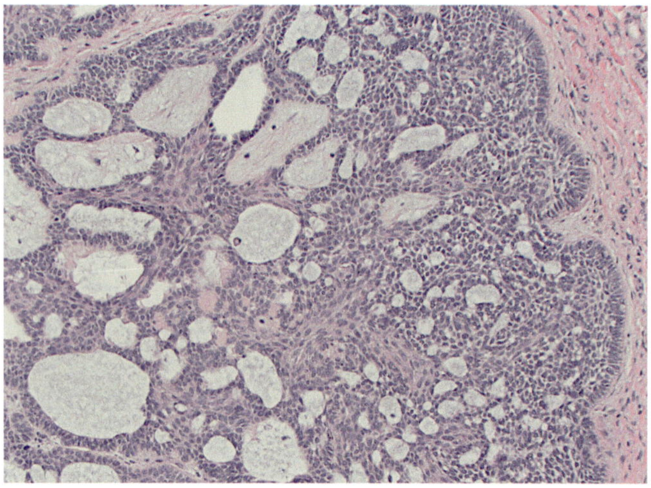

Fig. 10.27 Peripheral palisading of basaloid cells (100×)

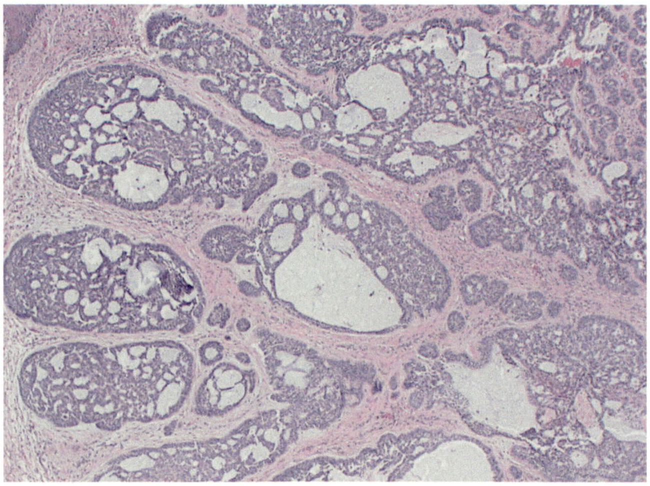

Fig. 10.28 Central cyst formation due to excessive mucin (pseudoglands) (40×)

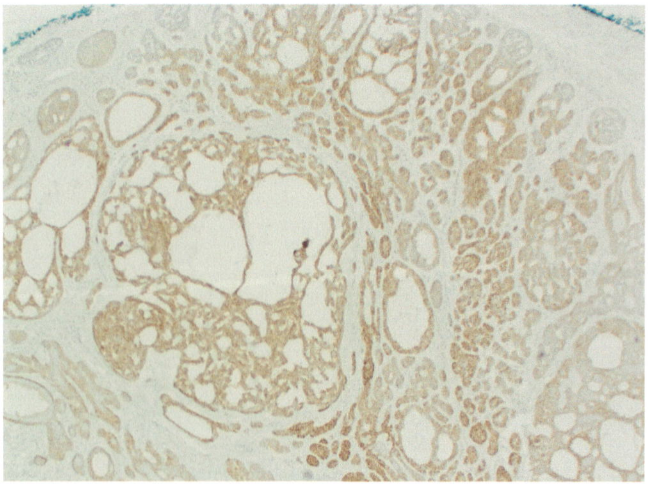

Fig. 10.29 Immunostain for BerEP4 is positive (40×)

10.9.1.3 Differential Diagnosis for Nodular/Adenoid Subtype of BCC

- Adenoid cystic carcinoma
  - Deep dermal tumor with subcutaneous extension.
  - Nests of basaloid cells with cribriform and tubular patterns and associated abundant mucin or basement membrane material within cysts.
  - Perineural invasion is frequent (100% in one case series) [51].
  - EMA, CK7, CEA, and CD117 are positive in ductal structures, and p63, calponin, and SMA are positive in the myoepithelial cells.
  - Not associated with HPV infection [52, 53].

10.9.1.4 Clinical Significance

- In a recent series ($n = 19$), patients with larger tumors (> 20 mm) have worse clinical outcomes. A surgical margin of <3 mm is associated with recurrences. The histological subtype does not have an impact on survival [49]. Rare vulvar BCC metastasizes to regional lymph nodes [54].

10.10 Differentiated Vulvar Intraepithelial Neoplasia (dVIN) (HPV-Independent VIN)

10.10.1 A 72-Year-Old Woman with Vulvar Itching

10.10.1.1 Key Diagnostic Features

- The epithelial thickness varies from hypertrophic/acanthotic epithelium with elongated and fused rete ridges to atrophic epithelium. Parakeratotic foci on the surface are frequently present (Fig. 10.30).
- The diagnosis depends on abnormal cytological features of keratinocytes in the lower one-third of the epithelium. A significant cytological atypia (Fig. 10.31) is the key to diagnosis. The nuclei are enlarged, pleomorphic with open chromatin, or relatively small, hyperchromatic, and angulated.
- The mitotic figures, including atypical forms, are usually present in the lower one-third of the epithelium.
- Keratinocytes in the upper layers (middle and upper one-third) of the epithelium have abnormal maturation with abundant cytoplasm, well-defined cell borders, and prominent intercellular bridges. An abrupt keratinization (keratin pearls) can be present (Fig. 10.31).
- The skin appendages can rarely be involved by dVIN [55].

10.10.1.2 Ancillary Studies

- Immunostain for p53 might support the diagnosis of dVIN [56]. The basal/parabasal cells can have a strong

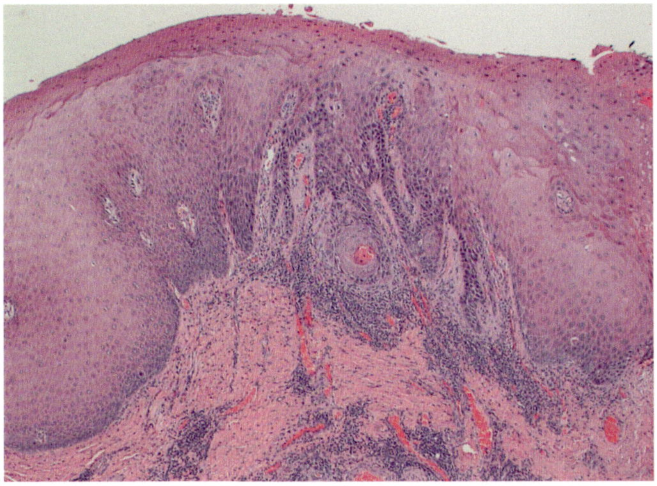

Fig. 10.30 Hypertrophic epithelium with elongated and fused rete ridges. There is parakeratosis on the surface. The keratinocytes in the upper two-thirds of the epidermis have abundant pink cytoplasm and well-defined cell borders (40×)

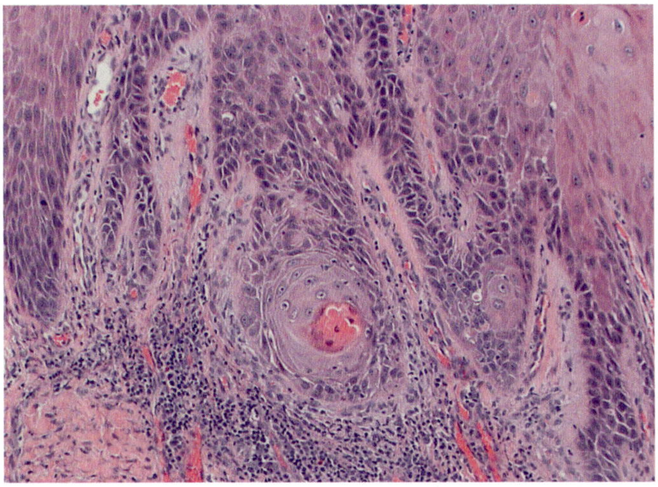

Fig. 10.31 The lower third of the epithelium has keratinocytes with significant cytological atypia. The nuclear-cytoplasmic ratio is high, nuclei are hyperchromatic, and mitotic figures are present. Paradoxical maturation and keratin pearl formation are prominent in this field (200×)

and diffuse staining pattern with p53 or have a complete absence of staining (null type) [57]. A moderate to strong basal staining with p53 ($\geq$70%) can also be present in other dermatoses, including lichen sclerosus, lichen planus, and spongiotic dermatitis. The positive staining is limited to the basal layer, and any staining in the parabasal layers is patchy in these entities [58]. Reportedly, diffuse, moderate-to-strong, full epithelial expression of CK17 or SOX2 is highly specific for dVIN and might contribute to the diagnosis [59]. P16 is negative in dVIN [60].

10.10.1.3 Differential Diagnosis

- Lichen simplex chronicus (LSC)
  - There might be basal cell atypia and disturbance of maturation in LSC [61]. Intense chronic inflammation makes it very challenging to rule out dVIN, but the reactive atypia should not be more than a mild degree. In some samples, p53 immunostain might be contributory to the diagnosis.
- Atrophic dVIN versus lichen sclerosus (LS)
  - A thin epidermis with underlying homogenization of the stroma is the characteristic morphological feature of LS. The nuclear pleomorphism is minimal, and disturbances in cell maturation are absent in most LS samples. LS can progress to squamous cell carcinoma but does not meet the criteria for dVIN [62].
- Lichen planus (LP)
  - Hyperkeratosis, acanthosis, and civatte bodies (eosinophilic spherical structures)
  - The presence of wedge-shaped hypergranulosis, artifactual cleft formation between the epidermis and papillary dermis, and pigment incontinence support the diagnosis of LP.
  - LP might be associated with VIN [63].
- HPV associated VIN with superimposed LSC [64]
  - The epithelium has changes such as hyperkeratosis, hypergranulosis, acanthosis, hypercellularity, abnormal maturation, hyperchromasia, and basal atypia.
  - Parabasal and mid-epithelial staining by p53 without involvement of the basal layer is a characteristic finding in HPV-associated VIN with superimposed LSC.

10.10.1.4 Clinical Significance

- dVIN can progress to keratinizing and nonkeratinizing invasive squamous cell carcinoma. The keratinizing type is more common [65].

10.11 Deep (Aggressive) Angiomyxoma (AA)

10.11.1 A 46-Year-Old Woman with Pelvic Fullness/Pressure

10.11.1.1 Key Diagnostic Features

- Hypocellular proliferation of spindle and ovoid cells within a loose and myxoid stroma with infiltrative margins [66] (Fig. 10.32).
- Extension into surrounding tissue results in entrapment of adipose tissue, muscle, and nerve bundles (Figs. 10.33 and 10.34).
- Numerous variable-sized vessels are present. Myoid bundles or collagen wrap around the vessels (Fig. 10.35).

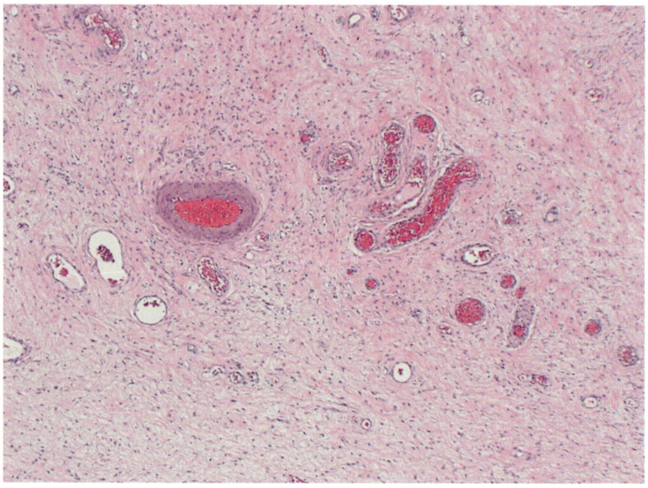

Fig. 10.32 Spindle cell proliferation within a myxoid stroma. The cells have bland nuclei and scant cytoplasm. Numerous blood vessels with varying caliber are in the field (40×)

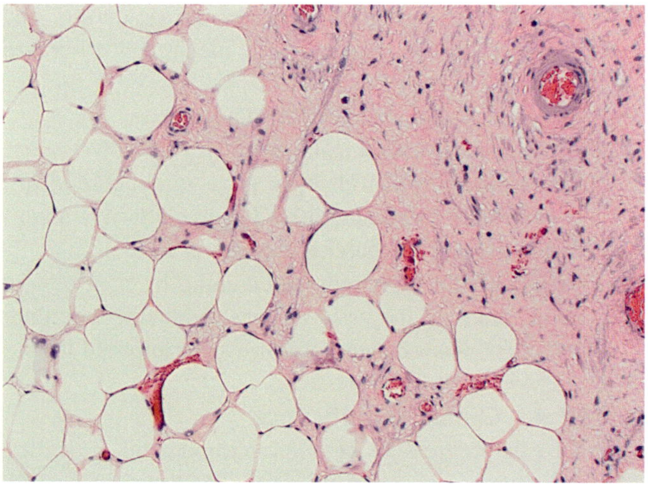

Fig. 10.33 The margins are infiltrative into surrounding adipose tissue (100×)

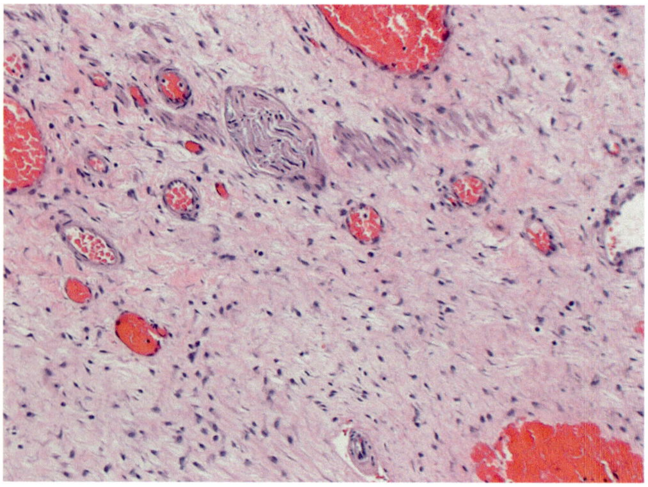

Fig. 10.34 Entrapped benign nerve bundle and smooth muscle (100×)

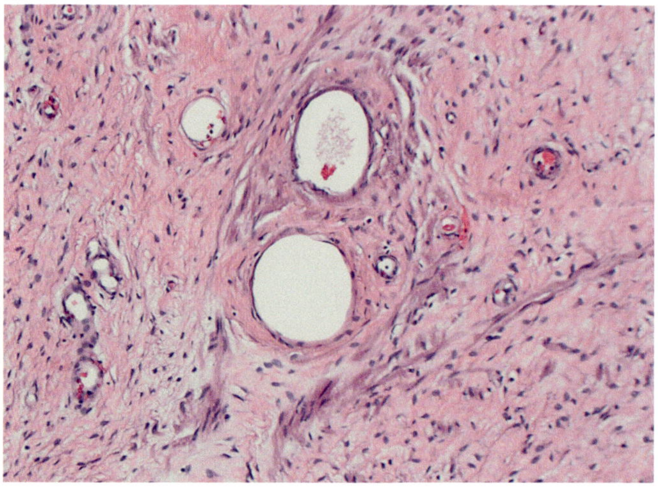

Fig. 10.35 Capillaries are surrounded by collagen and myoid bundles (100×)

- The neoplastic cells are oval to stellate with scant cytoplasm or with cytoplasmic processes.
- No mitotic activity is present.

10.11.1.2 Ancillary Studies

- Desmin and SMA are positive in the myoid cells around the blood vessels.
- ER/PR: positive [67].
- S100: negative.
- Rearrangements of *HMGA2* can be detected in one-third of the tumors [68].

10.11.1.3 Differential Diagnosis

- Superficial angiomyxoma [26, 69]
  - Usually dermal location
  - Multinodular myxoid lobules without infiltrative borders
  - Composed of bland spindle or stellate cells and thin-walled curvilinear blood vessels
- Myxoma
  - Intramuscular lesions
  - Overall hypocellular with slightly more cellular at the periphery with collagenized capsule
  - Lacks typical vasculature of AA
- Low-grade myxoid liposarcoma [70]
  - Paucicellular with monomorphic, stellate, or fusiform-shaped cells without cytological atypia.
  - Delicate thin-walled arborizing capillaries form a network reminiscent of chicken wire fencing.
  - Numerous signet ring lipoblasts, particularly at the periphery of the lobule.
  - S100 is positive.
- Myxoid neurofibroma
  - Slender wavy nuclei are positive for S100 (neural origin).
  - Lacks typical vasculature of AA.

- Low-grade myxofibrosarcoma [71]
  - Alternating hypocellular and hypercellular areas. The lesion is more fibrous than myxoid with an abrupt or gradual transition from one to another.
  - Curvilinear vascular pattern with perivascular condensation of tumor and inflammatory cells.
  - Collagen rosettes or epithelioid areas can be present.
  - Trichrome highlights background collagenous stroma.

10.11.1.4 Clinical Significance

- Locally aggressive tumors without metastatic potential. Local recurrences are associated with incomplete resections.

10.12 Pseudovascular Squamous Cell Carcinoma (Pseudoangiosarcomatous Carcinoma)

10.12.1 A 57-Year-Old Woman with a Large Ulcerated Vulvar Mass

10.12.1.1 Key Diagnostic Features

- Presents as an ulcerated or crusted nodule (Fig. 10.36).
- Cords of polygonal or flattened cells line pesudovascular spaces [72, 73].
- Pseudolumina/internal spaces contain detached tumor cells and erythrocytes. The neoplastic cells are polygonal with prominent one or more nucleoli (Figs. 10.37 and 10.38).
- Typical keratinizing squamous cell carcinoma can be focal in the same sample (Fig. 10.39).

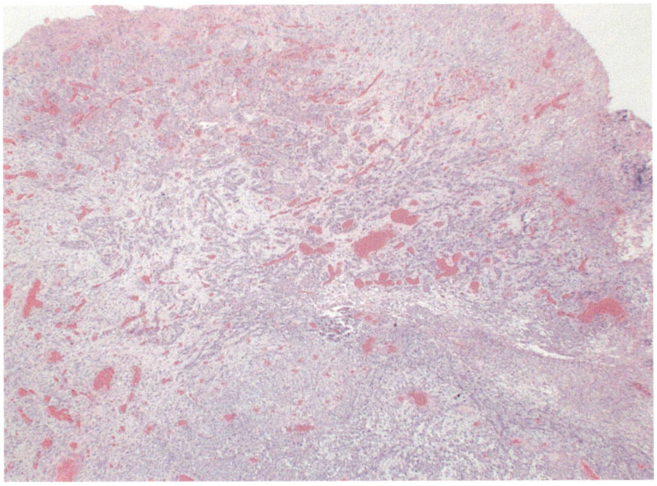

Fig. 10.36 The surface of the lesion is ulcerated (20×)

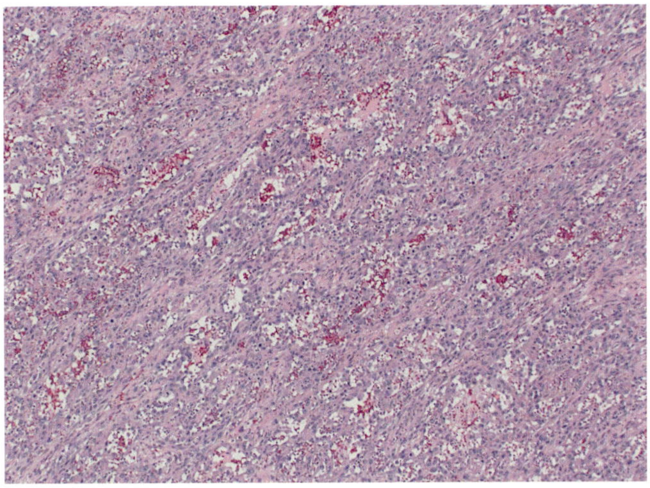

Fig. 10.37 The blood fills the anastomosing spaces (pesudoglandular areas) (40×)

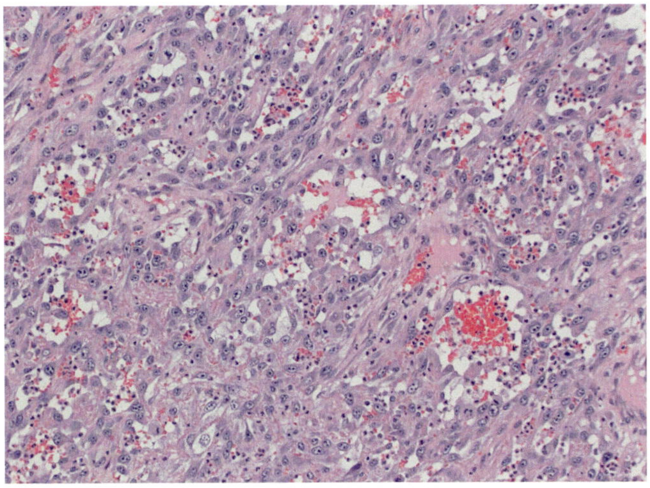

Fig. 10.38 Polygonal cells with internal pseudolumina and detached cells (100×)

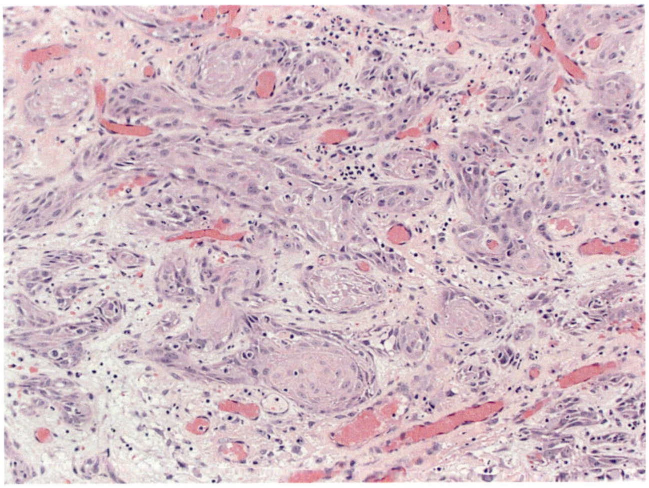

Fig. 10.39 Squamous differentiation is present under the ulcerated area in high-power examination (200×)

10.12.1.2 Ancillary Studies

- Cytokeratin cocktails, p63, p40, EMA: positive
- Vascular markers (CD34, CD31, factor VIII): negative
- P16/HPV: can be positive or negative [73, 74]
- E-cadherin: negative in pseudosarcomatous component [75]

10.12.1.3 Differential Diagnosis

- Angiosarcoma
  - The epithelioid cells are arranged in nests, clusters, or papillae and line irregularly shaped anastomosing vascular channels in well-differentiated lesions. A solid growth pattern dominates in poorly differentiated angiosarcoma.
  - Tumor cells are typically plump, pleomorphic, and mitotically active.
  - Cytokeratin might be positive in some lesions [76].
  - Vascular markers (CD31 and CD34) support the diagnosis.
- Malignant melanoma
  - Might have acantholytic or discohesive changes [77].
  - Subepidermal cleft formation with separation of the epidermis and underlying melanocytes at the dermal-epidermal junction.
  - Melanoma markers such as Melan A, HMB45, and S100 are positive.

10.12.1.4 Clinical Significance

- Aggressive clinical behavior with a high mortality rate [78, 79]

10.13 Epithelioid Hemangioendothelioma (EHE)

10.13.1 A 40-Year-Old Woman with Vulvar Lesion

10.13.1.1 Key Diagnostic Features

- The epithelioid cells are organized in strands, solid nests, and cords within a collagenous or myxohyaline stroma (Figs. 10.40 and 10.41).
- The neoplastic cells contain eosinophilic cytoplasm and intracytoplasmic vacuoles (Fig. 10.42).
- Usually, the mitotic activity is low, and cytological atypia is minimal.
- EHE can be stratified into two risk groups with different clinical course. Patients in high-risk groups have tumors with >3 mitotic figures/50 high-power fields and tumor size >3.0 cm [80].
- Rarely, neoplastic cells may organize in a cribriform growth pattern and mimic invasive carcinoma.

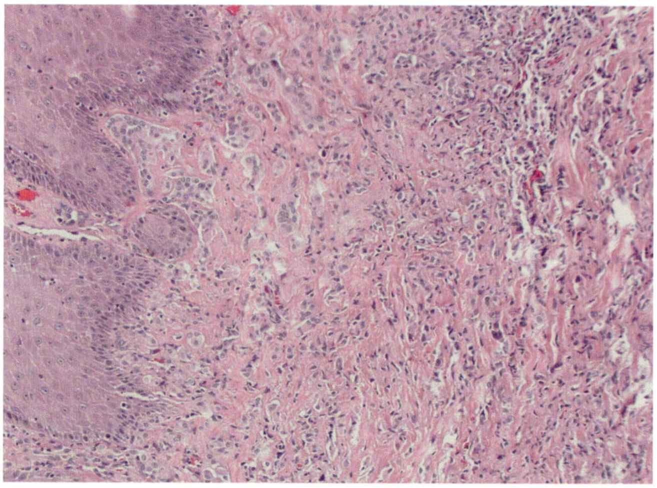

Fig. 10.40 Diffuse proliferation of epithelioid cells within the dermis. They are forming small groups and cords (40×)

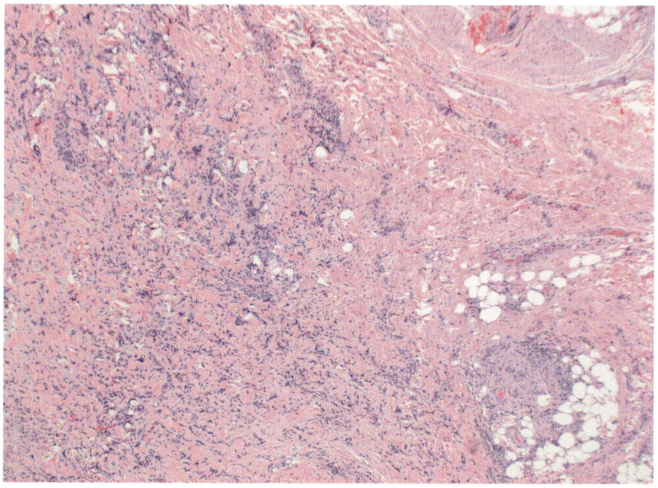

Fig. 10.41 The lesion infiltrates into adipose tissue (20×)

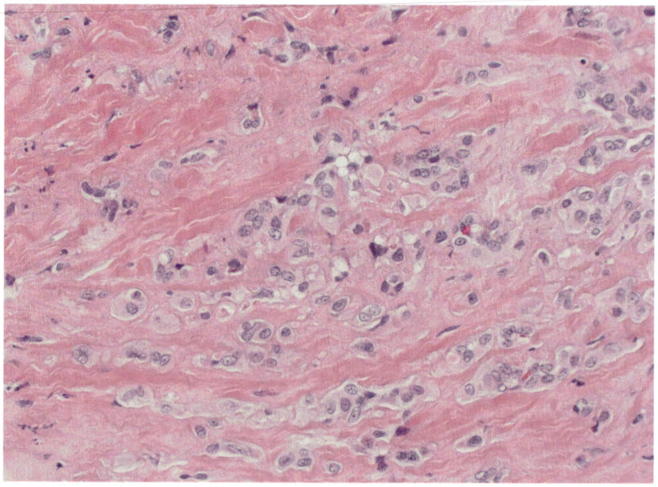

Fig. 10.42 The neoplastic cells have mild nuclear atypia and abundant eosinophilic cytoplasm. They lack mitotic activity. Rare intracytoplasmic vacuoles are in the field (central and right lower quadrants) (200×)

10.13.1.2 Ancillary Studies

- EHE expresses endothelial differentiation markers such as CD31, ERG (Fig. 10.43), CD34, and FLI-1.
- EHE is molecularly characterized by *WWTR1-CAMTA1* (90%) or *YAP1-TFE3* (10%) gene fusions [81, 82].
- CAMTA1 immunohistochemistry is a good surrogate to detect *WWTR1-CAMTA1* translocation (Fig. 10.44), whereas TFE3 is less specific, and therefore molecular confirmation is essential [83].
- Focal cytokeratin expression can be seen in less than 30% of lesions [84].

10.13.1.3 Differential Diagnosis

- Epithelioid angiosarcoma
  - Irregular sinusoidal vascular channels.
  - The presence of striking cytologic atypia, elevated mitotic count, and necrosis is relatively more common in epithelioid angiosarcoma.
  - CAMTA1 or TFE3 expression is negative in angiosarcoma [85].
- Epithelioid sarcoma (ES)
  - Nodules of medium-sized, rounded epithelioid cells that surround necrotic debris and collagen.
  - Cells are polygonal and blend with the collagen.
  - ES might express CD34 and ERG, but CD31 is consistently negative.
  - Loss of INI1 expression in ES [86].
- Malignant melanoma
  - The presence of an in situ component in the epidermis is contributory to the diagnosis.
  - The cytological atypia and mitotic activity are prominent.
  - S100, SOX10, Melan A, and HMA45: positive.
- Metastatic carcinoma
  - Significant cytological atypia and high mitotic activity.
  - Clinical correlation is necessary to rule out primary disease.
  - Negative for endothelial markers.

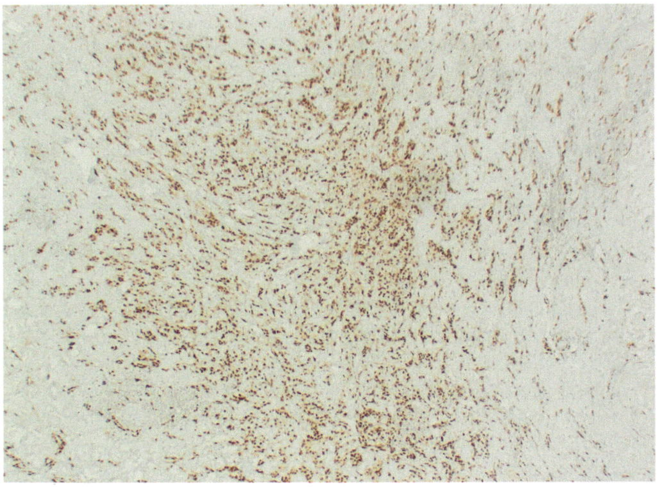

Fig. 10.43 A vascular marker, ERG is positive in neoplastic cells (40×)

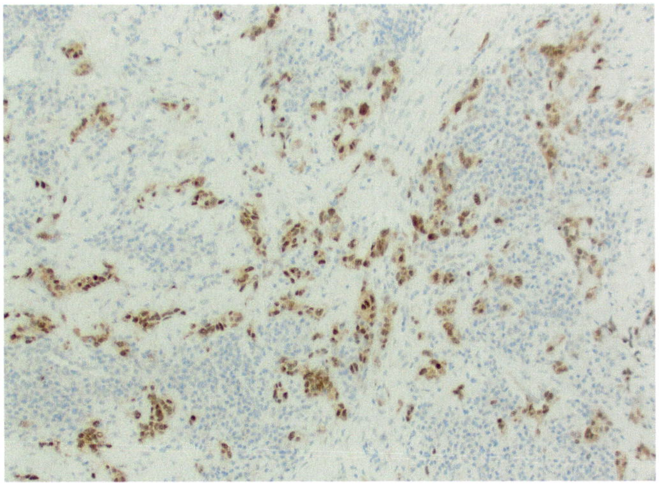

Fig. 10.44 CAMTA1 nuclear positivity confirms the diagnosis (100×)

10.13.1.4 Clinical Significance

- EHE is a low-grade malignant vascular tumor with an intermediate clinical behavior. Patients with *WWTR1-CAMTA1* fusion-positive EHE have a less favorable outcome in comparison to the *YAP1-TFE3* subset. The 5-year overall survival is 59% and 86%, respectively [87].

References

1. Koenig C, Tavassoli FA. Nodular hyperplasia, adenoma, and adenomyoma of Bartholin's gland. Int J Gynecol Pathol. 1998;17(4):289–94.
2. Santos LD, Kennerson AR, Killingsworth MC. Nodular hyperplasia of Bartholin's gland. Pathology. 2006;38(3):223–8.
3. Tseng YA, Lawrence WD, Slater SE. Nodular hyperplasia of the Bartholin gland, a benign mimicker of aggressive angiomyxoma: a case series and literature review. Int J Gynecol Pathol. 2018;37(6):554–8.
4. Barcellini A, Gadducci A, Laliscia C, Imparato S, Vitolo V, Preda L, et al. Adenoid cystic carcinoma of Bartholin's gland: what is the best approach? Oncology. 2020;98(8):513–9.
5. Helmi Z, Nori W, Ghani Zghair MA, AbdulrahmanHadi BA. Bartholin gland carcinoma: a case report. J Pak Med Assoc. 2021;71(Suppl 9)(12):S86–8.
6. Bhalwal AB, Nick AM, Dos Reis R, Chen CL, Munsell MF, Ramalingam P, et al. Carcinoma of the Bartholin gland: a review of 33 cases. Int J Gynecol Cancer. 2016;26(4):785–9.
7. Wang W, Chen H, Guo H, Chen L, Zhu M, Zhu Y. Adenoid cystic carcinoma of the Bartholin's gland is easily misdiagnosed: a case report and literature review. Medicine (Baltimore). 2022;101(45):e31744.

8. Scinicariello F, Rady P, Hannigan E, Dinh TV, Tyring SK. Human papillomavirus type 16 found in primary transitional cell carcinoma of the Bartholin's gland and in a lymph node metastasis. Gynecol Oncol. 1992;47(2):263–6.
9. Nazeran T, Cheng AS, Karnezis AN, Tinker AV, Gilks CB. Bartholin gland carcinoma: clinicopathologic features, including p16 expression and clinical outcome. Int J Gynecol Pathol. 2019;38(2):189–95.
10. El-Khoury J, Renald MH, Plantier F, Avril MF, Moyal-Barracco M. Vulvar hidradenoma papilliferum (HP) is located on the sites of mammary-like anogenital glands (MLAGs): analysis of the photographs of 52 tumors. J Am Acad Dermatol. 2016;75(2):380–4.
11. Konstantinova AM, Michal M, Kacerovska D, Spagnolo DV, Stewart CJ, Kutzner H, et al. Hidradenoma papilliferum: a clinicopathologic study of 264 tumors from 261 patients, with emphasis on mammary-type alterations. Am J Dermatopathol. 2016;38(8):598–607.
12. Sington J, Chandrapala R, Manek S, Hollowood K. Mitotic count is not predictive of clinical behavior in hidradenoma papilliferum of the vulva: a clinicopathologic study of 19 cases. Am J Dermatopathol. 2006;28(4):322–6.
13. Goto K, Maeda D, Kudo-Asabe Y, Hibiya T, Hayashi A, Fukayama M, et al. PIK3CA and AKT1 mutations in hidradenoma papilliferum. J Clin Pathol. 2017;70(5):424–7.
14. Pelosi G, Martignoni G, Bonetti F. Intraductal carcinoma of mammary-type apocrine epithelium arising within a papillary hydradenoma of the vulva. Report of a case and review of the literature. Arch Pathol Lab Med. 1991;115(12):1249–54.
15. Kim GY, Solanki MH, Guo R. Vulvar apocrine hidradenocarcinoma arising in a hidradenoma papilliferum-A case report. J Cutan Pathol. 2021;48(8):1085–7.
16. Brown ST, Nalley JF, Kraus SJ. Molluscum contagiosum. Sex Transm Dis. 1981;8(3):227–34.
17. Sand FL, Thomsen SF. Skin diseases of the vulva: infectious diseases. J Obstet Gynaecol. 2017;37(7):840–8.
18. Epstein WL. Molluscum contagiosum. Semin Dermatol. 1992;11(3):184–9.
19. Chen W, Koenig C. Vulvar keratoacanthoma: a report of two cases. Int J Gynecol Pathol. 2004;23(3):284–6.
20. Misago N, Inoue T, Koba S, Narisawa Y. Keratoacanthoma and other types of squamous cell carcinoma with crateriform architecture: classification and identification. J Dermatol. 2013;40(6):443–52.
21. Orosz Z, Lehoczky O, Szoke J, Pulay T. Recurrent giant fibroepithelial stromal polyp of the vulva associated with congenital lymphedema. Gynecol Oncol. 2005;98(1):168–71.
22. Piqué-Duran E, Palacios-Llopis S, Moreno-Ramis P, Pérez-Cejudo JA, Martínez-Martín MS. Comparative study of pagetoid dyskeratosis between acrochordons and soft fibromas. Am J Dermatopathol. 2006;28(6):478–81.
23. Nucci MR, Young RH, Fletcher CD. Cellular pseudosarcomatous fibroepithelial stromal polyps of the lower female genital tract: an underrecognized lesion often misdiagnosed as sarcoma. Am J Surg Pathol. 2000;24(2):231–40.
24. Nucci MR. Mesenchymal lesions of the lower genital tract. Surg Pathol Clin. 2009;2(4):603–23.
25. Schoolmeester JK, Fritchie KJ. Genital soft tissue tumors. J Cutan Pathol. 2015;42(7):441–51.
26. Calonje E, Guerin D, McCormick D, Fletcher CD. Superficial angiomyxoma: clinicopathologic analysis of a series of distinctive but poorly recognized cutaneous tumors with tendency for recurrence. Am J Surg Pathol. 1999;23(8):910–7.
27. Furlong MA, Fanburg-Smith JC, Miettinen M. The morphologic spectrum of hibernoma: a clinicopathologic study of 170 cases. Am J Surg Pathol. 2001;25(6):809–14.
28. Le BH, Boyer PJ, Lewis JE, Kapadia SB. Granular cell tumor: immunohistochemical assessment of inhibin-alpha, protein gene product 9.5, S100 protein, CD68, and Ki-67 proliferative index with clinical correlation. Arch Pathol Lab Med. 2004;128(7):771–5.
29. Schoolmeester JK, Michal M, Steiner P, Michal M, Folpe AL, Sukov WR. Lipoblastoma-like tumor of the vulva: a clinicopathologic, immunohistochemical, fluorescence in situ hybridization and genomic copy number profiling study of seven cases. Mod Pathol. 2018;31(12):1862–8.
30. McCluggage WG, Ganesan R, Hirschowitz L, Rollason TP. Cellular angiofibroma and related fibromatous lesions of the vulva: report of a series of cases with a morphological spectrum wider than previously described. Histopathology. 2004;45(4):360–8.
31. Chen E, Fletcher CD. Cellular angiofibroma with atypia or sarcomatous transformation: clinicopathologic analysis of 13 cases. Am J Surg Pathol. 2010;34(5):707–14.
32. Maggiani F, Debiec-Rychter M, Vanbockrijck M, Sciot R. Cellular angiofibroma: another mesenchymal tumour with 13q14 involvement, suggesting a link with spindle cell lipoma and (extra)-mammary myofibroblastoma. Histopathology. 2007;51(3):410–2.
33. Panagopoulos I, Gorunova L, Bjerkehagen B, Andersen K, Lund-Iversen M, Heim S. Loss of chromosome 13 material in cellular angiofibromas indicates pathogenetic similarity with spindle cell lipomas. Diagn Pathol. 2017;12(1):17.
34. McCluggage WG, Perenyei M, Irwin ST. Recurrent cellular angiofibroma of the vulva. J Clin Pathol. 2002;55(6):477–9.
35. Agaram NP, Prakash S, Antonescu CR. Deep-seated plexiform schwannoma: a pathologic study of 16 cases and comparative analysis with the superficial variety. Am J Surg Pathol. 2005;29(8):1042–8.
36. Meyer A, Billings SD. What's new in nerve sheath tumors. Virchows Arch. 2020;476(1):65–80.
37. Azurah AG, Grover S, McGregor D. Plexiform schwannoma of the clitoris in a young girl: a case report. J Reprod Med. 2013;58(7–8):365–8.
38. Cohen JN, Yeh I, LeBoit PE. Melanotic schwannoma of the vulva: a case report and review of the literature. Am J Dermatopathol. 2020;42(1):46–51.
39. Hirose T, Tani T, Shimada T, Ishizawa K, Shimada S, Sano T. Immunohistochemical demonstration of EMA/Glut1-positive perineurial cells and CD34-positive fibroblastic cells in peripheral nerve sheath tumors. Mod Pathol. 2003;16(4):293–8.
40. McMenamin ME, Fletcher CD. Expanding the spectrum of malignant change in schwannomas: epithelioid malignant change, epithelioid malignant peripheral nerve sheath tumor, and epithelioid angiosarcoma: a study of 17 cases. Am J Surg Pathol. 2001;25(1):13–25.
41. Petrilli AM, Fernández-Valle C. Role of Merlin/NF2 inactivation in tumor biology. Oncogene. 2016;35(5):537–48.
42. Liao X, Liu X, Fan X, Lai J, Zhang D. Perianal Paget's disease: a clinicopathological and immunohistochemical study of 13 cases. Diagn Pathol. 2020;15(1):29.
43. Liao X, Mao W, Lin A. Perianal Paget's disease co-associated with anorectal adenocarcinoma: primary or secondary disease? Case Rep Gastroenterol. 2014;8(2):186–92.
44. Al-Obaidy KI, Kao CS, Idrees MT. P16 expression in extramammary Paget's disease of the vulva and scrotum is not human papillomavirus related. Int J Surg Pathol. 2018;26(7):617–20.
45. Konstantinova AM, Shelekhova KV, Stewart CJ, Spagnolo DV, Kutzner H, Kacerovska D, et al. Depth and patterns of adnexal involvement in primary extramammary (anogenital) Paget disease: a study of 178 lesions from 146 patients. Am J Dermatopathol. 2016;38(11):802–8.

46. Konstantinova AM, Kazakov DV. Extramammary Paget disease of the vulva. Semin Diagn Pathol. 2021;38(1):50687.
47. van der Linden M, Oonk MHM, van Doorn HC, Bulten J, van Dorst EBL, Fons G, et al. Vulvar Paget disease: a national retrospective cohort study. J Am Acad Dermatol. 2019;81(4):956–62.
48. Namuduri RP, Lim TY, Yam PK, Gatsinga R, Lim-Tan SK, Chew SH, et al. Vulvar basal cell carcinoma: clinical features and treatment outcomes from a tertiary care centre. Singap Med J. 2019;60(9):479–82.
49. Flipo R, Bani MA, Rejaibi S, Talhi N, Sastre-Garau X. Vulvar basal cell carcinoma: clinical and histopathologic features. Int J Gynecol Pathol. 2022;41(1):86–92.
50. Santos M, Montagut C, Mellado B, García A, Ramón y Cajal S, Cardesa A, et al. Immunohistochemical staining for p16 and p53 in premalignant and malignant epithelial lesions of the vulva. Int J Gynecol Pathol. 2004;23(3):206–14.
51. Zhu J, Yin L, Wang Q, Wu X, Ke G. Clinicopathologic and survival analysis of patients with adenoid cystic carcinoma of vulva: single-institution experience. Int J Clin Oncol. 2020;25(12):2144–50.
52. Xing D, Schoolmeester JK, Ren Z, Isacson C, Ronnett BM. Lower female genital tract tumors with adenoid cystic differentiation: P16 expression and high-risk HPV detection. Am J Surg Pathol. 2016;40(4):529–36.
53. Nieuwenhuyzen-de Boer GM, Dasgupta S, Ewing-Graham PC, Van Bockstal MR. Adenoid cystic carcinoma of the Bartholin gland is not HPV-related: a case report and review of literature. Pathol Res Pract. 2020;216(6):152968.
54. Winkelmann SE, Llorens AS. Metastatic basal cell carcinoma of the vulva. Gynecol Oncol. 1990;38(1):138–40.
55. Mulvany NJ, Allen DG. Differentiated intraepithelial neoplasia of the vulva. Int J Gynecol Pathol. 2008;27(1):125–35.
56. Yang B, Hart WR. Vulvar intraepithelial neoplasia of the simplex (differentiated) type: a clinicopathologic study including analysis of HPV and p53 expression. Am J Surg Pathol. 2000;24(3):429–41.
57. Singh N, Leen SL, Han G, Faruqi A, Kokka F, Rosenthal A, et al. Expanding the morphologic spectrum of differentiated VIN (dVIN) through detailed mapping of cases with p53 loss. Am J Surg Pathol. 2015;39(1):52–60.
58. Liu YA, Ji JX, Almadani N, Crawford RI, Gilks CB, Kinloch M, et al. Comparison of p53 immunohistochemical staining in differentiated vulvar intraepithelial neoplasia (dVIN) with that in inflammatory dermatoses and benign squamous lesions in the vulva. Histopathology. 2021;78(3):424–33.
59. Dasgupta S, Koljenović S, van den Bosch TPP, Swagemakers SMA, van der Hoeven NMA, van Marion R, et al. Evaluation of immunohistochemical markers, CK17 and SOX2, as adjuncts to p53 for the diagnosis of differentiated vulvar intraepithelial neoplasia (dVIN). Pharmaceuticals (Basel). 2021;14(4).
60. Heller DS, Day T, Allbritton JI, Scurry J, Radici G, Welch K, et al. Diagnostic criteria for differentiated vulvar intraepithelial neoplasia and vulvar aberrant maturation. J Low Genit Tract Dis. 2021;25(1):57–70.
61. Medeiros F, Nascimento AF, Crum CP. Early vulvar squamous neoplasia: advances in classification, diagnosis, and differential diagnosis. Adv Anat Pathol. 2005;12(1):20–6.
62. van de Nieuwenhof HP, Bulten J, Hollema H, Dommerholt RG, Massuger LF, van der Zee AG, et al. Differentiated vulvar intraepithelial neoplasia is often found in lesions, previously diagnosed as lichen sclerosus, which have progressed to vulvar squamous cell carcinoma. Mod Pathol. 2011;24(2):297–305.
63. Bradford J, Fischer G. Management of vulvovaginal lichen planus: a new approach. J Low Genit Tract Dis. 2013;17(1):28–32.
64. Watkins JC, Yang E, Crum CP, Herfs M, Gheit T, Tommasino M, et al. Classic vulvar intraepithelial neoplasia with superimposed lichen simplex chronicus: a unique variant mimicking differentiated vulvar intraepithelial neoplasia. Int J Gynecol Pathol. 2019;38(2):175–82.
65. Dong F, Kojiro S, Borger DR, Growdon WB, Oliva E. Squamous cell carcinoma of the vulva: a subclassification of 97 cases by clinicopathologic, immunohistochemical, and molecular features (p16, p53, and EGFR). Am J Surg Pathol. 2015;39(8):1045–53.
66. Granter SR, Nucci MR, Fletcher CD. Aggressive angiomyxoma: reappraisal of its relationship to angiomyofibroblastoma in a series of 16 cases. Histopathology. 1997;30(1):3–10.
67. McCluggage WG, Patterson A, Maxwell P. Aggressive angiomyxoma of pelvic parts exhibits oestrogen and progesterone receptor positivity. J Clin Pathol. 2000;53(8):603–5.
68. Medeiros F, Erickson-Johnson MR, Keeney GL, Clayton AC, Nascimento AG, Wang X, et al. Frequency and characterization of HMGA2 and HMGA1 rearrangements in mesenchymal tumors of the lower genital tract. Genes Chromosomes Cancer. 2007;46(11):981–90.
69. Laskin WB, Fetsch JF, Tavassoli FA. Angiomyofibroblastoma of the female genital tract: analysis of 17 cases including a lipomatous variant. Hum Pathol. 1997;28(9):1046–55.
70. Fritchie KJ, Goldblum JR, Tubbs RR, Sun Y, Carver P, Billings SD, et al. The expanded histologic spectrum of myxoidliposarcoma with an emphasis on newly described patterns: implications for diagnosis on small biopsy specimens. Am J Clin Pathol. 2012;137(2):229–39.
71. Hollowood K, Fletcher CD. Soft tissue sarcomas that mimic benign lesions. Semin Diagn Pathol. 1995;12(1):87–97.
72. Nappi O, Wick MR, Pettinato G, Ghiselli RW, Swanson PE. Pseudovascular adenoid squamous cell carcinoma of the skin. A neoplasm that may be mistaken for angiosarcoma. Am J Surg Pathol. 1992;16(5):429–38.
73. Horn LC, Liebert UG, Edelmann J, Höckel M, Einenkel J. Adenoid squamous carcinoma (pseudoangiosarcomatous carcinoma) of the vulva: a rare but highly aggressive variant of squamous cell carcinoma-report of a case and review of the literature. Int J Gynecol Pathol. 2008;27(2):288–91.
74. Giordano G, D'Adda T, Merisio C, Gnetti L. Vulvar acantholytic squamous carcinoma: a case report with immunohistochemical and molecular study. Int J Gynecol Pathol. 2005;24(3):303–6.
75. Bayer-Garner IB, Smoller BR. The expression of syndecan-1 is preferentially reduced compared with that of E-cadherin in acantholytic squamous cell carcinoma. J Cutan Pathol. 2001;28(2):83–9.
76. Meis-Kindblom JM, Kindblom LG. Angiosarcoma of soft tissue: a study of 80 cases. Am J Surg Pathol. 1998;22(6):683–97.
77. Kartono F, Shitabata PK, Magro CM, Rayhan D. Discohesive malignant melanoma simulating a bullous dermatoses. J Cutan Pathol. 2009;36(2):274–9.
78. Nagore E, Sánchez-Motilla JM, Pérez-Vallés A, Martínez-Lahuerta C, Alegre V, Aliaga A. Pseudovascular squamous cell carcinoma of the skin. Clin Exp Dermatol. 2000;25(3):206–8.
79. Kiyohara T, Miyamoto M, Shijimaya T, Nagano N, Nakamaru S, Makimura K, et al. Pseudovascular squamous cell carcinoma: a review of the published work and reassessment of prognosis. J Dermatol. 2018;45(12):1448–51.
80. Deyrup AT, Tighiouart M, Montag AG, Weiss SW. Epithelioid hemangioendothelioma of soft tissue: a proposal for risk stratification based on 49 cases. Am J Surg Pathol. 2008;32(6):924–7.
81. Antonescu CR, Le Loarer F, Mosquera JM, Sboner A, Zhang L, Chen CL, et al. Novel YAP1-TFE3 fusion defines a distinct subset of epithelioid hemangioendothelioma. Genes Chromosomes Cancer. 2013;52(8):775–84.
82. Errani C, Zhang L, Sung YS, Hajdu M, Singer S, Maki RG, et al. A novel WWTR1-CAMTA1 gene fusion is a consistent abnormality

in epithelioid hemangioendothelioma of different anatomic sites. Genes Chromosomes Cancer. 2011;50(8):644–53.
83. Stacchiotti S, Miah AB, Frezza AM, Messiou C, Morosi C, Caraceni A, et al. Epithelioid hemangioendothelioma, an ultra-rare cancer: a consensus paper from the community of experts. ESMO Open. 2021;6(3):100170.
84. Miettinen M, Fetsch JF. Distribution of keratins in normal endothelial cells and a spectrum of vascular tumors: implications in tumor diagnosis. Hum Pathol. 2000;31(9):1062–7.
85. Righi A, Sbaraglia M, Gambarotti M, Gibertoni D, Rovira MP, Benini S, et al. Primary vascular tumors of bone: a monoinstitutional morphologic and molecular analysis of 427 cases with emphasis on epithelioid variants. Am J Surg Pathol. 2020;44(9):1192–203.
86. Hornick JL, Dal Cin P, Fletcher CD. Loss of INI1 expression is characteristic of both conventional and proximal-type epithelioid sarcoma. Am J Surg Pathol. 2009;33(4):542–50.
87. Rosenbaum E, Jadeja B, Xu B, Zhang L, Agaram NP, Travis W, et al. Prognostic stratification of clinical and molecular epithelioid hemangioendothelioma subsets. Mod Pathol. 2020;33(4):591–602.

Index

O. Saglam, *Challenging Cases in Gynecologic Surgical Pathology*, https://doi.org/10.1007/978-3-031-51656-6

GPSR Compliance

The European Union's (EU) General Product Safety Regulation (GPSR) is a set of rules that requires consumer products to be safe and our obligations to ensure this.

If you have any concerns about our products, you can contact us on ProductSafety@springernature.com

In case Publisher is established outside the EU, the EU authorized representative is:

Springer Nature Customer Service Center GmbH
Europaplatz 3
69115 Heidelberg, Germany

Batch number: 10756390

Printed by Printforce, the Netherlands